Liberty and Insanity in the Age of the American Revolution

Liberty and Insanity in the Age of the American Revolution

Sarah L. Swedberg

LEXINGTON BOOKS
Lanham • Boulder • New York • London

Published by Lexington Books
An imprint of The Rowman & Littlefield Publishing Group, Inc.
4501 Forbes Boulevard, Suite 200, Lanham, Maryland 20706
www.rowman.com

6 Tinworth Street, London SE11 5AL, United Kingdom

Copyright © 2021 The Rowman & Littlefield Publishing Group, Inc.

All rights reserved. No part of this book may be reproduced in any form or by any electronic or mechanical means, including information storage and retrieval systems, without written permission from the publisher, except by a reviewer who may quote passages in a review.

British Library Cataloguing in Publication Information Available

Library of Congress Cataloging-in-Publication Data

ISBN: 978-1-4985-7386-3 (cloth)
ISBN: 978-1-4985-7388-7 (pbk)
ISBN: 978-1-4985-7387-0 (electronic)

Contents

Introduction		1
1	Insanity and Confinement in an Age of Liberty	17
2	The Many Madnesses of Colonial Protest	47
3	Impolitic Madmen: Dividing into Enemy and Friend	77
4	The Folly and Madness of War, 1775–1783	107
5	"The Whole Country Is Now in a State of Madness": Life and Government during Wartime	135
6	An Irrational State, 1783–1787	161
7	"The Temple of Tyranny Has Two Doors," 1787–1791	183
8	Party Politics and Foreign Policy, 1792–1796	211
Epilogue		235
Bibliography		243
Index		261
About the Author		269

Introduction

What follows are stories of people experiencing war and upheaval, about how nervous that war and upheaval made them, and how they saw madness everywhere. They saw madness in government policies, in protests, in price gouging, in battles, in their households, and everywhere else they looked. This should not surprise us for their world shifted and changed rapidly and the medical language of disease and mental illness helped them make sense of it. When Americans changed their relationships to government through a war for independence, some of them believed they would create a government and society that functioned better than the one they left behind. However, in the first decade after the war they experienced many hardships that were reminiscent of the ones that came before and their household dynamics continued to shift and change. In the new nation, Americans continued to take up arms against their government or to take up arms to protect their government. In addition, they got drawn into world wars and frontier wars in uncomfortable ways. Their stories are stories of freedom and unfreedom, of rationality and irrationality, of trying to tip governments toward freedom and rationality but often letting the darkness of unfreedom and irrationality win out for all the reasons people have always let them win out. Their language was often beautiful. Their intentions were often pure. In the end, they created an imperfect union that was more or less imperfect than the one they had left, depending on who told the stories.

This book focuses on the dual concepts of liberty and insanity in the age of the American Revolution. While historians have examined the history of the changing psychological beliefs and practices in the eighteenth and early nineteenth centuries and have detailed efforts to create asylums to house and treat the mentally ill, we have not fully examined the ways that the discussion about mental illness intersected with society, law, and politics. Insanity exposed fractures in family, community, and institutions and raised difficult questions about the nature of governance. Anglo-Americans translated their concerns about the world around them through the medical language of mental illness. Each of the following chapters focuses on at least one of three main ways medical language worked its way into political discourse.

The first way is that medical doctors and laypeople believed that change and conflict increased the incidents of madness. Medical doctors determined that madness could come from very ordinary causes, but extraordinary times or events increased the possibilities of joy, sorrow, grief, or loss leading to insanity. In his *Zoonomia, or, the Laws of Organic Life*, first published in the late eighteenth century, Erasmus Darwin believed the "furious insanities" were caused by "pride, anger, revenge, [and] suspicion."[1] In the chapters that follow, we can see all of these emotions at work, and particularly anger and suspicion. Even before the war broke out, American colonists often found themselves in a frenzy of anger against the policies of King and Parliament and sometimes suspicious to the point of paranoia about men and power and their intentions. In a time and place where the world was unsettled, it followed that individuals' minds were also unsettled, leading them to depression of spirits, mania, frenzy, delusion, or fanaticism, all species of insanity according to the doctors.

In addition, as I discuss in chapter 4, military conflict brings madness to both the battlefield and the home front. Today we recognize post-traumatic stress syndrome (PTSD) in war veterans and others who experience traumatic events. Those who study PTSD in soldiers find that both witnessing and participating in violence has an effect on their mental health or illness. Even when the state sanctions wartime violence against clearly knowable enemies, "killing another human being is the single most pervasive, traumatic experience of war" with observation of violence close behind.[2] In the era of the American Revolution, men and women did not have the diagnosis or understanding of PTSD but, throughout the period of military conflict, they wrote about the folly and madness of war and worried about the effects on themselves and their polities. Even after Americans had left some of the folly and madness of warfare behind them in 1783, they still engaged in military actions. Chapter 6 includes stories about one of these small-scale military conflicts, Shays's Rebellion in Massachusetts, with a particular focus on the ways the sometimes-violent-conflict played out in the language of rationality and irrationality. Even absent military conflict, the world continued to confound and trouble Americans who subsequently accompanied their political innovations with heated arguments. Chapters 7 and 8 focus on postwar political arguments, the divisions those arguments created, and the ways Americans deployed medical metaphors throughout. Their experiments in government never worked perfectly, debts went unpaid on individual and national levels, and political actors continued to use their power in what many believed were corrupt and nefarious ways.

Secondly, whether British and British-American men and women supported holding onto older forms of government or experimenting with new ones, most of them agreed that their governments should be rational. By the 1770s, American politicians moved toward creating governments based on the social contract. The social contract was not a new idea, of course, as the language had found its way into compacts, charters, and agreements, but it became everywhere apparent in the attempts to build new state and national governments during the American Revolution. It can be found in the new constitutions, political speeches, tracts and pamphlets, and declarations. For instance, the second sentence of the 1780 Massachusetts Constitution stated, "The body-politic is formed by a voluntary association of individuals: it is a social compact, by which the whole people covenants with each citizen, and each citizen with the whole people, that all should be governed by certain laws for the common good." Building governments based on the social contract increased the anxiety over madness for these governments could work well only if there were rational actors in place. For stability to be achieved, for relationships among colonists or American citizens to work, for a common good to be defined, many believed there needed to be some general consensus about roles and functions for individuals. In *A Letter to the Citizens of Pennsylvania*, George Logan wrote: "In a state of civil Society, man must be considered as a Member of a great political Family. He is connected with his Fellow-citizens, by ties of interest and *benevolent* attachment; and his social affections must extend to the whole Community which he is a Member. He should feel the Safety and the common Welfare, intimately connected with his own."[3] In other words, people needed to be good social individuals, understanding their positions and occupying them fully according to the norms. Otherwise, they created dangerous situations for themselves, their families, communities, and even their governments.

For adherents to this world view, lunatics posed a problem. Lunatics had lost their ability to reason and to govern themselves. The most insane raved, covered themselves with their own excrement, said inappropriate things, held delusions about their social positions, or acted violently. In the post-Revolution world, culture and society emphasized rationality as one of the cornerstones of good government. In his gubernatorial inaugural address in 1800, Pennsylvanian Thomas McKean argued that important attributes for "all who are employed in the business of Government," were "wisdom, moderation, and fortitude." Only these attributes would help Americans work toward "preserving social order, confidence, and concord."[4] In this conception of society, lunatics—whether governors or simply citizens—did not possess wisdom, moderation, or fortitude and therefore disrupted society by creating a weak link between the people and the people's government. Edward Cutbrush, in his 1794 medical dissertation on insanity, made this connection plain: "an uninterrupted use" of reason "is absolutely necessary for the well-being of all societies, both civil and religious."[5]

Lastly, men and women deployed the language of insanity to create boundaries between those considered friends and those considered enemies. In 1792, William Pargeter wrote that the "distempered fancy" of the madman "transforms his best friends into the bitterest enemies, and he views them with an implacable aversion."[6] If this were true, many of those whom I studied and wrote about operated with distempered fancies. The transformation of former friends and neighbors into enemies is the particular but not exclusive focus of chapter 3. Americans, bitterly divided in every stage of the era of the American Revolution by their actions and political beliefs, often argued that those like them were sane and rational but that those who opposed them were lunatics or madmen. Educated or uneducated, invested or uninvested with power, the men and women who people these pages created ideologies though the endless process of othering. They could point at those on the other side of whatever view divided them and say that those people over there have been worked into a frenzy but look at us here, taking the rational course of right action. This endless othering sometimes allowed them to justify illegal or violent actions against their enemies even off the battlefields, claiming that they acted for the greater good of society or in support of liberty against deluded people who posed a threat to society and government.

In these ways, as they defined the world around them as a world gone mad, Americans in the period of the American Revolution and early republic tapped into popular understandings of health and illness that permeated the political culture of the time. Popular medical understanding worked its way into language at every turn. When they looked around them, Britons and Americans diagnosed mental and physical disorders in the world they observed and proposed medical solutions. The world was sick from inflammation, cancer, madness or other diseases. Politicians and laypeople alike wanted to act as doctors to the body politic, but their diagnoses and proposed cures diverged wildly from one another. The examples are woven in the following chapters showing how George Cressener proposed bleeding for the inflammation of colonial protests and Henry Strachey lamented that the whole American nation had lost its mind. Over and over again people turned to what they knew, and what they knew was a popular understanding of the working of health and illness and a desire for a cure.

Varieties of knowledge ranging from folk remedies to formal medicine occupied the spaces of medical understanding. Formal and informal as well as cross-cultural medical knowledge moved through the familiar networks of sociability and trade. Colin Calloway explained that Europeans, already attuned to herbal remedies "often were inclined to see Indian healers as at least equal in ability to European physicians."[7] In western Maine, Abenaki Molly Ockett was one of the best-known healers. Anglo-American Henry Tufts apprenticed himself to Ockett after she cured him of a knife wound and he went on to "pass himself off as a physician" when he returned to his community.[8] As Europeans used Native American medical knowledge and brought it back into their communities, they also sought the care of a host of other healers to a far greater extent than they did trained male physicians. Even wealthy George Washington first sought a bleeder in his last days and, according to the physicians who attended him at the very end of his life, "he would not by any means be prevailed upon by the family to send for the attending physician till the following morning."[9]

In North America, only a small minority of men styling themselves physicians had formal education. Many of them had served as apprentices, learning medicine in the boundaries of an established physician's formal practice. In the eighteenth century, physicians wanted to position themselves as experts and to control the medical marketplace often publicly denouncing other healers. Early in the century, during the Boston inoculation controversy, Dr. William Douglass worked hard toward that end, "defending the integrity of the medical profession against the interference of those whom he considered to be credulous laymen."[10] He was particularly appalled by the fact that Cotton Mather had learned about smallpox inoculation initially from enslaved people and slave traders. While Douglass came to believe inoculation could be efficacious, he insisted that it needed to be regulated by the Massachusetts legislature "and carried out by 'abler hands, than *Greek old Women, Madmen and Fools.*"[11] It is unclear whether he considered Mather an old woman, a madman, or a fool, but his triad is telling. Trained practitioners of medicine and legislators, the patriarchs of the society, were the only ones who could decide about medical practices in his opinion. He and other male physicians wanted to establish the unquestionable right to regulate access to medicine and thus presented all other options as unmitigated madness.

At the beginning of the next century, Benjamin Rush lectured his medical students about their duties in society. Although he believed physicians were the ones best charged with dispensing medicine he told his audience that quacks sometimes had accidentally discovered "our most useful remedies." Quacks did not know how to properly dispense the medications they had discovered, he said. Nonetheless, he believed that physicians could learn from them, taking the folk knowledge out of the hands of the ignorant and applying it. In addition, he told his students to "converse with nurses and old women" for they passed along knowledge that would be useful to physicians. "Even negroes and Indians have sometimes stumbled upon discoveries in medicine."[12] The "stumbled upon" is key here, as Rush believed while these others might have accidentally developed medicine or discovered cures, they had not done it through observation and rational experimentation as physicians had. The difference, for Rush, was that while he and his students could certainly benefit from folk knowledge, none of what physicians did should be the result of accident. Many Americans seeking medical care, however, did not make the distinction that Rush did and trusted the wisdom, observation, and often-proven benefits of the remedies offered by other healers. Therefore, they continued to call on a wide variety of men and women to tend to their illnesses and bought prepackaged remedies based on a recommendations of a host of healers without seeking the advice of a trained physician.

In this medical marketplace, many Americans also turned to home remedies and to cheaply-printed self-help medical guides written by either doctors or laypeople. Dr. William Buchan published the inexpensive and enormously popular *Domestic Medicine.* As Charles Rosenberg has shown, Buchan did not mean his work to become a medical self-help guide for the masses for he believed they needed to be under the care of the better sort, but nonetheless, believed that keeping medical knowledge from the elite was "injurious to the true interests of society." In order to prevent the spread of diseases, he believed widespread medical knowledge was necessary and that "men of every occupation and condition of life might avail themselves of a degree of medical knowledge."[13] Unlike Buchan, other doctors fought a mostly losing battle in keeping knowledge from the public. If doctors were not willing to publish self-help medical guides, the gap was filled in by others such as the founder of Methodism, John Wesley. In "Pills for the Poor: John Wesley's *Primitive Physic*," Samuel J. Rogal explained that Wesley could author an authoritative medical self-help guide because, "medical knowledge was neither voluminous or complicated, [and] the majority of educated individuals believed that they could dispense 'practical physick' with as much confidence, if not actual competence, as any surgeon, physician or apothecary."[14]

Practical physic applied not just to individual bodies but also to the body politic. In the eighteenth century, Americans conceived of the political world as sharing characteristics with the human body. The body politic thrived or grew diseased, aging and declining in mental and physical capacity. The political world also needed healing, but while it was useful for individuals to observe their own ailments and apply non-harmful, non-heroic, and simple home remedies, it could be dangerous when those same individuals diagnosed the body politic from positions of prejudice and political leanings. When they looked around them they saw a world sick from inflammation, cancer, madness, or other diseases, diseases caused by the actions and wrong thinking of their political opponents. They then tried to act as doctors to the ailing world but not only did their diagnoses and proposed cures diverge wildly from one another but also these political doctors often evinced desires to apply harsh and heroic measures as a cure instead of the gentle home remedies they might try first on themselves. These examples are woven into the following chapters as people accessed medical knowledge to understand and explain their frightening and changing world.

What did this physic Americans turned toward look like, practical or otherwise? As I show in the following chapters, humoral theory still held a firm place in both medical and political writings. Doctors and writers of medical tracts believed that bleeding, purging, or blistering could help balance the humors and cure illnesses in individuals' bodies while political commentators urged the same measures for the body politic. Physicians and others applied these remedies to both physical and mental illness. By the eighteenth century, the idea of madness as demonic possession had largely gone by the wayside and doctors and others looked toward rational explanations and cures for mental illness.

Increasingly, doctors also believed that rational approaches could cure some forms of mental illness. In the mid-eighteenth century, Dr. William Battie was one of the doctors who found the carceral treatment of the mentally ill in the famous Bethlem Hospital irrational and inefficacious. He advocated that the first course of treatment should involve removing the madmen or women from their surroundings and then turning to gentle practices that included conversation, good diet, fresh air and exercise, and freedom from chains. Battie criticized the fact that doctors turned first to "Antimonial vomits, strong purges, and Hellebore," believing that they were too chary with their information, withholding observations and experiments that could aid their profession in order to shore up their own reputations.[15] With better and shared knowledge, doctors could effect more cures and restore patients' sanity. Battie, however, did not reject heroic measures. If the gentle cures did not work, doctors could then try a number of different techniques including "vesicatories, caustic, vomits, rough cathartics, an errhines."[16]

Despite criticism of Battie, most famously from Dr. John Monro the physician to the Bethlem Hospital, Battie's analysis, together with other writings and practices that advocated for a more humane approach to madness, took hold, forming the basis of what would become called moral medicine later in the century. By 1796, Quaker reformers had opened the York Retreat in England to provide moral medicine to suffering Quakers, becoming a model (in theory anyway) for asylums and hospitals on both sides of the Atlantic Ocean, working to restore the suffering to rationality and therefore creating a stable social order. The mind and body of the individual were intimately connected to the mind and body of the body politic.

As healers treated mental illness, one of their concerns was that the conditions present in societies with good government had the potential to create an excess of emotion which then made people sick. In a late seventeenth-century text, *Every Man His Own Doctor*, court physician John Archer postulated that "the perturbations of the Mind do much hurt to the Body, as No Physitian will deny." He went on to caution that "there are some men in perfect Health that will fully take upon them such a habit or custome [*sic*] of Anger, that not only disturbs their own House and Relations, but thereby brings into their own Bodies Sickness and Death."[17] The custom of anger could come from many different places in a person's life. On a personal level, a failed business or romance, a harsh word from a friend or neighbor, the accidental death of a loved one, among other distressing circumstances might spark anger. On a political level, societies that created space for disputation, contention for office, and choice in everything from consumer goods to religious denominations also sparked anger and other passions and therefore had the potential to lead to emotional distress.[18]

In the aftermath of the American Revolution, Benjamin Rush noted that a new "species of insanity" had emerged that he called *Anarchia*. This insanity had been caused by an "excess of the passion for liberty," which had been further "inflamed by the successful issue of the war." Madness came from a "sense of freedom," Alexander Anderson wrote in his 1796 Columbia College dissertation. "In despotic governments raving madness is less frequent, because slavery tends to depress the mind."[19] Dr. Johann Spurzheim agreed. In his 1812 *Observations on the Deranged Manifestations of the Mind, or Insanity*, he hypothesized that there were more insane people in England than anywhere else because there "every thing finds opposition, and opposition naturally excites the feelings."[20] Spurzheim wrote that large-scale and oppositional political participation meant increased cerebral function. Increased cerebral function was one of the idiopathic, or spontaneous, causes for insanity. Two decades later, in an appendix to an American edition of Spurzheim's study, Dr. Amariah Brigham insisted, "insanity prevails most in those countries where people enjoy civil and religious freedom, where every person has liberty to engage in the strife for the highest honors and stations in society, and where the road to wealth and opportunity is equally open to all."[21] Republics in particular bred insanity because the freedom of choice present in republican forms of government meant that citizens needed to exercise their minds extensively. The very nature of societies marked by liberty brought about the increased possibility of mental or physical illness.

Therefore, with liberty came threat and danger. Many of these threats and dangers are developed in the chapters that follow but it is worth noting in this introduction that Americans used the word *madness* or its cousins (insanity, lunacy, and frenzy among others) to capture them. For example, unchecked liberty allowed for anarchy which was seen as an expression of madness. Madness could make itself apparent in mobbing, in petitions for political change, in calls for boycotts, and in many of the actions taken by individuals working to define or redefine their relationships to structured power. More frighteningly, the actions of the men and women who had become mad through personal or political strife threatened to destabilize the orderly commonwealths Anglo-Americans sought to maintain or create. If an individual's body was wracked by illness, and an individual body was one element of the larger political or social body, that element threatened the whole. Therefore, the liberty that Anglo-Americans praised in their political worlds had the potential to create dangerous conditions in the body politic. Speakers and writers returned to the theme of society and government imperiled by unchecked liberty.

Using this shared medical and political understanding of the world as its basis, this book intervenes in the conventional telling of a well-known political and military timeline by focusing on the fears of a maddened body politic. This is not a forced or artificial imposition. On both sides of the Atlantic Ocean, men and women used the language of health and illness in referring to the world around them, and frequently used the language of mental health and illness. This brings home, again, how much eighteenth-century Anglo-Americans truly believed that illness and medicine operated in the same ways in the individual as they did in government and society. The body of the body politic was one with a mind, heart, limbs, skin and bones, and blood, and like a human being it could evince health and vigor or illness and lethargy. In the eighteenth century, medical knowledge helped people make sense of the world around them.

Health, disease, and medicine have never existed separate from political considerations and machinations and always lay bare social, economic, and other inequalities. This is not the main focus of this book but it is one historians and readers need to always keep in mind. The starkest examples come from slave communities where regular medical care could be sought or denied based on the whim of the master or, as one story of my next chapter shows, where enslaved people could be declared mad and placed in or taken out of hospitals. Rana A. Hogarth has recently shown us the ways the medical doctors participated in the process of constructing race by "identifying the so-called tangible traits unique to black people's bodies." They did not do this to justify or defend slavery but "to advance the standing of medical polities in the Atlantic World and expand white prerogatives."[22] White men and women claim these prerogatives throughout this book using the language of madness and of a metaphorical slavery that bore no relationship to chattel slavery. Gender inequality is also part of the very landscape of conflict and nation-making. In her work on Stephen and Mary Girard and financial speculation, Brenna Holland examined the ways the "male physicians increasingly attempted to root diseases of the mind in the bodies of women and people of color."[23] One cannot understand any aspect of American history without understanding the ways these inequalities were constructed or shored up through multiple avenues and, in the case of my study, show up not only in the questions of who could be a part of the body politic but also in the medicine that helped explain Americans' worldviews.

Knowingly or unknowingly, medical practitioners have often participated in the creation of knowledge that served political power structures. Whether they simply accepted what was considered a known truth or they employed the scientific method in ways that confirmed what they thought they knew, then and now physicians, apothecaries, and others have participated in the political world. Physicians or scientists might believe they operate outside of politics, evaluating data objectively and systematically, but physicians, like any social scientist or historian, can end up finding what they think they are going to find. Paradigm shifts happen far less frequently than they should. This was as true in the eighteenth century as it is for us in the twenty-first century. When some of the diagnoses and proposed cures of the eighteenth century seem extraordinary, dangerous, or laughable to us, it is worth remembering that in our century, physicians and scientists are still shaped by the world around them and respond accordingly. Then, as now, followers of powerful leaders or adherents to a political party sometimes dismissed reason, experiment, and tested conclusions as they became seduced by the leader's or party's message. And then, as now, both good and bad medical knowledge shaped the language used to help explain politics, society, war, and other events, crises, or phenomenon.

The intersection of politics and medical language is at the crux of this book. I relied heavily on written records for my evidence, combing through the collections at the Massachusetts Historical Society, the Library Company of Philadelphia, the Historical Society of Pennsylvania, the William L. Clements Library, and as many print or digital sources as I could find. Whenever possible, I read into the cracks to bring in some of those who are largely absent from those records. As with any history, there are many gaps, suppositions, and silences that still need to be filled by other brave souls. In addition, although I organized this book chronologically, I never tackled the whole of any one period covered by a chapter. The examples used stand in for other examples, for moments when the world itself was disordered, the body politic deranged, or when the fears of what came next caused Americans to despair of their present and their future.

Through each of the chapters, it is apparent that Americans claimed, defined, and contested rights. They raised questions about government, society, and personal relationships and answered them in flawed and incomplete ways. Political leaders could boldly assert that they had come up with a perfect answer to a question, but their fellow Americans often disagreed. They often judged the foibles and limitations of their fellow subjects or citizens. In the most intense times of crisis, those in power often deserted their principles and grossly violated the rights of others. As the following chapters show, they justified these violations in a variety of ways ranging from a plea of temporary insanity to the claim of war necessity.

The generation of Americans who experienced the American Revolution and the beginnings of a new nation worried a lot about what they had wrought. They held deep-seated concerns that their experiments in government would not last. History was certainly against them; they held up their experiment against the historical examples offered by Greece and Rome and concluded that they, too, may be doomed to fail. They worried about regionalism and the potential for disunion. The most pessimistic were sure the United States would soon break asunder. The pessimists were right, of course. Americans faced the threat of secession and civil war throughout the first decades of the nineteenth century and then actual secession and civil war in the 1860s. The Americans in this book and those who came later were and remain a contentious and squabbling bunch with differing ideological and political views.

What the founding generation shared were concerns that irrational actors could bring devastation to the new nation. When I started this project in 2011, their concerns intrigued me, but by that time the nation had managed to navigate a lot of irrationality and a good deal more war. It seems less a thought-exercise as I write these words in the first month of 2020 after experiencing four years of what seems to me and many others an era of chaotic, irrational rule from the Executive Branch, absent the checks and balances that James Madison believed would come from the Legislative and Judicial Branches. Sometimes government seems broken in exactly the ways the founding generation worried it might be. While this keeps me up at night, there is also some comfort in studying earlier periods of chaos like the early 1790s when some Americans feared that the French had interfered in their elections and that their political opponents were unhinged. The fears of Americans in the last decades of the eighteenth century can sometimes seem distant. In many ways, their world was so different from ours, it seems almost a foreign country as David Lowenthal posits.[24] My own fears in the present day, shared with a good number of Americans, however, create empathy and understanding for those men and women in the past. The echoes of that time sound a little louder for me now, and I find both terror and solace in the records they left behind.

My terror and solace has been shared by many, and I want to end my introduction by thanking a host of family members, friends, and colleagues across the nation. First and foremost to my wife and life partner Adele Cummings who cheered this endeavor on from the very beginning. At one point, as I grew closer to the end point of writing and editing I asked, "Did you ever think I was just lying, and I wasn't writing a book at all?" She looked at me as if I were a lunatic and told me, "Of course not." I was glad to have someone to tell stories from the archives, many of which did not make it into this book. My parents, to whom this book is dedicated, encouraged my intellectual curiosity from a young age and did not stop loving me even when, at the age of twenty, I told them I was dropping out of college and moving to San Francisco. (It helps to be low in the birth order.) I wish they had lived to see the book in print. My six siblings also shaped this manuscript through now-more-than-five decades of connection. In particular, George and I spent a lot of time sending each other direct messages about patriotism and loyalism as I wrote what became chapter 3. I am a better person because of all of them (in birth order): Erika, Anne, Lisa, John, George, and Matt. They also chose wonderful spouses and have amazing children. I always enjoy the times we were able to get together, share stories, or sometimes just be weird, quiet, introverts together.

This project was born in Philadelphia in the summer of 2011 during a National Endowment for the Humanities seminar on the problem of governance in the early republic. I will forever be beholden to Dr. John Larson and Dr. Michael Morrison who gave me a chance to participate despite the fact that my greatest accomplishment at that point was to teach large numbers of wonderful, squabbling and contentious students year after year. After over a decade with a heavy teaching load, I had lost my faith in my capacity as a scholar but I found my voice again in interacting with the others in the seminar who valued my input and found the initial stages of this project fascinating enough that I continued. Dr. Larson in particular wrote letter of support after letter of support for mostly-failed fellowship applications. At another low point, my fellow FREACs encouraged me in my project and gave me valuable feedback on an early attempt at writing. Similarly, writing for the scholarly history-of-medicine blog, Nursing Clio, gave me confidence in my writing. Thank you so much to the Executive Editor Jacqueline Antonovich who, once upon a time, was a student in several of my classes at Colorado Mesa University, and to all the editors who have been so kind and supportive: Cassia Roth, Elizabeth Reis, Laura Ansley, Sarah Handley-Cousins, R. E. Fulton, Carrie Adkins, Laruen MacIvor Thomson, and Averill Earls, as well as others.

The archivists, librarians, and staff at the Massachusetts Historical Society, Library Company of Philadelphia, and the Historical Society of Pennsylvania lent me their ears and their expertise, steering me toward sources and providing quiet spaces to discover and ponder. My best trip to a library ever, however, was my trip to the William L. Clements Library at the University of Michigan in the Spring of 2019. The Howard H. Peckham Fellowship on Revolutionary America allowed me to spend three weeks in their collections. Jayne Ptolemy provided a lengthy list of potential sources, many of which found their ways into these pages, Cheney Schopieray talked enthusiastically about Henry and Jane Strachey during tea, and Clayton Lewis introduced me to the Satiric Prints which mostly (to my great sadness) did not make their way into this book. The other staff there were always willing to provide kind words and support. The other financial aid that I received came from an anonymous donor in the wake of my disappointment at being an alternate for a long-term fellowship and my fears of running out of money during my half-salary sabbatical year. I think we came up with a clever name for her "fellowship" but I can no longer remember it. She will know I appreciated her kindness in a low time. Hillary Faccio, a friend for all of my adult life, also provided me with the equivalent of financial support by giving me a temporary home in Boston for my research trips, making it possible for someone who teaches at an institution with almost no travel funding to continue to search for the perfect primary sources.

My past and present colleagues at Colorado Mesa University have been an invaluable source of support. Steve Schulte never turned down a request for a letter of support, Brenda Wilhelm has shared laughter and tears, Kristen Hague invited me to participate in a panel of captivity that helped shape my thinking, Erika Jackson provided me with inspiration to keep writing, and Carol Christ never failed in her using her superpower (human connection). Reenie Neal provided me with valuable feedback on chapter 1. I never did take up Jennifer Hancock's offer to read my manuscript because I was always too busy trying to get the words down on the page but I appreciated the offer very much. This book would not have been possible if I had not been granted a sabbatical for the academic year 2018–2019 and without the great work of the Tomlinson Library librarians who find ways to get me books and access to materials despite their limited budget. Thank you, too, to my friends who offer needed distractions, including all the members of the Lesbian Drinking Group, Robyn Parker, Claudette Konola, Caleb Ferganchick, and the members of the newly formed social justice group Right and Wrong who let me tag along and help when I can even though I am at least 20 years older than everyone but Shannon. Lastly, to all my students past and present who challenge and inspire me. Even if this book had never seen the light of day, my connection to the undergraduates who have participated in the work of creating knowledge has made my career more than worthwhile.

NOTES

1. Erasmus Darwin, *Zoonomia; Or, the Laws of Organic Life. In Three Parts* (Boston: Thomas and Andrews, 1803), 300.

2. Alan Fontana and Robert Rosenheck, "Traumatic War Stressors and Psychiatric Symptoms among World War II, Korean, and Vietnam War Veterans," *Psychology and Aging* 9, no. 1 (1994): 30, doi:10.1037//0882-7974.9.1.27.

3. George Logan, *A Letter to the Citizens of Pennsylvania* (Philadelphia: Patterson & Cochran, 1800), 8–9.

4. Thomas M'Kean, *The Inaugural Address of Thomas M'Kean* (Lancaster, PA: Dickson, 1800), 4.

5. Edward Cutbrush, *An Inaugural Dissertation on Insanity: Submitted to the Examination of the Rev. John Ewing, S.T.P. Provost; The Trustees and Medical Professors of the University of Pennsylvania; for the Degree of Doctor of Medicine, On the Nineteenth Day of May, A.D. MDCCXCIV* (Philadelphia: Zachariah Poulson, Jr., 1794), 5, https://archive.org/details/2548037R.nlm.nih.gov.

6. William Pargeter, *Observations on Maniacal Disorders* (Reading, 1972). https://archive.org/details/b21522388/page/n151.

7. Colin G. Calloway, "Indians, Europeans, and the New World of Disease and Healing," in *Major Problems in the History of American Medicine and Public Health* (Boston: Houghton Mifflin, 2001), 42.

8. Calloway, "Indians, Europeans, and the New World of Disease and Healing," 43.

9. "Illness and Death of George Washington," *The New Hampshire Journal of Medicine* 8, no. 1 (January 1858): 103.

10. John B. Blake, "The Inoculation Controversy in Boston: 1721–1722," *New England Quarterly* 25, no. 4 (December 1952): 503, doi:10.2307/362582.

11. Blake, "Inoculation Controversy," 504.

12. Benjamin Rush, *Observations on the Duties of a Physician, and the Methods of Improving Medicine. Accommodated to the Present State of Society and Manners in the United States* (Philadelphia: Prichard & Hall, 1789), 10. Evans Early American Imprint Collection.

13. William Buchan, *Domestic Medicine: Or a Treatise on the Prevention and Cure of Diseases, by Regimen and Simple Medicine. To Which Is Added, Characteristic Symptoms of Diseases, from the Nosology of the Late Celebrated Dr. Cullen of Edinburgh* (Newcastle: K. Anderson, 1812), xxii, collections.nlm.nih.gov.

14. Samuel J. Rogal, "Pills for the Poor: John Wesley's *Primitive Physic*," *Yale Journal of Biology and Medicine* 51 (1978): 82, https://www.ncbi.nlm.nih.gov/pmc/articles/PMC2595647/.

15. William Battie, *A Treatise on Madness* (London: J. Whiston and B. White, 1763), 2, doi: 10.1136/bmj.39297.741644.94.

16. Battie, *A Treatise on Madness*, 85.

17. John Archer, *Every Man His Own Doctor* (London, 1673), 71, https://books.google.com/books?id=I83Mzl0q2qMC.

18. Nicole Eustace, *Passion Is the Gale: Emotion, Power, and the Coming of the American Revolution* (Chapel Hill: University of North Carolina Press, 2008), 97–98.

19. Anderson, *Inaugural Dissertation*.

20. Spurzheim, *Observations on the Deranged Manifestations of the Mind*, 124.

21. Amariah Brigham in Spurzheim, *Observations on the Deranged Manifestations of the Mind*, 236.

22. Rana A. Hogarth, *Medicalizing Blackness: Making Racial Difference in the Atlantic World, 1780–1840* (Chapel Hill: University of North Carolina Press, 2017), 2–3.

23. Brenna Holland, "Mad Speculation and Mary Girard: Gender, Capitalism, and the Cultural Economy of Madness in the Revolutionary Atlantic," *Journal of the Early Republic* 29, no. 4 (Winter 2019): 650, https://muse.jhu.edu/article/740242.

24. David Lowenthal, *The Past Is a Foreign Country* (New York: Cambridge University Press, 1985).

Chapter 1

Insanity and Confinement in an Age of Liberty

In 1850, Dr. Jenks S. Sprague asked the Medical Society of the State of New York, "What condition of mind disqualified an individual for the enjoyment of his *civil rights*—the rights of property and personal liberty?"[1] For well over a century, doctors, lawmakers, and those suffering from mental illness had been asking that question. Indeed, eighteenth-century British and American subjects and citizens raised the question repeatedly. This should not surprise us. As many scholars have detailed, Anglo and Anglo-American men and women in the eighteenth century thought deeply about the questions of power, liberty, and constraint. This chapter examines those questions, the medical knowledge of the day, and the language of liberty in relationship to the commitment of those deemed insane by individuals or medical professionals. Those who were put into institutions or otherwise confined helped highlight the tensions between liberty and tyranny, or as Anglo and Anglo-Americans often phrased it, liberty and slavery. We can still hear some of the voices of those who protested against their confinement. Other voices are mute but legal or medical records about their confinement also tell us stories.

In 1850, Sprague answered his own question in the way his predecessors had, that all individuals should be allowed to exercise those rights "so long as such exercise neither interferes with, nor *endangers* the rights of others." Only when "the rights of civil society are rendered *insecure* by the acts of an insane individual" could that individual be "deemed *disqualified* for the enjoyment of such rights."[2] By the time Sprague published his observations, English immigrants and their descendants, together with others, had been building communities in North America for over two centuries, working to hold in balance the rights of individuals against the idea of the common good. For example, the seventeenth-century leaders of Jamestown, the first English community to establish itself permanently in North America, leaned toward coercion rather than liberty, but even they claimed the coercive laws were for the common good, or the "advancement of the good . . . and felicity" of the colony.[3] These laws *secured* the rights of civil society.

Even sane people could sometimes interfere with and endanger the rights of others if left with too much liberty. As John Trenchard and Thomas Gordon had outlined in the early eighteenth century in a series of essays on British liberties published under the name *Cato's Letters,* Britons rejected "boundless liberty" which would only lead to chaos. Instead, Gordon argued in letter number 33, they "quitted part of their natural liberty to acquire civil security."[4] These were the ideas embraced by Americans in their local forms of government throughout the colonial period and into the United States. In his 1967 classic study on the ideological origins of the American Revolution, Bernard Bailyn wrote, "Liberty . . . was the capacity to exercise 'natural rights' within limits set not by the mere will or desire of men in power but by non-arbitrary law."[5] Security meant giving up some natural liberty; however, in order for true liberty to prosper, this could not be done without consent. Government should not be arbitrary or tyrannical. The people made choices about how they were ruled and, to a certain extent, by whom they were ruled. These principles underpinned the governments of Britain and its colonies, leading Britons to celebrate their systems as the best on the face of the earth.

Of course, liberty is easy to call for and hard to define and to hold. For many eighteenth-century thinkers, in the mythical state of nature, all people had been free to do whatever they pleased regardless of consequences or the effects on their neighbors. All people had been created equal but had been rent by schisms and evil behavior. Government had emerged to check the worst impulses of people in the state of nature and to work toward a common good. While people had crafted governments to bring order and stability to the world, governments also came with danger. With government came positions of power and the abuse of power by the men who held those positions. The pages of English history were filled with authoritarian movements and countermovements and the mid-eighteenth century would be no different.

Where was the line between liberty and tyranny? The answer depended on many factors including race, gender, social standing, and perceived sanity or insanity. The treatment of men and women deemed insane and the debate over their treatment gave one measure of where that line between liberty and freedom was drawn. The sometimes arbitrary diagnosis of people highlighted the dangers of power in the hands of tyrants. In a system that tied the individual to the whole—the body to the body politic—the expanse or limits of bodily autonomy help us examine the expanse or limits of other kinds of autonomy. The qualifications for the enjoyment of civil rights rested on traits or concepts often defined by men in power not for the common good but for their own self-interest. Of course those in power always claimed they acted for the good of the whole, but those who were denied rights and liberties contested such claims. If illness can act in the same ways on the body and the body politic, then the treatment of those who suffer from illness help unpack the ideological origins of those who battled over ideology and governmental policies.

The problem of whether someone was insane enough to be denied access to their rights and liberties was exacerbated by the belief that good governments bred insanity. This presented a further conundrum for if good government made people insane it would also exclude people from the body politic for not being rational enough to participate. In governments built on the consent of the governed, it was necessary to determine who was capable of consent. This was fodder not just for politicians and lawmakers but commenters on and critics of the systems that politicians and lawmakers created. At the end of the eighteenth century, author Charles Brockden Brown put questions about who was capable of consent into the mouth of his character, Alcuin. At a party, Alcuin asks Mrs. Carter, "Shall the young, the poor, the stranger, and the females, be admitted, indiscriminately, to political privileges? Shall we annex no condition to a voter than he be a thing in human shape, not lunatic, and capable of locomotion?"[6] One potential set of answers to those questions, one that Alcuin ultimately rejects, was that political privileges should extend to all rational humans with the ability to move. However, even if rationality was one of the only limits imposed, who would make the determination about the rationality of the potential voter? After all, what were the markers for a reasonable being? There were no easy answers to those questions.

The answers were difficult because sanity and insanity, rationality and irrationality have always been relative and culturally defined and the definitions have always been in flux more often than stable. Britons in the eighteenth century recognized the wisdom of the question Montaigne had asked in the sixteenth century, "Is there anyone who does not know how imperceptible are the divisions separating madness from the spiritual alacrity of a soul set free, or from actions arising from supreme and extraordinary virtue?"[7] People recognized that some of the historical and scientific figures they admired had been deemed madmen or women by their contemporaries. They also recognized that they lived in a world of constant negotiation where rules could and did change. After all, by the eighteenth century, Britons' sense of self remained tied up with the English Civil War, the Reformation, the Restoration and all of the attendant confusion. Their ancestors had experienced drastic changes in political systems and allegiances. In British North America, colonists were not that far distant from the time when their governments had been forced to change allegiance from Crown to Commonwealth and then back to Crown. Certainly the social memory of that time continued to mold the policies made in the colonies. Particularly in New England, the social memory of unpopular and tyrannical governments being forced upon their ancestors continued to resonate.

All of this is to say that the ideas of social construction of health and illness did not spring fully formed into existence at the end of the twentieth century; it is not an idea discovered in our own lifetimes. In his dissertation, Alexander Anderson wrote that, "It is difficult to define that state of the intellectual faculties which may be said to constitute a reasonable being; for, so various are the sensations of different people, and their conclusions from them—so imperceptible the gradations from a slight error in reasoning to fatuity, that we can scarcely say where rationality ends and folly begins." There were plenty of people then, as now, who could not conduct conversation easily, who were shy, who might commit faux pas in company, who were awkward, or who disagreed with social conventions. Should these people have been considered insane? Anderson balked at that. "Some have made the characteristic of *madness* to consist in a mode of thinking and acting different from the generality of mankind: But this, if admitted, would evidently include every great genius, who, in the pursuit of truth, dares to differ from others."[8] Anderson argued that people had to allow for oddness and even seeming insanity in order to also allow for thinkers and doers who could change society for the better. At the very least, reasonable people would agree that social norms were hard to pin down and negotiate.

The "furiously mad" were the exception; they were the ones easy to eliminate from the body politic. In North America, governments had been doing so since the seventeenth century. Massachusetts Bay Colony passed a law that allowed imprisoning any person "lunatic and so furiously mad as to render it dangerous to the peace or the safety of the good people for such a lunatic person to go at large."[9] Concerned citizens in Pennsylvania petitioned the Provincial government to create an avenue for care for "Lunatics" who were "a Terror to their Neighbours, who are daily apprehensive of the Violences they may commit."[10] Virginia Governor Francis Fauquier had asked for a lunatic hospital to house "a poor unhappy set of People who are deprived of their Senses, and wander about the Country, terrifying the Rest of their Fellow Creatures."[11] Weighing the good of the whole against the good of the individual, colonists created laws and institutions meant to confine those whose madness made them a danger.

The danger of the furiously mad was real. Dr. Johann Spurzheim did not exaggerate when he wrote that some suffering from derangement "feel a ferocious inclination to commit to the flames every thing of a combustible nature, or to imbrue their hands in human blood."[12] At their most violent, the actions of the furiously mad could result in violence and murder. Because of this danger, lawmakers and others contended that confinement of the furiously mad was a necessary step to protect families and communities. Using this evidence

Michel Foucault argued, in his groundbreaking *Madness and Civilization: A History of Insanity in the Age of Reason,* that by the eighteenth-century doctors, lunatic asylums, and medical hospitals had become instruments for social control and that deviance became less tolerated than it had been previously. He wrote, "Tamed, madness preserves all the appearances of its reign. It now takes part in the measures of reason and in the labor of truth."[13] While Foucault's analysis remains provocative, he was a better philosopher than historian. As David Rothman pointed out in his 1971 classic, *The Discovery of the Asylum: Social Order and Disorder in the New Republic*, Foucault's categories "seem rigid (are reason and unreason mutually exclusive?), and there remains too little room for other considerations."[14]

Looking carefully through the historical record, the analysis of Rothman holds more weight than that of Foucault. Bent on a sweeping analysis, Foucault saw only instruments of social control. And while it is true that eighteenth-century medical practitioners did sanction confinement, they were not men bent on creating social conformity for they recognized genius in many non-conformists. Many of them also very genuinely wanted to help those who were harmful to themselves or others and to cure them if possible.[15] They believed, like medical student Edward Cutbrush, that "an uninterrupted use" of reason "is absolutely necessary for the well-being of all societies, both civil and religious," and they wanted to restore people to reason and full enjoyment of their rights, if possible.[16] They understood, as Rothman explained, that reason and unreason were not mutually exclusive, nor were desires for a well-ordered society and a genuine concern for the ill.

Although laws and customs excluded the furiously mad from the body politic, the question still remained if others were lunatic at all or if they were simply harmless lunatics. To complicate this further, distinguishing between dangerous and harmless lunatics was far from an exact science and thus fraught with peril. In his *Treatise on Insanity*, Philippe Pinel detailed five species of mental derangement, but within each of the five there were ranges (from mild to profound) and variations. For example, Pinel wrote that "melancholia with delirium, presents itself in two very opposite forms. Sometimes it is distinguished by an exalted sentiment of self-importance, associated with chimerical pretensions to unbounded power or inexhaustible riches. At other times, it is characterized by great depression of spirits, pusillanimous apprehensions and even absolute despair."[17] If one "mental derangement," as Pinel characterized it, could present in two opposite forms, diagnosing the mad was difficult. If madness separated people from their rights and some forms of madness were difficult to diagnose, doctors and community members needed to tread carefully.

Doctors did not always tread carefully for, like actors on the political stage, doctors could err in their judgment or be corrupted by power. One way they asserted their power was through diagnosis. By diagnosing someone as furiously mad or delirious, they could disqualify the diagnosed from access to the rights of civil society. Sometimes the evidence of derangement was clear but other times the moral or value judgment of the doctor was based on hearsay or behavior that was odd but not necessarily dangerous. Although doctors' authority could be contested, diagnosis gave them power because their declaration that someone was mentally ill often came with the ability to sentence him or her to confinement or recommend a course of treatments ranging from mild to brutal. By diagnosing people as mad, the doctor transformed them from adults into dependent children, thus strengthening their authority over them and denying them access to the rights that were the birthright of white men and women. Paul Starr wrote about this power in *The Social Transformation of American Medicine*, that "As gatekeepers into and out of various institutions, professionals acquire means of ensuring compliance quite independent of any belief in the moral basis of their authority."[18] This meant that men and women could be confined against their will solely on the word of a doctor who was capable of error.

Confining men and women and depriving them of rights of property and personal liberty proved problematic, even in those cases when an argument could be made that the confinement was for the good of society, because in an age where people demanded liberty, confinement clearly took their liberty away. Confinement became more problematic when the argument for confinement did not rest on solid medical knowledge. In England, men and women were placed in madhouses, including in those run for profit, often on the affidavit of one physician only and even when other physicians disagreed with the diagnosis. Married women, who had no legal voice, could be put into private madhouses by their husbands. Daniel Defoe wrote that men sent "their Wives to mad-Houses at every Whim or Dislike," and that they did this to "be more secure and undisturb'd in their Debaucheries."[19] In North America, family members or friends could petition to get their loved ones declared *non compos mentis* to confine them, to take away their ability to control their estates, or both. In Pennsylvania, hospital admittance was allowed only after a physician certified a person's insanity, but doctors like Benjamin Rush could simply write a note like, "James Sproul is a proper patient for Pennsylvania Hospital;" no other proof was needed.[20] Once admitted the patient had few avenues for appeal. According to the historical record, unscrupulous family or community members sometimes followed no official protocol and could use bribery to achieve their ends. In the end, whether the mental illness was real, suspected, or manufactured, the practice of confinement raised as many or more questions than it solved.

The historical record has left us stories, both fictional and non-fictional, of those confined for mental illness. These stories show people both ill and well forced into confinement often against their will for various reasons and they show the abuses in the system that mirrored the abuses in the political system. Many of the stories detailed men or women who were tricked or forced into confinement. Roy Porter noted about this era, "As confinement grew, a patient's protest literature emerged with it. Cries went up from former asylum inmates vindicating their sanity and alleging victimization by sinister foes."[21] This protest literature shared a narrative arc with political pamphlets, speeches, and other writings in its emphasis on the tyrannical capriciousness of those in power who could deny liberty on a whim. These stories were also a form of the increasingly popular captivity narrative that told stories of people whose liberty was taken away as they were thrust into worlds where they could assert little control over their own lives. If they had been subjects or citizens, they now were captives, absent the rights they had previously enjoyed. Captivity narratives appealed to eighteenth-century readers because those who chafed at acts of Parliament or royal decrees drew parallels between the political world that contained them and the literal captivity detailed in the stories. Captivity narratives asked their readers to travel with the protagonists into their time of bondage, or, in the words of Charles Fitz-Geffrey's seventeenth century sermon, for the reader to "Make their bondage your thralldom, their suffering, your own smarting." Fitz-Geffrey asked his hearers to "Have a fellow-feeling with [the captives], as being members of the same body."[22] The narratives asked the readers to place themselves in the body of the writer as he or she experienced captivity in order to understand what it meant to have one's liberty taken away in an arbitrary manner. This was not difficult for an audience primed to see threats to liberty everywhere they looked, who experienced governmental practices as a loss of liberty, and who deeply feared the men in power who could exert extraordinary control over their lives.

Because of the doctors' power of diagnosis, once confined as madmen or women, captives found it difficult or impossible to prove that they were not insane. In 1830, Dr. John Connolly wrote, "Once confined, the very confinement is admitted as the strongest of all proofs that a man must be mad."[23] Or, as James A. Holstein wrote, commenting on late-twentieth-century court-ordered insanity, "The mental illness assumption consistently undermined patients' credibility," that people "are reluctant to rely upon claims made by 'crazy' people, claims that cannot be trusted or believed."[24] Writers in the eighteenth century confirmed this. Confined against his will in London, Alexander Cruden, whose story I will come back to later in this chapter, tried to free himself by using his power of reason on anyone who would listen. At one point, he wrote that he had asked the maid who waited on him in the private madhouse where he was imprisoned, "what signs of madness she had found in him." According to Cruden, "She could not instance any, but only foolishly mentioned his peremptory Refusal to see *Wightman, Oswald* and his Wife," the very people who had put him in the madhouse against his will. We have no corroborating evidence from the maid. We do not know how she would have told the story, but in Cruden's version she did not see madness in him but did not doubt the others who had told her Cruden was mad.[25] That presumptive evidence of madness—that people are mad because they are in a madhouse—speaks to one of the aspects of danger inherent in confining anyone not furiously mad.

It also speaks to the power of the language of madness for in the world outside the madhouse, calling one's political opponent a lunatic often enough might make that presumption of lunacy stick, particularly if the speaker were powerful enough and the person to whom the language was directed eccentric enough. For men in political power, the end goal of the use of this language was the metaphorical equivalent of putting his opponent in the madhouse. If he could make his opponent seem like a madman, he could also discredit him. If he could get enough others to believe the charge of lunacy, he did not need a straightjacket or a madhouse keeper because his accusation served to discredit his opponent, confining him in reputation if not in real life. There was often great power in the language of lunacy although, as demonstrated below in the story of James Otis, sometimes literal madmen continued to hold onto power even after confinement. While it might be an imperfect weapon, it was nonetheless wielded with great frequency. It worked best against those who already had less power, reifying the structural inequalities of race, gender, and social status. It might be possible for a powerful, articulate, and well-connected white man to climb back out of the metaphorical madhouse even if his opponent had been successful in slandering his name, but it was almost impossible for those without the same access to structural power. Losing reputation as a sane and rational person, someone with whom it was worthwhile to interact or conduct business, pushed people already on the margins even further out.

The point here is twofold. First, it was hard for people to demonstrate their rationality if they had been confined for madness. Second, tyranny could exist in the medical as well as the political realm. Because of this, those confined against their will for madness used the political language of their world to make dual points about the injustice done to them as individuals and about greater injustice in their societies that their individual stories revealed. The madhouse or the straightjacket acted on the body, just like laws or proclamations acted on the political body politic. Without just cause, and without evidence of wrongdoing, medical or political leaders punished others in order to increase their own power and deny it to deserving others. Both captivity narratives of those confined against their will and other political writings used a common language, railing against "the machinations of some designing persons . . . who are grasping at power and the property of their neighbors."[26] While that particular language comes from the American Political Society in Worcester during upheavals in Massachusetts in 1774, the same charges came from the pens of the chroniclers of the injustices in the medical world. In *The Ideological Origins of the American Revolution*, Bernard Bailyn laid out the "belief that what lay behind every political scene, the ultimate explanation of every political controversy, was the disposition of power."[27] This study shows that what lay behind every medical scene, every confinement, every admittance to a madhouse was also the disposition of power. The medical was both personal and political.

ENGLISH STORIES

The stories of the machinations of designing persons, of madness, of freedom and unfreedom that follow span the Atlantic Ocean. Although there were significant differences in institutional care in Britain and in the colonies, Britons on both sides of the ocean shared the concern that their liberty could be taken away. The political, medical, and other cultures in North America remained rooted in Britishness well into the nineteenth century. Many in the colonies read and paid close attention to any story that highlighted abuses of power or pointed toward a troubled world. Their government was a shared government and, although the ocean could serve as a barrier, it more often served as a conduit that carried everything from goods to British officials to the potential for tyranny.

The first story here, although it does not come first chronologically, is the story of James Tilly Matthews. I start with this story because it highlights the problems in the power of diagnosis and the question of whose voice got heard in cases of lunacy. Matthews was a London tea broker who was also delusional. At the beginning of the French Revolution, he believed he could be an agent of peace between Great Britain and France. Instead, the French suspected him of being a double agent and imprisoned him for three years before determining he was a lunatic and sending him home. Once back in London he saw political conspiracies everywhere he looked and made a public spectacle of himself by interrupting a House of Commons debate by shouting, "Treason," from the public gallery. He was held first in a house of corrections before being transferred to Bethlem Hospital. His family contested his diagnosis as a maniac and appealed to Lord Kenyon who agreed with the doctors rather than the family after witnessing Matthews's erratic behavior. Matthews was both clearly mad and, often, a model inmate of Bethlem. Today, doctors believe that he suffered from schizophrenia. In his sane moments, he helped design the new Bethlem and was an arbiter for disputes. When in the throes of his illness, however, he believed that a gang in London used a device called the Air Loom to engage in acts of villainy. Among other things, Matthews believed they used this device to steal ideas or to kill people by using the magnetic atmosphere to interfere with their organs or to use the fluids in a person's brain as an electrical conduit.

In 1809, however, Matthews's family tried again to get him released and enlisted the help of two doctors, George Birkbeck and Henry Clutterbuck, who examined Matthews six times and declared that he was sane. John Haslam, the apothecary for both Bethlem Hospital and several private madhouses, published a pamphlet in defense of keeping Matthews confined and disagreed with the critics who believed Matthews was sane enough or safe enough (if actually insane) to be freed. In his pamphlet, Haslam dismissed his opponents, writing, "if one party be right, the other must be wrong: because a person cannot correctly be said to be *in* his senses and *out* of his senses at the same time."[28] Haslam used most of the pamphlet in his attempt to prove that he was the party in the right and that the doctors Birkbeck and Clutterbuck, who believed Matthews should be released, were the party in the wrong. Or, as historian Roy Porter noted, Haslam, in his pamphlet, "seeks to vindicate the right of the Bethlem medical staff to speak authoritatively upon insanity, indeed to act as public guardians of rationality."[29] Haslam painted himself as not just an expert in diagnosis, but also a guardian of the public. "There are already too many maniacs allowed to enjoy a dangerous liberty," he wrote, "and the Governors of Bethlem Hospital . . . were not disposed to liberate a mischievous lunatic to disturb the good order and peace of society."[30]

Haslam's use of "dangerous liberty" is telling. Allowing a madman or woman to live outside of the walls of an institution put the liberty of the wider community at risk. Haslam weighed the balance between liberty and security and came down on the side of security. He insisted Matthews was both insane and that he posed a threat to the safety of others. This moment tells us not just about an apothecary asserting his authority to guard the public from a dangerous lunatic, but about other deep divisions that existed in the eighteenth century. As shown in later chapters, the insistence of a perfectly clear division between right and wrong figured in the political world as well. If Haslam was right, then Birkbeck and Clutterbuck were wrong; in Haslam's mind, there was no place for more than one truth. Similarly, in the years leading up to the American Revolution, many of the actors and observers did not see shades of gray. For example, nothing could dissuade some Britons from their belief that Americans wanted independence in the first years of the 1770s despite all evidence to the contrary. They believed that their reading of situation was right and that anyone who stated otherwise was wrong and perhaps even crazy.

This insistence on a clear determination of right or wrong frustrated those confined for madness against their will for, as presumed lunatics, it was hard for them to convince others that they were right. They tried, nonetheless, to change public opinion. Those who were able to, made the case that they were sane and that they had the evidence to prove it. To them, any doctor or madhouse keeper who said otherwise was clearly in the wrong. For Matthews's family, it was clearly wrong that he remained in Bethlem and they insisted that Haslam's tyranny was not based on right, not based on rational evidence, but based solely on the power exerted over their loved one's life and well-being. For them the wrong was unequal power and their lack of voice for change.

Others were denied the very privilege of speaking up or out because they did not have the social standing that allowed their words to be published. The horror of people confined against their will, however, haunted the Anglo and Anglo-American imagination enough so that writers of fiction took up their tales, highlighting not only the tyranny apparent in the unjust confinement of sane people but sometimes, also, the tyranny inherent in the patriarchal system that denied a legal voice to most women. These works of fiction gave voice to female protagonists, already stripped layers of protection by English common law, who were then stripped of protection again by unjust confinement. These fictional accounts of women confined lay bare not just the corrupting influences of political or medical power but the dangers of a world in which women's decisions about their lives and bodies could be easily taken away.

In 1726, Eliza Haywood published *The Distress'd Orphan, or Love in a Madhouse*. In this tale, Annilia, an orphan, is set to inherit a fortune when she comes of age. Because of this, her guardian and uncle, Giraldo, determines she should marry Horatio—his son and her cousin—to keep the money in the family. When she falls in love with and wants to marry Colonel Marathon instead, Giraldo tries to change her mind and then threatens her. She is not moved by pleading or by threat, and answers, "The Love of Liberty is natural to all, and I should have more reason to regret than be pleas'd with the large Fortune left me by my Father, if it must subject me to eternal slavery."[31] Annilia's language reflects the growing claim by Britons that liberty was their birthright and that while they gave up some of that liberty for the greater good, no one could be made a slave through unjust law, or, in Annilia's case, through a forced marriage.[32] Variations on the language Haywood appropriated in this tale would continue to resound through the following half century or more, realizing itself in many forms, including in the rhetoric employed during the war for independence in North America.

In *The Distress'd Orphan*, when Giraldo discovers Annilia trying to move out of his house in order to preserve her freedom, he first imprisons her in her room and then promises her freedom if she marries Horatio. When she continues to refuse, Giraldo resolves to send her to a private madhouse, where "he had often been told, that for a good Gratification, the Doors would be open as well for those whom it was necessary, for the Interest of their Friends, to be made Mad, as for those who were so in reality."[33] In the middle of the night, Annilia is awakened by three strangers, seized, forced into a hackney coach, and confined in a private madhouse. Giraldo is correct that if he pays enough money, it does not matter if his niece is mad or not and that the conditions there might very well drive her mad. Here, too, Haywood's fiction reflected a reality for women in particular. Women dependent on fathers, guardians, or husbands had no legal voice under the laws of coverture making it relatively easy to remove them from their homes on trumped-up charges of insanity. Private madhouses could be corrupt institutions, run solely for financial gain. They existed outside of the law and provided space for individuals removed when they proved problematic for family members, business partners, or anyone else with whom they had found themselves in conflict.

Although works like *The Distress'd Orphan* were written as fictional stories of families, romance, and corruption, they can also be read as meditations on the body politic. Haywood wrote Annilia's story, but Annilia's story could just as easily been a story of the continued tensions between claims for natural liberty and assertions of power on a political level, or those between heads of households and other family members on a familial level. Britons conceived of political relationships as family relationships. Giraldo could be a minister or a king abusing power for gain. Giraldo puts his niece away for interfering with his plans, Parliament passed an emergency riot act and suspended the writ of habeas corpus to keep political opponents from interfering with their plans, and women had no legal voice under coverture leaving them as potential victims on multiple levels. The fictional corruption in Haywood's story reflected that within the political and familial worlds in which real people lived.

If fiction is one reflection of the body politic, real-life stories are another. From the distance of two hundred years or more it is often impossible to tell whether the real-life people who were confined in madhouses or hospitals were sane or whether they were justly or unjustly confined. While that determination mattered greatly for both the confined and the confiners, it matters less for the purposes of this study. Regardless of their sanity or insanity, those who found themselves confined against their wills challenged the political systems directly and called on liberty both on the personal level (they wanted to be free from confinement) but also on the political level (they believed their story reflected more widely on society and culture). Alexander Cruden could not free himself from the madhouse by using the power of reason but he could write about it after he escaped, leaving descriptions of some of his madhouse experiences for the historical record.

Determined he was insane, his friends and family members had him confined more than once. In a pamphlet published in 1739 about one of these experiences, he claimed that he had been set up by men who wished him ill and had tricked him into confinement. After a series of strange and sometimes violent encounters that involved a widow he was courting, friends, and his landlady, he was home at work on his papers when some "foolish people" barged into his room and convinced him to get into a hackney coach. Cruden wrote that he did enter the coach willingly for he believed he was simply being taken to Robert Wightman's house for conversation. However, as the hackney coach took a direction away from Wightman's house and toward Bethlem Royal Hospital, Cruden became suspicious. When he realized he had been tricked, "he expostulated with them in the following manner: 'Oh! what are you going to do with me? I bless God, I am not mad." He then asked, "Are you going to carry me to *Bethlehem?*" Despite his protest, he was taken to a private madhouse on Bethnal Green where he continued to insist that his keepers "had no Power over him in Law, Equity or Consanguinity."[34]

Throughout his experience of capture and confinement, Cruden insisted he was not mad. Indeed he believed his confinement violated legal and moral principles. The law should have protected him from being confined against his will, he was descended from the same people as his confiners, and he held the same religious principles as they did. When he finally managed to escape the madhouse, he published his pamphlet in an attempt to shine a light into the darkness of madhouse practices and to prove he was sane. The darkness of the practices included being denied writing implements, a practice that Cruden claimed was "worse than any in a *Spanish Inquisition*."[35] Self-consciously using the markers of difference that invoked societies that were considered tyrannical, five paragraphs later he accused Matthew Wright, the madhouse keeper, of treating the occupants of his private madhouse "worse than Galley-slaves" and being "like a *Turkish Bashaw*." Wright's servants who helped take care of the madhouse inmates were "obsequious Cannibals." In page after page, Cruden raised the specter of those foreign governments and powers Britons considered most oppressive. He compared the private madhouse to places where arbitrary force rather than liberty was the guiding principle, calling on all the tropes available to him. Cruden's narrative did what it was intended to do which was to raise hackles. Whether his story was true or not, he posited himself within a tradition that focused on the travesty of free and independent men and women who had their liberty taken away by designing others.

Cruden's voice was but one in a growing crescendo of British voices in the eighteenth century that equated false confinement with lost liberty. As long as lawmakers refused to respond, it was a story that would not die. Each year increased the pressure to enact some sort of reform in a system that could be argued was for personal or financial gain rather than protection of society or the treatment and cure of the insane. In 1774, thirty-five years after Cruden's publication, Samuel Bruckshaw published an account of his imprisonment for insanity, called *One More Proof of the Iniquitous Use of Private Madhouses*; even his title made it clear that all the evidence that had come before was not enough, that the public and those in power needed *one more* piece of evidence, and perhaps many more, before changes would be made. In this account, Bruckshaw claimed he had been imprisoned when his neighbors resented his purchase of a parcel of land. Like Cruden, he emphasized the contrast between ideas of liberty and the fact of captivity, frightening his readers by reminding them that the "oppression which crushes me today, may fall on my neighbor tomorrow, nor can anyone assure himself he shall be able to escape."[36] In 1796, a similar story was published by William Belcher who had also been imprisoned against his will in a private London madhouse. Belcher published a letter he had written to the doctor who had "restored [him] from legal death," freeing him from his captivity. He, too, worried about what his imprisonment meant not just for himself as an individual but for society. Belcher wrote that what had happened was "a horrible disgrace to government and to society," and that he had a duty "to God, my country, and humanity to speak."[37]

Perhaps these men had actually been mad and their confinement justified. Regardless, these and other similar stories by those confined under the charge of madness reminded readers of the tension between freedom on one hand and what they called slavery on the other. The 1791 London newspapers published a piece entitled "Mad Houses" in which the author wrote that the public should keep a "very strict eye" on "these gaolers of the mind; for if they do not find a patient mad, their oppressive tyranny soon makes him so."[38] Foucault argued that in the Middle Ages, "the madman . . . reminds each man of the truth," serving as instruments of social criticism. In the eighteenth century, falsely confined madmen and women reminded others that in a free society, corrupt individuals could deprive others of their rights and freedoms. Whereas Foucault argued that, by the eighteenth century, "confinement is explained, or at least justified, by the desire to avoid scandal," for Bruckshaw and Belcher, the scandal had not been avoided by their confinement.[39] Instead, they had been imprisoned by men warped by their own self-interest; imprisonment exposed rather than avoided scandal. Porter was right when he wrote that, "Every age gets the lunatics it deserves."[40] In these cases, each one of these stories helped to focus the paranoia of people, already ready to see conspiracies against their liberty everywhere they looked, on the dangers that lurked in their societies. The combination of publicity and concern led to Parliament to pass the Madhouses Act in 1774 requiring all madhouses to be licensed by a committee of the Royal College of Physicians. It did not stop all abuses, of course, but it was a step toward reform of a dangerous system that threatened British liberties.

AMERICAN STORIES

Americans were fortunate to be absent the institution of the privately-run and profit-making madhouses that existed in England, but like Britons everywhere they faced the tension between liberty and confinement and between inclusion and exclusion from the body politic. In the colonies, the stories of the mad and the confined added an additional layer to the conversation. The protagonists were not only situated within a liberty-loving culture but also in colonies where, by the very nature of imperial power, men and women had different relationships to government and society. By the mid-eighteenth century, the stories of madmen and women took place against a backdrop of growing tensions between the colonies and the mother country, a growing resistance, and eventually outright rebellion. And, as if to prove the doctors correct that liberty caused madness, some of the most ardent lovers of liberty were themselves mad or had mad family members.

James Otis, Jr. could have stepped out of any mad doctor's case file as someone driven insane by engagement in political opposition and high levels of mental activity. In the 1760s, Otis came into view as an early voice against the new policies that tried to tie the colonies more tightly to the empire. He emerged into the spotlight in 1761 when, as a lawyer, he challenged the constitutionality of the writs of assistance. Early in his five-hour speech, he proclaimed the writs were "the worst instrument of arbitrary power, the most destructive of English liberty and the fundamental principles of law, that ever was found in an English law-book."[41] When Parliament passed the Sugar Act in 1764, Otis responded in a pamphlet, *The Rights of the British Colonists Asserted and Proved*. While Otis acknowledged that Parliament had the power with which to tax the colonies, he believed using that power violated the rights of those living in the colonies, that "the supreme power cannot take from any man any part of his property without his consent in person, or by representation."[42]

While Otis earned a reputation as a spokesman for liberty, he also demonstrated erratic behavior and speech. Peter Oliver, the Chief Justice of the Massachusetts Superior Court, complained to John Adams that Otis was "forever abusing the Court." Adams agreed with Oliver, noting that Otis was often "distracted." "It is a pitty," Adams said to Oliver, that Otis "was not better guided. He has many fine Talents."[43] Otis's friends did attempt to guide him and to tame his madder impulses but those efforts had little effect.[44] Oliver responded to Adams, "I have known him these twenty years, and I have no opinion of his head or his heart. If Bedlamism is a talent, he has it in perfection."[45] To Oliver, Otis seemed like one of the mad confined in London's Bethlem Royal Hospital. Otis was not confined at that time, however; instead he freely brought his madness into the public political arena. He seemed a madman to Oliver but Bostonians elected him to the General Court as a representative, and elected him again even as his behavior became more and more erratic. Otis was not always sane but the men of Boston wanted him as a representative because of his willingness to go toe to toe with the political elite. Perhaps his madness allowed him to overcome deferential barriers that would have prevented him from doing so, creating space for resistance in ways that a fully sane and rational individual might not have been able to.[46]

In May 1768, opposing Thomas Hutchinson's election to the Massachusetts assembly's upper house, Otis created a scene in the House chamber. According to Hutchinson, "Our great incendiary was enraged and ran about the House in a fury."[47] In her biography of Mercy Otis Warren (Otis's sister), Rosemarie Zagarri wrote that, "Members reacted to Otis's breach of decorum with shock, repulsion, and dismay."[48] His actions and his words transformed some of his fellow subjects into enraged enemies. The next year, Otis was attacked with a cane by one of these men, John Robinson, a member of the American Board of Customs Commissioners. The blow to his head that Otis received from Robinson worsened his mental health. By 1770, Otis was removed from Boston for care only to return a few months later. At some points he was sane and rational, and at others, "he raved, jumped out of windows and was pitifully bewildered to find his clients seeking other assistance."[49]

If doctors like Anderson, Spurzheim, and Brigham were correct in their later hypotheses, Otis's big brain and oppositional nature might have been what had driven him mad in the first place. His madness embarrassed some of his allies and observers, but it was also one element that made his fiery protests so effective. Absent some of the social niceties that kept others from breaching the rules of decorum, Otis could speak and publish what others kept private, helping to give voice to a nascent protest movement. Despite his own unease with Otis's behavior, Adams remembered him fondly in later years. In 1818, Adams defended Otis against his detractors once again, writing, "I have been young and now am Old, and I solemnly Say, I have never known a Man whose Love of his Country was more ardent or Sincere; never one, who Suffered So much; never one whose Services for any ten years of his Life, were So important and essential to the Cause of his Country as those of Mr Otis from 1760 to 1770."[50] Otis's mental illness prevented him from doing more, but if Adams's assessment were correct, he had been an essential actor in the push for revolution, a cause that sane and rational men could take up after mad Otis had thrown down the gauntlet.

Unfortunately, we cannot know how Otis experienced his mental illness. Was it freeing or enslaving? By the mid-1770s, insanity changed the workings of Otis's mind in ways that sometimes interfered with his ability to reason and argue. In addition, Otis's insanity led to his confinement which was, at the very least, physically uncomfortable at times and psychically uncomfortable in his rational moments. Hutchinson wrote that in December of 1771, Otis was carried out of Boston bound hand and foot. Even if those who confined him tried to carry him away in a discreet fashion, what a spectacle this must have made for those who did witness it: one of the great liberty men was bound and had his liberty taken away temporarily. If he had some of his rationality intact at that moment, how terrifying and humiliating it must have been as well. Mercy Otis Warren spent a great deal of time worrying about her brother and what she interpreted as the trap that was his irrational mind. To her acquaintance, Sarah Walter Hesilridge, Warren wrote "that her heart was bleeding" for her brother. "It is indeed hard to submit calmly to see those abilities which once equaled and even surpassed many of the first characters, clouded, shattered and broken: to see the mind of a man so superior, thus darkened." She hoped that God would "restore again to usefulness, a man so capable and so willing to promote the happiness of his fellow man."[51]

In 1783 when Warren reported on Otis's death to his daughter, Elizabeth Otis Brown, she wrote that the attack by Robinson had given Otis "that irreparable wound which broke the energetic power of reason, & almost shook from the throne that distinguishing Characteristic of the human Soul." She continued that her brother wanted to be released from the trap of irrationality and "often invok'd the messenger of death to give him a sudden release from a Life become burdensome in every Sense." Perhaps, in an age of liberty, Otis had recognized that he had made a slave to insanity. Warren certainly thought so. She considered that when he died, "His great soul was instantly set free (from a thraldom in which the Love of his country & of mankind had invok'd him) by a flash of Light'ning." She thought her newly established country "is more indebted" to Otis "for the investigation of her rights & the defence of her Liberties than perhaps to any other Individual." She saw her brother as "a martyr to his beloved Country."[52] In his biography of Thomas Hutchinson, Bernard Bailyn characterized Otis as "an extraordinary perceptive intellectual." Bailyn wrote that Otis "tore and dove and raged in half-lunatic indignation," but that "he was capable, as perhaps no one else of the time, of seeing the deep issues and of relating them to practical and personal politics."[53] Perhaps the times created Otis's madness and Otis's madness helped create the times. Otis suffered from his mental illness in a tumultuous time that invited irrationality.

With Otis's impassioned words as one entrance, in the 1760s and 1770s American colonists began to negotiate British ideology, shifting interpretations to suit their emergent belief systems. Early protests against tax policies became a concerted cry of "no taxation without representation." Throughout the colonies, British subjects called on their British liberties, but also located these liberties into an American geography and grammar. Their distance from the metropolitan center of the British empire, for instance, meant that they believed that the new laws, designed to raise revenue, violated their British liberties for only the colonial assemblies had the right to raise revenue. By 1767, John Dickinson situated the colonists' rights as existing not solely within the realm of the British Empire but additionally within the soil under the colonists' feet. Were colonists to obey the Townshend Acts, "the tragedy of American liberty is finished," Dickinson wrote.[54] Madness dogged their heels at every turn.

In Virginia, Patrick Henry was one of the men who worked to shift and negotiate Americans' ideology, pressing his listeners to insist on their natural liberties and to resist British policies, eventually calling for a war to do just that. As Henry made a name for himself as an advocate for liberty, his wife, Sarah Shelton Henry, lost her mind. By 1770, she had, according to Dr. Thomas Hinde, the family physician, "lost her reason and could only be restrained from self-destruction by a strait-dress."[55] She was then confined in a basement room. We don't know much about her illness or care since we mostly have the stories of later generations that insist the basement room was sunny and that the family was loving and engaged. According to the family, her husband tended to her when he was home, but most of her care, as well as the care of five of the Henry children, fell to their eldest daughter Martha Fontaine and the Henry family enslaved people.[56] Martha's husband, John Fontaine, managed the plantation while Patrick pursued his career and political ambitions. If other families' surviving narratives are an indication, Martha and John Fontaine did all of this willingly, but certainly not without their own grievances or without occasionally feeling as if Sarah had unjustly taken away some of their own liberty of movement or action. The enslaved people, of course, had no liberty to object to their burden of care.

Henry may well have grieved for his wife's condition, but his reliance on his daughter, son-in-law, and enslaved people meant that his wife's mental illness did not get in the way of his own freedom or ambition. Unconfined, by 1774 he had been elected as a delegate to the First Continental Congress. While he attended Congress, his wife attempted to die by suicide. Even after Henry returned home, he continued to pursue his primary goal which was not to care for his wife but to organize a volunteer company. In Hanover, Virginia he addressed the men of the town "in a very animated speech, pointing out the necessity of our having recourse to arms in defense of our rights."[57] Meanwhile Sarah was locked in a basement room, stripped of rights both by the laws of coverture and by her confinement. A few months later, in February 1775, Sarah Shelton died. Various accounts have her dying by suicide but the record is unclear. The next month, Henry attended the Second Virginia Convention as a delegate where he gave his most famous speech. In the speech he asked, "Is Life so dear, or peace so sweet, as to be purchased at the price of chains and slavery?" He then answered, "Forbid it, Almighty God! I know not what course others may take, but as for me, give me liberty or give me death!"[58] Perhaps his wife had weighed this equation and had chosen death over the chains of mental illness that kept her locked away from society.

Henry's speech focused on the political and military crisis at that moment and not the recent death of his wife. Looking back, however, the confluence of those events showcase the various points of access to liberty or confinement. As Sarah suffered from mental illness, losing her reason and her freedom of movement, confined in a (sunny?) basement room and cared for mostly by enslaved people, her husband pursued a course of action that helped lead down the road to war and American independence. His eloquence and call to action maintain a mythological place in American history. Sarah's unhappiness and misery are largely missing from the historical record. Patrick Henry emerged as the "lion of liberty"; his wife, in her last days, was the madwoman in the basement.

The story bends even further for those not fully vested with rights as British subjects. Within the system of freedom and both ideological and chattel slavery that the Henry's story evokes, further questions need to be raised when enslaved men and women were declared insane. From the very beginning of its existence, the Pennsylvania Hospital admitted and treated enslaved people. "Dr. Moore's Negro man, a Lunatick, was received 3rd Mo. 26th, 1753. His master promised payment. 1st Mo. 23d. 1754. Admitted Negro Adam, a Lunatick and pay patient belonging to Mrs. Margaret Clymer, under the care of Dr. Thos. Bond. 2nd Mo 16th, 1754. Black Adam, at ye request of his Mistress Margaret Clymer, was this day discharged."[59] These records tell a story but most of the story remains hidden from view. Would the admitting physicians question a slave owner if he or she promised payment in exchange for confining an enslaved person in the hospital? Had "Black Adam" been ill? Was he really a lunatic? If he had been ill, when Mrs. Clymer had him discharged from the hospital had he been cured, or did she simply need him for work or show? If nothing else, Adam's diagnosis of lunacy disproved the medical theory that slavery so suppressed the mind that enslaved people were incapable of madness. Of course that assertion was absurd because the conditions of slavery and the racism that justified slavery, the denial of freedom and the separation of families caused anxiety, depression, grief, and fear, all of the very things doctors believed drove white men and women mad. It is more than possible that Adam was both a enslaved person and a madman and equally possible that Clymer had simply used the existing system to suit her own needs.

Already absent liberty and civil rights, further constraints on enslaved people's lives could come at the whim of their owners. In 1751, the same year the Pennsylvania legislature voted to fund the hospital, South Carolina passed a law regarding "slaves that may become lunatic, belonging to poor persons who may be unable to provide" for them. This law, too, gave lie to doctors' assertions of the absence of madness in enslaved men and women and supports the claim that the system of slavery instead drove them mad. By this law, a justice of the peace was required "to cause such lunatic to be secured in some convenient place in the parish . . . to prevent his or her doing any mischief."[60]

With black men and women, and particularly enslaved people, the long-ago language of "doing any mischief" raises even more questions for historians. Mischief, of course, could be a catch-all category for any of the ways slaves asserted agency or expressed their humanity. A century after the South Carolina law allowing justices of the peace to confine "lunatic" slaves, the southern physician Samuel Cartwright came up with a new name for what he believed to be a disease. *Drapetomania*, according to Cartwright, was the mental illness that led enslaved people to run away. Instead of a desire for freedom it was "a disease of the mind as any other species of mental alienation, and much more curable, as a general rule."[61] Enslaved people's quests for freedom or autonomy, the very same ideals a revolutionary generation valued, were punished in a system predicated on either keeping black people enslaved, or, if freeing them, making sure they remained among the lower sort. It would not be surprising in a system of slavery if back talk or feigned illness, some of the markers of slave resistance, were not also read as mental illness.

In addition to enslaved people, other unfree people make brief appearances in the historical records of insanity. In 1765, the redemptioner Conrad Döer petitioned the managers of the Pennsylvania Hospital for the return of his thirteen-year-old daughter, Mary Elizabeth. When Döer's wife and another child—Mary Elizabeth's mother and sister—died, Mary Elizabeth was, according to Döer, "seized with so violent a Grief as would not yield to any Comfort." Döer agreed to have Mary Elizabeth admitted to the hospital as he was assured by Captain Ralph Foster that "her Cure and Maintenance should not cost me a Penny." Döer made his arrangements for paying off the passage for his family, but when he went to pick up his daughter at the hospital, he "was told that the Managers would deliver up the Girl to the Owners of the Ship who had assumed to pay for her cure and Accommodation and that these Merchants would sell her for the Charges of the Hospital."[62] Mary Elizabeth was mad with grief at the death of her family members and admitted to the hospital for a cure but the hospital charges meant that she was no longer attached to her father, but would be sold, separately, into an indenture.

The hospital claimed to be blind to financial need and instead to be focused on the care of the indigent. Their mission was to restore the insane to sanity and claimed that "a beggar, in a well regulated Hospital, stands an equal chance with a prince in his palace for a comfortable subsistence, and an expeditious and effectual cure of his diseases."[63] While the doctors and hospital managers may have been committed to this in theory, the scraps of stories of enslaved people and redemptioner children who came through their doors tell us that, in practice, the commitment to comfortable subsistence and effectual cures of diseases was secondary. Enslaved people who could be pulled out of treatment at their owners' whim and children who could be taken away from their parents tell us about one brutal underside of medical care in the eighteenth century. Their stories, only partly told in these historical records, are stories of tyranny winning out over liberty and stories of full exclusion from the body politic. We can only patch them together without the benefit of the voices of those who suffered.

Only those with the privilege of literacy, wealth and status could tell their own stories. Like Cruden or Bruckshaw in England, those who could tell their stories in America highlighted the themes of liberty deserved and liberty denied. John Macpherson's story is particularly interesting because it involves Macpherson, a colorful war hero, and John Dickinson who, in the year Macpherson was confined for insanity, was one of the most ardent spokesmen for British liberty in the American context. The story takes place in Philadelphia, which was and still is sometimes known as "the cradle of liberty." It brings us back, directly, to Sprague's question from the beginning of this chapter, "What condition of mind disqualified an individual from the enjoyment of his *civil rights*--the rights of property and personal liberty?"

Macpherson gained fame as a privateer during the Seven Years' War. He had lost his arm when a French cannonball struck him, but that did not keep him from privateering (and making a fortune for himself). In 1770, when he published the letters that outlined his story of confinement for insanity, he referred to his service. He wrote, "To serve the land I live in, I would bear a greater load of chain and torments." Although he had his liberty denied, he continued, "Thank God, I live in a land of liberty, in a land (I must take the liberty to say) I have served."[64] In 1769, Dickinson was best known for his *Letters from a Farmer in Pennsylvania* that he had written and published to protest the Townshend Acts. Although the letters had been published anonymously, by the time Macpherson was confined, Dickinson's identity as author was known. In the first of these letters, he had claimed that human welfare "can be found in liberty only, and therefore her sacred cause ought to be espoused by every man, on every occasion, to the utmost of his power."

He also penned "The Liberty Song," first published in the *Boston Gazette* in 1768. The lyrics of the song included, "Come, join hand in hand, brave Americans all,/ And rouse your bold hearts at fair Liberty's call; / No tyrannous acts shall suppress your just claim, / Or stain with dishonor America's name."[65] If one is to believe Macpherson, the same man who wrote the lyrics, "No tyrannous acts shall suppress your just claim," was the man who, without any just claim, and for his own honor and glory, kept Macpherson imprisoned for insanity.

The basic outline of the story is this: by his own account, in May 1769, Macpherson was seized in the garden of his Philadelphia mansion, put into a "mad shirt," taken into one of the outbuildings, and chained against his will for three months before regaining his freedom. Macpherson's wife, Peggy, together with Macpherson's friend, John Dickinson, were convinced this was for his own good. Dickinson later wrote to Macpherson, "I am persuaded that your reason was injured." In this letter, he told his friend that this diagnosis of madness was confirmed by Dr. Thomas Cadwalader. If his reason was truly injured, Macpherson was incapable of self-government and therefore a danger to himself, his family, and society. Dickinson tried to reason with his friend, "What should make so many men of sense adopt this opinion, unless there was some foundation for it?" Should not Macpherson want to be restored "to that remarkable strength of understanding that used to give pleasure to all your acquaintance"? Dickinson begged Macpherson to understand that he was "still beloved by your family and friends" and asked him to cease to believe their attempts at aid "are cruelties practices upon you."[66]

In a later letter, Dickinson tried again, "The fever with which you have been afflicted, was so violent, as greatly to alarm those who most affectionately love you; and I beseech you that you will not permit the least resentment to dwell in your mind against any of your family, or me, to whom your anger will be a great misfortune."[67] Whether or not Macpherson was insane, his behavior was eccentric and he leveled violence or the potential of violence against his family members who crossed him. It is impossible to know, now, what happened in that household, but it is likely that his wife and other residents of his household feared him. Macpherson, however, did not see his confinement as an act of benevolence; instead he called it "worse than Indian cruelty."[68] As Cruden had done with his references to the Spanish Inquisition, galley slaves, and the like, Macpherson called on a rich and growing narrative source that contrasted the true liberty of Great Britain and its subjects with savage others. His audience was well familiar with the narrative of "Indian cruelty" that included details of the slow torture of male captives—both Indian and European—by other Indians. In the midst of the Seven Years' War, *The British Magazine* published, "The History of Canada" which told of French missionaries who were "often killed, sometimes taken and tortured to death by the most hideous torments."[69]

It is interesting, of course, that Macpherson referenced this trope, and it speaks, perhaps, to anxieties over manhood as well as loss of liberty. Indian men, enduring torture by their enemies, proved their manhood by remaining brave and stoic. European men admired and tried to emulate this behavior. Perhaps that demonstration of manhood was what Macpherson would have preferred. Instead, he had been emasculated when he was put into the mad shirt. Because others determined him to be mad, he lost his ability to act and to make decisions for himself and his family, and because he was restrained, he lost his freedom of movement. In Myra Glenn's microhistory of another sailor, Horace Lane, she showed that "a male was manly if he exerted agency, control, over his life and successfully defended his freedom."[70] Macpherson had lost the ability to exert agency and control over his life, and his published letters were an attempt, once he regained his freedom, to defend his sanity and his manhood, and to try to rebuild his good name.

In addressing the "Impartial Public" in 1770, Macpherson claimed that he had never been mad and asked an important eighteenth-century question. What did it mean for both his body and the body politic if "my unhappy story, become precedent in these young countries? ... [W]here will then be the liberty we pretend to contend for, when the hands of doctors and divinity and physic, are the only persons entrusted with it?"[71] As Bailyn has shown, to eighteenth-century thinkers, power "meant the dominion of some men over others. . . Most commonly the discussion of power centered on its essential characteristic of aggressiveness: its endlessly propulsive tendency to expand itself beyond legitimate boundaries."[72] This is the lens through which Macpherson saw his story. Those who abused legitimate power were numerous, but the worst abusers were his wife Peggy and his friend Dickinson. To Macpherson, his wife was duped and therefore duplicitous. However, he lay the worst blame at the feet of his friend as he became convinced that Dickinson had ulterior motives. As he sent letters out into the world from his place of confinement, Macpherson defended himself. When he got no satisfaction from those he blamed, he kept writing, even after freed, and then published some of his correspondence.

The first letters to his wife were mild. In the very first one he published in his account, he accepted that she might have been alarmed by his behavior, and wrote, "I beg you will inform me on whom my liberty depends?" He hoped that she would work with others toward his release and pleaded, "If you love me, don't let me live in torment any longer."[73] He even begged to be put into a hospital instead of chained in a building on his own grounds. Peggy's side of the story remains a mystery. She visited her husband in his confinement but may have been glad of his straightjacket. Of her communications with her husband during his confinement verbally or through a letter, he included little in his published account. There is one hint in a letter to Peggy dated November 2, 1769 that read, "Your very extraordinary behavior to me yesterday, makes me despair of a reconciliation." She had obviously expressed a desire to move from Mount Pleasant, their house, but he denied this request. "I presume you will not think it hard in me to keep you as long at Mount-Pleasant from this day, as you keep me in chains for lunacy."[74] Peggy may not have been frightened of her husband at all times, but at one point she had been frightened enough to agree with his capture and confinement. If he did not physically threaten her, he used the powers given to him under coverture—even during his period of confinement—to deny her the one thing she wanted: to move to a safer place and win a little peace of mind. Can she be read as a woman abused physically or mentally? It is not outside of the realm of possibility.

By 1770, the couple was separated, never to be reconciled. In a letter dated April 23, 1770, Macpherson chastised Peggy, "The conduct of my dear sons this morning . . . convinces me, that your heart is a stranger to tenderness and mercy; but you may depend your barbarities will recoil upon yourself. . . I desire to know, in writing, your terms, as I am fix'd on a separation." He did print her reply, "I received yours . . . and as the desire of a separation is yours, I apprehend the offer of terms should be yours also. . . May God give you his blessing, which is the wish of her who is still willing to be Your affectionate and dutiful Wife."[75] It is clear that Macpherson no longer believed Peggy was his affectionate and dutiful wife, and that she had broken the covenant they had made when they married.

Macpherson believed his wife had been led to this point of betrayal particularly by his friend Dickinson. In his publication, Macpherson went back to 1768, and the anonymous publication of *Letters from a Farmer in Pennsylvania*. He included a poem that he had written and published as "An American Mariner" in one of the pamphlet versions of Dickinson's letters that began, "Hail worthy Farmer! Liberty's best friend!" According to his 1770 publication, Macpherson had been one of Dickinson's greatest advocates. What, then, had gone wrong? Macpherson implied that he had been confined under the direction of John Dickinson because Dickinson had received sole credit for his writings that, perhaps, Macpherson or another man had had a hand in producing. Macpherson charged that Dickinson was invested in making people believe that his former friend had lost his mind. He began merely with hints, "My principal enemy . . . is John Dickinson, Esq.; who wrote the *Farmer's Letters*, or rather has got the credit of them."[76] In a later letter to a lawyer, Macpherson implied that he would publicly expose Dickinson, "Everlasting infamy hangs over his head, which I will let fall at a proper time."[77] In May 1770, Macpherson wrote to Dickinson himself, "Was it not natural for a man of your stamp (for I now know it) to wish the world would believe me mad, when you well knew that your very existence, as a man of sincerity, or veracity, depended upon my tongue? . . . To raise a friend to the highest pinnacle of fame, *I* have deceived the Public."[78]

According to Macpherson, Dickinson was acting duplicitously for his own fame and fortune. This violated eighteenth-century ideals of virtuous behavior, as he was putting his own gain before the commonweal. More personally, for Macpherson, Dickinson had built up his own good name and fortune at the expense of Macpherson's reputation, freedom, and manhood. Macpherson, the one-armed war hero and lover of liberty, determined to fight back. Unfortunately, for Macpherson, the annals of history have erased his challenge to Dickinson's veracity and authority. Of course, Dickinson's own historical reputation was tarnished in other ways, particularly by his refusal to sign the Declaration of Independence and for having continued to advocate for peace in 1776. Nonetheless, Dickinson still exists in our American narration as a man inspired to stand up against taxation without representation despite his later weaknesses. But Macpherson is nowhere to be found in the same American narration.

Macpherson deserves a place in this narration if only for the important questions his story raises. For a period of time he was denied his civil rights on the word of a few individuals. Within the confines of a straightjacket, he had no recourse except to plead for mercy with the very people who had confined him. Although he eventually regained his civil rights and continued in his profitable business, his story adds an additional layer to the American story. In an age praised for its liberty it remained too easy to take that liberty away. It had been taken away, at least temporarily, from Otis and Macpherson because of their insanity or alleged insanity. It was taken away even more easily from countless others often on the word of only one or two people. Americans remained concerned by the potential answers to Macpherson's question in a modified form. Where was the liberty they contended for when a few people in power were entrusted with it? They needed to answer that question for it was key to crafting governments based on rational principles during a time of the chaos and confusion of war and its aftermath.

NOTES

1. Jenks S. Sprague, "Observations on Various Subjects in Forensic Medicine" *Transactions of the Medical Society of the State of New-York, During its Annual Session, Held at Albany, February 5, 1850* (Albany: Weed, Parsons & Co., 1850), 211, https://hdl.handle.net/2027/mdp.39015076629271.

2. Sprague, "Observations," 212.

3. "Articles, Lawes, and Orders, Divine, Politique, and Martiall for the Colony in Virginea," Virtual Jamestown, http://www.virtualjamestown.org/exist/cocoon/jamestown/laws/J1056.

4. John Trenchard and Thomas Gordon, *Cato's Letters, or Essays on Liberty, Civil and Religious, and Other Important Subjects*. Four volumes in Two, edited and annotated by Ronald Hamowy (Indianapolis: Liberty Fund, 1995), https://oll.libertyfund.org/titles/1237#Trenchard_0226-01_777.

5. Bernard Bailyn, *The Ideological Origins of the American Revolution*, enlarged ed. (Cambridge: Belknap Press of Harvard University Press, 1992), 77.

6. Charles Brockden Brown, *Alcuin: A Dialogue* (New York: T & J Swords, 1798), 66. Evans Early American Imprint Collection.

7. Quoted in Michel Foucault, *History of Madness*, ed. Jean Khalfa, trans. Jonathan Murphy and Jean Khalfa (New York: Routledge, 2006), 34.

8. Alexander Anderson, *An Inaugural Dissertation on Chronic Mania* (New York: T. and J. Swords, 1796), 5, urn:oclc:record:1046641738.

9. Quoted in Isaac Ray, *A Treatise on the Medical Jurisprudence of Insanity* (London: G. Henderson, 1839), 429, https://books.google.com/books?id=sFwqJ0hFrvgC.

10. "To the honourable House of Representatives of the Province of Pennsylvania, The Petition of Sundry Inhabitants of the Said Province," in Thomas G. Morton, *The History of the Pennsylvania Hospital, 1751–1895* (Philadelphia: Times Printing House, 1895), 8, https://books.google.com/books?id=W85XAAAAMAAJ.

11. Quoted in John C. Burnham, *Health Care in America: A History* (Baltimore: Johns Hopkins University Press, 2015), 57.

12. J. G. Spurzheim, *Observations on the Deranged Manifestations of the Mind, or Insanity*. First American Edition (Boston: Marsh, Capen & Lyon, 1833), 2. Library Company of Philadelphia.

13. Foucault, *Madness and Civilization*.

14. David J. Rothman, *The Discovery of the Asylum: Social Order and Disorder in the New Republic* (Boston: Little, Brown and Company, 1971), 36.

15. Rothman, *Discovery of the Asylum*, xviii.

16. Cutbrush, *An Inaugural Dissertation on Insanity*, 5.

17. Philippe Pinel, *A Treatise on Insanity, in Which Are Contained the Principles of a New and More Practical Nosology of Maniacal Disorders Than Has Yet Been Offered to the Public . . .* (Sheffield: W. Todd, 1806), 143, https://books.google.com/books?id=E4FIAAAAYAAJ. Lest we put this down simply to primitive and inaccurate medical knowledge, currently the fifth edition of the *Diagnostic and Statistical Manual of Mental Disorders* (DSM) published in 2013 runs 991 pages with additional proposals listed on the American Psychiatric Association's website. A perusal of just a few pages of the DSM highlights the many grey areas involved with mental illnesses and the continued socially constructed nature of those illnesses.

18. Paul Starr, *The Social Transformation of American Medicine: The Rise of a Sovereign Profession and the Making of a Vast Industry* (New York: Basic Books, 1982), 11.

19. Quoted in Leonard Smith, "'The Keeper Must Himself be Kept': Visitation and the Lunatic Asylum in England, 1750–1850," *Clio Medica* 86 (2009): 201.

20. Quoted in Thomas S. Szasz, *The Manufacture of Madness: A Comparative Study of the Inquisition and the Mental Health Movement* (Syracuse: Syracuse University Press, 1970), 147.

21. Roy Porter, "Reason, Madness, and the French Revolution," *Studies in Eighteenth-Century Culture* 20 (1991): 56.

22. Charles Fitz-Geffrey, *Compassion toward Captives, Chiefly toward Our Brethren and Country-Men Who Are in Miserable Bondage in Barbarie* (Oxford, 1637), quoted in Linda Colley, *Captives* (New York: Pantheon Books, 2002), 154–155. Emphasis in the original.

23. John Connolly, *An Inquiry Concerning the Indications of Insanity, with Suggestions for the Better Protection and Care of the Insane*, quoted in Thomas S. Szasz, ed. *The Age of Madness: The History of Involuntary Mental Hospitalization Presented in Selected Texts* (New York: Jason Aronson, 1973), 11.

24. James A. Holstein, *Court-Ordered Insanity: Interpretative Practice and Involuntary Commitment* (New York: Aldine de Gruyter, 1993), 136.

25. Alexander Cruden, "The London-Citizen Exceedingly Injured," in Allan Ingram, ed., *Voices of Madness: Four Pamphlets, 1683–1796* (Thrupp: Sutton Publishing Limited, 1997), 48. In a later part of his published narrative, Cruden attributed the maid's reluctance to declare him sane solely on her economic need for employment.

26. Ray Raphael, "Blacksmith Timothy Bigelow and the Massachusetts Revolution of 1774," in Alfred F. Young, Gary B. Nash, and Ray Raphael, eds, *Revolutionary Founders: Rebels, Radicals, and Reformers in the Making of the Nation* (New York: Vintage Books, 2001), 38.

27. Bailyn, *Ideological Origins*, 55.

28. John Haslam, *Illustrations of Madness*, ed. Roy Porter (London: Routledge, 1988), 15.

29. Porter, "Introduction," in *Illustrations of Madness*, xxx.

30. Haslam, *Illustrations of Madness*, 80–81.

31. Eliza Haywood, *The Distress'd Orphan, or Love in a Mad-House*, rev. ed. (1726; repr., New York: AMS Press, Inc., 1995), 32.

32. For instance, see the pamphlet attributed to Henry St. John, 1st Viscount Bolingbroke, *The Freeholder's Political Catechism* (Dublin, T. Moore, 1733).

33. Haywood, *Distress'd Orphan*, 39.

34. Cruden, "The London-Citizen Exceedingly Injured," 29.

35. Cruden, "The London=Citizen Exceedingly Injured," 67.

36. Samuel Bruckshaw, "One More Proof of the Iniquitous Abuse of Private Madhouses," in Ingram, *Voices of Madness*, 78.

37. William Belcher, "Belcher's Address to Humanity," in Ingram, *Voices of Madness*, 130–35.

38. Quoted in William Ll. Parry-Jones, *The Trade in Lunacy: A Study of Private Madhouses in England in the Eighteenth and Nineteenth Centuries* (London: Routledge and Kegan Paul, 1972), 222.

39. Foucault, *Madness and Civilization*, 66.

40. Roy Porter, "Reason, Madness, and the French Revolution," *Studies in Eighteenth-Century Culture* 20, no. 1 (1991): 73.

41. "Adams's 'Abstract of the Argument': Ca. April 1761," *Founders Online*, National Archives, accessed April 11, 2019, https://founders.archives.gov/documents/Adams/05-02-02-0006-0002-0003.

42. Quoted in Richard A. Samuelson, "The Constitutional Sanity of James Otis: Resistance Leader and Loyal Subject," *The Review of Politics* 61 (1999): 500, https://ww.jstor.org/stable/1408465.

43. Diary of John Adams, 5 June 1762. *Adams Papers Digital Edition*, https://www.masshist.org/publications/adams-papers/index.php/view/DJA01d332. This conversation appears as it was recorded in Adams's diary.

44. Otis's profile Clifford K. Shipton, *Sibley's Harvard Graduates,* Vol. 11 (Boston: Massachusetts Historical Society, 1960), 247–287.

45. Diary of John Adams, *Adams Papers Digital Edition*.

46. For example, in his article, "Disability Nationalism in Crip Times," Robert McRuer writes about "creative forms of resistance generated within and around cultural locations of disability." *Journal of Literary and Cultural Disability Studies* 4, no. 2 (2010), https://www.muse.jhu.edu/article/390397.

47. Quoted in James Kendall Hosmer, *The Life of Thomas Hutchinson: Royal Governor of the Province of Massachusetts Bay* (Boston: Houghton, Mifflin and Company, 1896), 135, https://books.google.com/books?id=KloYAAAAIAAJ.

48. Romemarie Zagarri, *A Woman's Dilemma: Mercy Otis Warren and the American Revolution* (Wheeling, IL: Harlan Davidson, Inc., 1995), 51.

49. Quoted in Mary Ann Jimenez, "Madness in Early American History: Insanity in Massachusetts from 1700 to 1830," *Journal of Social History* 20, no. 1 (Autumn 1986): 25.

50. John Adams to William Tudor, Sr., 25 February 1818, *Founders* Online, National Archives, https://founders.archives.gov/documents/Adams/99-02-02-6858.

51. Jeffrey H. Richards and Sharon M. Harris, eds, *Mercy Otis Warren: Selected Letters* (Athens: University of Georgia Press, 2009), 21–22.

52. Mercy Otis Warren to Elizabeth Otis Brown, 15 June 1783, in Richards and Harris, 172–73. Otis really did die after being struck by lightning.

53. Bernard Bailyn, *The Ordeal of Thomas Hutchinson* (Cambridge: The Belknap Press of Harvard University Press, 1974), 52.

54. John Dickinson, *Letters from a Farmer*, Letter II, in Paul Leicester Ford, *The Writings of John Dickinson*, Vol. 1 (Philadelphia: Historical Society of Pennsylvania, 1895), 320, https://books.google.com/books?id=2-kzAQAAMAAJ.

55. Quoted in Harlow Giles Unger, *Lion of Liberty: Patrick Henry and the Call to a New Nation* (Philadelphia: De Capo Press, 2010), 72.

56. In Unger's *Lion of Liberty*, he allows the family voice to be prominent, "Here she was in her own home with loyal and faithful servants giving her ever tender loving care" (72). The servants were enslaved people, and we cannot know how they felt.

57. Quoted in Unger, *Lion of Liberty*, 93.

58. Patrick Henry, "Give Me Liberty or Give Me Death," The Avalon Project, https://avalon.law.yale.edu/18th_century/patrick.asp.

59. Quoted in Thomas G. Morton and Frank Woodbury, *The History of the Pennsylvania Hospital 1751–1895*, facsimile ed. (New York: Arno Press, 1973), 127.

60. David J. McCord, ed., *The Statues at Large of South Carolina*, Vol. 7 (Columbia, SC: A.S. Johnston, 1840), 424, https://hdl.handle.net/2027/hvd.32044013334099.

61. La Marr Jurelle Bruce, "Mad Is a Place; or, the Slave Ship Tows the Ship of Fools," *American Quarterly* 69 (June 2017): 305.

62. "The Petition of Conrad I. Döer, the Father of Mary Elizabeth Döer, a Child about 13 years of Age, a Convalescent in your Hospital," reprinted in Thomas S. Szasz, *The Age of Madness: The History of Involuntary Mental Hospitalization* (Lanham, MD: Jason Aronson, Inc., 1974), 15–17.

63. *Some Account of the Pennsylvania Hospital* (Philadelphia: Office of the United States Gazette, 1817), 38.

64. John Macpherson, *Macpherson's Letters, &c.* (Philadelphia: 1770), iii–iv, http://opac.newsbank.com/select/evans/11713.

65. John Dickinson, "The Liberty Song," *Dickinson College Archives and Special Collections*. http://archives.dickinson.edu/sundries/liberty-song-1768.

66. John Dickinson to John Macpherson, 13 August 1769, in *Macpherson's Letters*, 11.

67. John Dickinson to John Macpherson, in *Macpherson's Letters*, 19–20.

68. Macpherson, iv.

69. Tara Goshall Wallace, "'About savages and the awfulness of America': Corruptions in Humphry Clinker," *Eighteenth Century Fiction* 18, no. 2 (Winter 2005–2006): 239, http://muse.jhu.edu/article/200591.

70. Myra C. Glenn, "Troubled Manhood in the Early Republic: The Life and Autobiography of Sailor Horace Lane," *Journal of the Early Republic* 26, no. 1 (Spring 2006): 70.

71. Macpherson, *Macpherson's Letters*, iv.

72. Bailyn, *Ideological Origins*, 56.

73. Macpherson, *Macpherson's Letters*, 4–5.

74. Macpherson, *Macpherson's Letters*, 21.

75. Macpherson, *Macpherson's Letters*, 73–74.

76. Macpherson, *Macpherson's Letters*, 42.

77. Macpherson, *Macpherson's Letters*, 47.

78. Macpherson, *Macpherson's Letters*, 86–87.

Chapter 2

The Many Madnesses of Colonial Protest

In 1763, colonists could not imagine the extent to which they would ask the question of who decided for their liberties in the years to come and how their desire for answers would lead to further conflict. After all, in that year, British North American colonists celebrated the official end to the Seven Years' War and proudly proclaimed themselves members of the most liberty-loving country in the world. Now that they were "safe from the griping hand of arbitrary Sway and cruel Superstition" that had threatened them because of the French presence in North America and the resultant conflicts that arose from that presence, their liberty needed to be guarded jealously.[1] The threats to liberty were everywhere; they could come from the corrupting influences of power in the hands of public officials or from the people. If liberty caused madness, American colonists were going to be in trouble. Their liberty had to be checked by legal constraints to keep good order in the colonies and to prevent, to the extent possible, licentious behavior that would break apart the social compact. The Reverend James Horrocks preached to congregants in Petsworth, Virginia, that Americans must watch their actions now more closely than ever. "It is Folly," he told his listeners, "nay it is madness to suppose that it is true Liberty, which allows Men to act as they please, just as their inflam'd Brains, or wild Imagination may urge them on."[2] Horrocks feared that the new opportunities afforded by the defeat of the French could destroy some of the needed restraints on men's actions allowing them to cause harm to themselves and others, and therefore damaging society.

In theory, laws guided Americans into civil liberty and away from the excesses of natural liberty. In practice, when colonists believed that laws, people, or customs stood in the way of their natural liberties, they disobeyed those laws, attacked those people, or ignored those customs. While England had a rich tradition of protest, those protests generally did not exceed the limits imposed by ideas of deference and the threat of punishment if protest was taken too far. However, in the 1760s and into the 1770s, Americans pushed those limits sometimes beyond their breaking point, creating conditions that made many fear that colonists were bent on disrupting the business of government and opening the door to anarchy. If John Macpherson wondered where liberty was when it was so easily taken away by doctors and scheming others, a number of British subjects wondered what happened when ordinary people took the liberty to disobey laws or to enact violence against their neighbors. Again and again, society seemed to tip away from the balancing point between civil and natural liberty and to open the doors to dangerous possibilities.

From homes, rostra, and pulpits, speakers and writers celebrated their belief that the war "hath given us the just, undisputed, and peaceful possession of a territory, whose value and extent we are not able to estimate."[3] Still remaining in that territory, however, were Indian tribes allied with the English colonial governments as well as powerful tribes that had not been defeated by British forces and continued to fight for their lands and autonomy. Increasingly, backcountry settlers refused to distinguish between peaceful or English-allied Indians and those who remained in conflict with white settlers pushing westward into new territories. In Pennsylvania, backcountry settlers painted all Indians with the same descriptive brush: they were threatening savages who attacked the settlements of innocent subjects of Britain who might appear peaceful but harbored enemies in their midst.

At the end of 1763, some of these Americans actively and savagely dismissed the rule of law in the backcountry of Pennsylvania. On December 14, armed with weapons and absent any expressed reservations about killing Indian men, women, or children, the self-styled Paxton Volunteers attacked a Conestoga village, murdering the residents they found there, scalping and otherwise mutilating their bodies, and then burning their cabins to the ground. The Volunteers claimed that the Susquehannocks who lived there were not peaceful residents who had proved their loyalty through long ties of trade and friendship, but were secret enemies who harbored hostile and French-allied Indians in their midst. Those Indians who escaped violence sought shelter in nearby Lancaster, where they were put in the workhouse for safety.

When the news reached Philadelphia, Governor John Penn expressed horror at the actions of his fellow white Pennsylvanians. He called on the forces of law and order to capture the so-called Volunteers, charge them with murder, and place them in jail to await trial. Instead, a group of 100 men rode to Lancaster, broke down the doors of the workhouse and slaughtered the Indian men, women, and children who had sought safety there, mutilating their bodies before riding home again. The Reverend John Elder wrote to Penn that while he had tried to argue with the Volunteers, he could do nothing "with men heated to madness." Despite Elder's words, it was likely that he did not plead too hard with the Volunteers for it is clear from the record that he might have hated their actions but not their motives. Elder placed the blame for the massacre squarely on the government for not enforcing a policy of removal "as was frequently urged without success." He defended the Volunteers as generally "virtuous and respectable—not cruel, but mild and merciful," and said, with time, their violence "shall be considered one of those youthful ebullitions of wrath caused by momentary excitement, to which human infirmity is subjected."[4] In other words, these men had been driven mad by a combination of anger and youth. Their anger excused their action and their youth exonerated them.

Penn remained horrified, despite Elder's attempt to excuse the Volunteers' actions. Less than two weeks later, he issued a proclamation that claimed the backcountry settlers had threatened "the Liberty and Security" of both individuals and the government, and charged again that the men who had perpetrated the violence and any of their accomplices needed to be apprehended and prosecuted for their crimes.[5] In order to protect other Indians allied with the Pennsylvania government from these threatening men, colonial officials brought them into Philadelphia placing them in a military barracks defended by British regulars for safety. If the government could not rein in the madness of the people, they would try to protect their allies from continued violence that went in the face of both man's law and God's law. No one could be safe in Pennsylvania if men like the Volunteers could take matters into their own hands in such a mad and brutal fashion.

For the Volunteers, the government's protection of Indians was one more proof that their government did not protect the safety or the liberty of its own people but enforced dangerous allegiances with savages who would unleash horrors against backcountry settlers. The Volunteers did not try to excuse their actions as those of men temporarily insane but rather presented themselves as rational actors behaving on principle. In their minds, they did not threaten the liberty and security of the colony but protected it particularly for white women, children, and men who lived in zones of conflict. For this reason, 250 men or so decided it was time to confront the government in its seat of power. In early February a militia marched toward Philadelphia on the Germantown Road.

The governor appointed a delegation headed by Benjamin Franklin to meet with the Volunteers as Philadelphia readied itself for an attack, mustering troops and blockading roads. When the Volunteers were intercepted by the delegation, they handed Franklin a petition that stated that the government had ignored the "Poor and Distressed Frontier Inhabitants." They called for government support for their efforts to work toward the removal of the Indians who had taken shelter in Philadelphia and stated that backcountry settlers were due "the common Feelings of humanity and Proper Tenderness and Regard for his Majesties Natural Subjects."[6] Nowhere did they express guilt or shame at their barbaric actions. In their eyes the Volunteers were not murderers or madmen, they were harmed subjects acting in rational fashion who deserved redress from their government rather than punishment. Franklin's delegation did not balk at meeting the Volunteers who had committed atrocities, instead it heard them out and then agreed to present their petition to the Pennsylvania government. The delegation brought a smaller group of the Volunteers into Philadelphia, not under arrest, not as violent madmen who threatened the stability of the backcountry and had threatened the Pennsylvania government but as "a set of very worthy men . . . who laboured under great distress."[7] For Franklin and some others the meeting revealed the Volunteers as rational fellow subjects who deserved their attention.

As these events unfolded, other colonists turned to their pens and presses either condemning or praising the backcountry settlers. For those who condemned the murders of the Indians, the so-called Paxton Volunteers were lawless madmen who spelled doom in a world that they had hoped had been moving toward peace and stability. As one pamphleteer wrote, "Madness in any Society of People is generally a Fore-Runner of their Destruction." For this writer, the murder of women and children in particular was a chilling reminder of what happened when people transgressed the boundaries set by law. He called for the Pennsylvania government to use military force to protect society against pending destruction and lawlessness.[8] Another writer called them "angry, giddy, violent and revengeful People" and wondered when they "would be persuaded to stop their mad Career."[9] This writer, too, feared the murder of innocent Indians was the first in a series of actions that would destroy the government in Pennsylvania. Unlike Elder, these writers did not excuse the actions of the Volunteers as temporary madness brought about by anger and youth, but saw their actions as a sign of an insidious mental disorder. The Volunteers wreaked havoc against peaceful Indians but also against white society. To inoculate against the disease element that the Volunteers represented and that threatened to spread, the government and people needed to stand for law and order to prevent further murders of innocent people.

In response to printed condemnations, the Paxton Volunteers published what they titled an apology which was not an apology at all but rather a justification of their actions. They claimed that the residents of the Conestoga village whom they attacked were not allies, but enemies who had fought with the French and protected other Indians who committed outrages against frontier settlements. They believed no one should condemn them for the killing of these Indians for they were protecting themselves and their family members from the perfidy of pretended allies. They reiterated the point that the real tragedy was that the Pennsylvania government, instead of protecting white subjects to the Crown, protected savages who blocked settlement and therefore progress and posed an ongoing threat.

This interpretation had a good deal of support from other Pennsylvanians. The author of a pamphlet entitled, *The Conduct of the Paxton Men, Impartially Represented*, agreed with Elder that the Paxton Volunteers had lost their minds, but excused their madness, explaining that they had been driven "*mad with Rage*," by the good treatment of "*Heathens*" and "*Traytors*" who murdered defenseless "*free-born Subjects of Britain*," in cold blood.[10] These men were indeed mad but for this pamphleteer the madmen spoke a truth that sane colonists did not dare to speak. The actions of the Volunteers were horrific but according to those who defended them, they were not to blame because the injustices inherent in government policy had left them to take matters into their own hands. Their defenders put themselves in the shoes not of the murdered Indians but of the murdering white men, finding sympathy for the backcountry residents who lived in constant danger and who, therefore, could be excused if those circumstances temporarily deranged them. In the end, this interpretation prevailed.

No matter how many others came to the defense of the murdered Indians or decried the savage actions of the backcountry settlers, in the end the madmen who had committed those actions did not find themselves confined against their will. They were never arrested, never put to trial, never convicted of crimes, and never put in prison cells, straightjackets, or chains. Writers who condemned (rather than excused) them as madmen had no power to take action to protect the larger society from their actions, and, in the end, the government decided with the Volunteers that the rights of the peaceful Indians mattered less than the claims of the backcountry settlers. A threat to the order of government was averted in large part because first the delegation who met the marchers on the Germantown Road and then the colonial government decided to sacrifice the rights of Indians to peace and liberty to the demands of free-born subjects of Britain.

In Pennsylvania, white settlers insisted on a world where their lives and liberty were valued more than Indians' lives and liberty, using force and the threat of force to alter the colonial government's relationship to the Susquehannocks and other allied Indians. Along the coastal regions, Indian lives and liberty largely existed in a more theoretical realm; for colonists there, the threat of the loss of liberty came from the government of the empire rather than the government of the colony. Throughout the North American colonies, free-born subjects of Britain increasingly demanded their own liberty, sometimes defining liberty in new ways while claiming old prerogatives. As Parliament passed new laws or tried to enforce old ones in attempts to pay off the war debt and strengthen their empire, the interests of the empire increasingly came in conflict with the interest of the North American colonists. More frequently, British subjects in North America claimed that Parliament exceeded the boundaries of their power and that body did not have the power to tax the colonists for it contained no colonial representatives. Americans, publicly and privately, accused Parliament of forging legal shackles designed to make free people into slaves. As shown below, all sides employed medical language but the protesters disagreed with the claims by Rush, Spurzheim, and other doctors that madness only thrived alongside liberty. In opposition to the medical writings, people on the ground believed "Oppression will make wise men mad."[11]

When Parliament passed the Sugar Act in 1764, the colony of New York petitioned the House of Commons. They claimed that they had no intention to be anything less than law-abiding citizens, but that the Sugar Act violated the "wholesome Laws of the Land" and threatened the liberty and property of the colonists. While the unwholesome law might not make them into madmen and women, the language of the petition paralleled the language of medical texts. In his *Medical Inquiries and Observations Upon the Diseases of the Mind*, Benjamin Rush would list "remote causes" of madness including "fear, grief, distress, . . . the loss of liberty" and "domestic tyranny." In similar language, the New York petition claimed that the Sugar Act would surely "dispirit the People, abate their Industry, discourage Trade, introduce Discord, Poverty and Slavery," and would harm both North America and the empire.[12] Not yet united in voice, colonists nonetheless wished to continue along their trade pathways in the patterns already established without the disruptions of new regulations. They argued that their trade already greatly benefited Great Britain and that no alternative in policy was needed.

While some colonists objected to the Sugar Act, the passage of the Stamp Act in 1765 worked to unify protest across the barriers of geography, ideology, and religion although disagreement over tactics worked to keep the barriers of economic status in place.[13] The idea of the Stamp Act was introduced in Parliament simultaneously to the debate and passage of the Sugar Act, but William Grenville suggested that time should be given for the colonial governments to consider the Stamp Act and respond. As Edmund Morgan wrote in *Prologue to Revolution: Sources and Documents on the Stamp Act Crisis, 1764–1766*, "Exactly what he proposed that the colonies do is difficult to determine, because no one recorded his exact words."[14] However, one reading of a letter from Charles Garth to the South Carolina Committee of Correspondence in June 1764 is that Grenville was determined to go ahead with the Stamp Act regardless of any measured considerations or objections from colonial governments. According to Garth, Grenville believed that "it was but natural for America to bear" part of the cost for the expense of maintaining a needed military force in North America, and that it was too unwieldy to continue to ask for appropriations from all twenty-six colonies in the Americas. Colonial legislatures might have some say in the rate of the tax, but that a stamp tax was too practical a solution to neglect to use.[15] If Garth's reading of the situation was correct, this is reminiscent of the stories of unjust confinement examined in chapter 1. The colonies became the presumed lunatic, begging for all the facts to be considered before being placed in a straightjacket or sent to the hospital, and Grenville becomes like John Haslam insisting that "if one party be right, the other must be wrong: because a person cannot correctly be said to be *in* his senses and *out* of his senses at the same time," or in this case said to be bearing the expense of military forces or not bearing the expense of military forces in the colony.[16]

While Grenville might have thought the Stamp Act a rational and practical solution to the costs of imperial power, some of the representatives of the Crown in North America expressed reservation about the proposed bill. Massachusetts Governor Francis Bernard worried to Richard Jackson that because the Massachusetts Assembly had never balked at imposing taxes in the colonies for the good of the empire, perhaps it would be the wiser course to continue to allow the colonies to tax themselves. The system was not perfect but it worked well enough. For those in North America, the French and Indian War had proved that the colonists invested themselves in the empire for they had provided men, supplies, and tax revenue in order to defeat the hated French and their Indian allies. As Royal Governor, Bernard wondered about the wisdom of changing a system to which no one in the colonies strenuously objected. It would be no different from changing a course of medicine that was already working a cure for an unknown and potentially dangerous alternative.

Bernard turned out to have accurately read the situation on the ground in his colony and others. Throughout North America, the proposed Stamp Act made the colonial governments nervous. Despite the fact that there was no clear instruction on how the colonial governments were supposed to respond, or even to what they were responding, Virginia, New York, and Massachusetts drew up petitions and sent them to Parliament through their agents. Agent Jasper Mauduit wrote that he was determined to get the Massachusetts Bay colony's petition onto the floor of the Parliament. When he wrote to the Massachusetts House of Representatives he assured them that he had been tireless in promoting their point of view and in removing prejudices in Parliament against "the humors and disposition" of the colony.[17] In other words, some members of Parliament believed that at least one of the elemental humors signaling illness had infected the Massachusetts body politic, but Mauduit worked hard to present the colonial government as sound and healthy with no need of corrective medicine.

It was clear, however, that Parliament remained suspicious about the mental and physical health of the colonial governments. No member of Parliament agreed to receive the petitions from Virginia or New York and despite the best efforts of Mauduit and others to accurately represent the temper and temperament of the colonial people and governments, the Stamp Act passed by a large majority of votes.

That Parliamentary majority might have expected a few complaints, like those they received in protest of the Sugar Act. The fierceness and immediacy of the resistance to the act by Americans of all social ranks and in various localities surprised and alarmed them. Elite men wrote letters and pamphlets and eventually gathered in New York at what they called the Stamp Act Congress to craft a unified but peaceful response. On the ground, ordinary men and women gathered in large numbers to first threaten violence and then sometimes to enact that threatened violence against the persons or properties of tax collectors, government officials, or those who spoke in support of the measure. Those resisting at all levels of society argued with their words and actions that liberty resists restraint, whether the restraint of the straightjacket or the restraint of unjust laws. Colonists unsettled society in ways from which it never recovered. Had the people gone mad? It certainly seemed so in the estimation of the King, some members of Parliament, and supporters of imperial government on both sides of the Atlantic. While the protesters believed they upheld liberty as it was threatened by tyranny, their detractors saw a threatening and disease-ridden madness. Each of the actions detailed below was read as either medicine or disease depending on the actors' or observers' interpretation of where the lines were drawn between their birthright of liberty, the just restraints on that liberty, and the implementation of tyranny.

The Virginia Assembly was the first colonial assembly to take action, passing resolutions to register their objections to the new law at the end of May 1765. The only resolution that failed stated that anyone supporting the Stamp Act "shall be deemed an Enemy to this his Majesty's Colony."[18] Virginia Governor Francis Fauquier wrote to the House of Lords that despite reasoned voices against the "rash heat" of opposition, he and others were only able to temper the resolutions, not prevent their publication.[19] Like the others examined here, Fauquier's letter reflected humoral medical understanding and the fear of excessive heat. Just a few years before he wrote about the rash heat of the Virginia Assembly, Dr. Benjamin Grosvenor wrote, *Health: An Essay on Its Nature, Value, Uncertainty, Preservation and Best Improvement*, explaining that "*Anger* ferments the whole Mass of Blood, throws it into a Fever" and cautioned his readers to "Keep your Eye upon the angry Man in his Fit, and you will see all the Symptoms of some of the most formidable Distempers, Madness, Frenzy and Convulsions."[20] Regardless of whether or not Fauquier had read Grosvenor, both men—one political and one medical—reflected the consensus opinion that fevered passions could throw the body and the body politic into mental and physical illness. And, just as fevers passed from body to body, the Virginia resolutions passed from colony to colony. In the eighteenth-century world of an active print sphere, other colonies reprinted the Burgesses's resolves, often including the rejected resolution. For Fauquier and others, it was clear that the rash heat had spread without the tempering influence of rational voices. Although the Burgesses declined calling the supporters of the Stamp Act enemies, protesting printers and people out of doors expressed no such qualms.

As eight more colonies passed resolves similar to those in Virginia, colonies also responded to the call from Massachusetts to meet in New York "to consult together on the present circumstances of the colonies."[21] Nine colonies selected members to attend the first meeting held on October 7, 1765. Virginia was notably absent, blocked from attending by Fauquier. The delegates adopted a Declaration of Rights and Grievances, an address to the King, a memorial to the House of Lords, and a petition to the House of Commons. In their declaration, they asserted their rights as British subjects and declared against any laws that "have a manifest tendency to subvert the rights and liberties of the colonists."[22] In each of the documents, they called for a repeal of the odious law and any others that had violated their liberties and made them captive to unjust authority.

In the colonies, voice after voice picked up this refrain, claiming that Parliament could not pass any tax laws that affected the colonies because the colonies had no voice in Parliament. In response to the idea of virtual representation put forward by some in Parliament, an idea that argued Americans were represented just as women, children, and servants were, A Plain Yeoman wrote to the *Providence Gazette*. "I wonder these subtle politicians had not shewn, that ideots, madmen, and cattle were not electors," he wrote, "and from thence infer that we are represented." For A Plain Yeoman, the argument itself was mad because American men were rational actors who participated in working colonial governments where their interests were considered alongside the needs of the empire. Americans were not idiots, madmen, or livestock, and because of that they could draw no conclusion except that Parliament punished them with no reason. This should alarm every rational subject of the King who should "begin to tremble for their own liberties."[23] Pennsylvanian John Dickinson wrote directly to William Pitt, former Parliamentarian and friend to America, for intercession. Employing weather and disease metaphors, Dickinson wrote that, "The Storm is now raging" in the colonies because of this law, and warned that the consequences would be felt in both England and America. He noted that "the Prosperity of the one cannot be infected, without the other's catching the Contagion."[24] If America fell ill because of the conduct of Parliament, that illness would not remained confined; the sickroom would expand through the empire.

As men of the upper sort convened in colonial legislatures and a colony-wide Congress and as they took up their pens to write pamphlets or letters, men and women of the lower sort took a different approach to the problem. They had no qualms about seeing supporters of the Stamp Act as enemies. They took actions against those they saw as enemies to the people despite the fact that they had no legal authority to do so. One sure way to rid themselves of the tyranny of an unjust tax was to make sure that the tax could never be collected, to use intimidation or actual violence to prevent the stamp distributors from doing their jobs. In Wilmington, North Carolina in October, a crowd of 500 people hung William Houston (the stamp distributor) in effigy and then burned his likeness on a bonfire. They then "went to every House in the Town, and brought all the Gentlemen to the Bonfire, and insisted upon their drinking to liberty and no stamps, and to wish "Confusion to Lord [Bute]," one of the despised members of Parliament, "and all his Adherents." When William Houston, the stamp distributor arrived in Wilmington on November 16, several hundred colonists with drums and flags confronted him to ask, "Whether he intended to execute his said Office, or not?"[25] Although he proclaimed himself opposed to enforcing this repugnant law, the crowd "carried him" to the courthouse where they forced him to sign a letter of resignation. The verb choice "carried" suggests gentleness, but one wonders, with crowds burning effigies of Houston, if his treatment was less-than-gentle. Even if they did treat him gently, at the very least he would have been terrified by the possibility of harsher and more violent treatment.

In Charlestown, South Carolina, colonists erected a gallows from which they hung effigies of George Saxby, the stamp distributor, and the devil, as well as "the Head of Lord [Bute], in a Boot."[26] They also threatened that anyone who dared to pull the effigy down did so at the threat of having a millstone tied around his neck before being thrown into the ocean. At the end of the day, the crowd cut down the effigies, carried them to Saxby's house where they broke his windows and then contined to the outskirts of town where they burned the effigies. In the face of this threat of violence, Saxby took the rational course of action and resigned from his office.

While the protests against the Stamp Act have been written into history as a unifying moment, the protests divided colonists in addition to unifying them. For those with access to the pen, the press, and formal political power, writing and speaking in measured tones was the answer. While they might secretly rejoice at the destruction of the stamp man's property, their words denounced the madness of the mobs. The elite were rational protesters and the members of the mob were disease elements or "rage intoxicated rabble," and while the elite sometimes made common cause with the lower sort, they did so only when politically expedient and only if they worked to keep their ties to destructive street actions secret.[27] They wanted the benefit of the rowdier and madder tactics but without a breakdown of deference and order.

In Philadelphia, John Hughes, the stamp distributor, wrote a series of letters to Benjamin Franklin in London. Although other stamp distributors had resigned, Hughes determined that he would hold onto his office and to perform his duty even in the face of opposition and even as he feared for his life. In September, Hughes wrote that each one of his letters could be his last "as the spirit or flame of rebellion is got to a high pitch among the North Americans." In his estimation, "a sort of frenzy, or madness, has got such hold of the people of all ranks." On September 12 and again on September 16, he wrote that he heard rumor that his house would be destroyed. In Philadelphia, however, he was somewhat protected by "sober and sensible" people, including the peace-loving Quakers. At midnight on the 16th, he wrote to Franklin that "several hundreds of our friends" were out in front of his house to protect him and his property, and at 5:00 the next morning he wrote that both he and his property remained safe.[28] Hughes was not Franklin's only informant. Joseph Galloway commented on the "present distracted state of the colonies." In Galloway's version of the same events Hughes described, almost 800 "sober inhabitants" in Philadelphia had managed to deter the mob set at intimidating Hughes.[29] While Hughes lived in fear for his life and property, in Philadelphia enough colonists were bent on law, order, and a less violent approach to political disagreement.

Franklin's wife, Deborah, also weighed in, writing to her husband that she feared that the Franklin property was a target for those unhappy with the Stamp Act. On September 22, she wrote that for nine days her friends urged her to move from their home. She did not leave but took precautions, sending their daughter Sally to stay with her brother William in New Jersey. Deborah stayed in their home and on a night where a number of Philadelphians were out in the streets threatening to harm the property of those who supported the Stamp Act, she accepted protection from male relatives and their guns in her husband's absence. She did not want to do anyone harm, "But if anyone Came to disturb me, I would show a proper resentment." She explained that she believed it was a Philadelphia merchant named Samuel Smith who had put her in harm's way, that he was "a setting the people a-mading by telling them that it was you that had planned the Stamp act."[30] Deborah Franklin's language is telling. In an atmosphere of heightened tension, the action of one man had infected the people with madness, unleashing the less rational forces of human nature, and opening the door to irrational and violent behavior, or people amadding. In the absence of other cures, self-protection became Franklin's inoculation.

The Franklins' friendship with the Hughes meant that Deborah felt protective toward John Hughes, his wife, and their children. In early October 1765, Deborah wrote to her husband to tell him that she had just visited Hughes who had been in a bad state. Philadelphians who continued to be opposed to the Stamp Act had raised a crowd and then sent messengers to tell him they were coming after him. This had "almost [terrified] his wife and children to death," and clearly terrified Hughes as well. If her library contained William Buchan's *Domestic Medicine*, she could turn to the page that read, "Fear and anxiety . . . pre-dispose us to diseases," and that "Sudden fear has generally violent effects."[31] In any case, she witnessed the negative effects fear had on the health of the members of the Hughes family. Deborah wrote that she despised the men who had the gall to praise themselves for stopping short of physical harm for terror damaged as well. Whatever Deborah thought about the Stamp Act, the actions of a lawless mob terrifying men, women, and children were unforgivable. She believed that most Philadelphians despised the violence done to the stamp distributors and others as much as she did, and that Samuel Smith might very well "kill himself with his own ill-nature."[32]

While Hughes, Deborah Franklin, and others could count on the restraint and intervention of the peaceable members of Philadelphia society, in Boston the people out of doors took control of the anti-Stamp Act protests. The stamp distributor, Andrew Oliver was one of the targets. As was the case in other cities, the people first hung Oliver in effigy and then took the effigy down, staging an elaborate act of street theater by using the effigy to stamp all goods that passed down Market Street. They then destroyed a building they believed was going to house the Stamp Office, carried Oliver's effigy to his residence where they burned and then destroyed the house, stable, coach houses, any other outbuildings, and all the movable property they could get their hands on. They also forced Oliver to the Liberty Tree where he publicly resigned from his office. Several years later, Andrew Oliver's brother Peter wrote that the mob had been seized by "the Frenzy of Anarchy." Their "political Enthusiasm," meant that even those who had previously been law-abiding citizens, "seemed to be wholly absorbed in the Temper of Riot."[33] The people had gone mad, and no political doctor could step in to inoculate against their enthusiasm.

Massachusetts Governor Bernard understood the anger of the people to an extent, even as he believed they had reacted unreasonably in their anger. He wrote to William Barrington, a member of Parliament who was adamant that the colonies should pay for their share of the war. Bernard assured him that this was a reasonable expectation but that the colonial governments were in heavy debt already because they had contributed to the war in ways that stretched them beyond their means. The people in Massachusetts paid "very burthensome Taxes" for this purpose and would continue to do so for four more years as that colony climbed out of its war debt. If Parliament had only waited those four years while working to strengthen colonial governments, he believed, colonists might not have been opposed to an additional tax imposed by Parliament.[34]

Since Parliament had not waited, Bernard despaired that reason could be injected as medicine into the inflamed minds of the people of Boston. As the events unfolded around him, he wrote that he expected the worst and tried to provide solutions for every exigency. However, he was like a man confined against his will, defenseless against the rule of the mob. "The Mob, both great & small, became highly elated" in the wake of the destruction of Oliver's house, "& all kinds of ill humours were set on float." The Stamp Act produced the equivalent in the body politic of yellow bile, the humor that led to aggression. In addition, the people's madness was contagious, creating an unregulated bedlam in Boston. Bernard wrote to the Earl of Halifax, "I consider myself only as a prisoner at large, being wholly in the power of the people." He had become governor in name only, unable to do anything to keep the madmen and madwomen from willfully and openly disobeying the laws.

Bernard worried that the poor had embarked on a campaign of "taking away the distinction of rich & poor," and worried even more that the better sort refused to step in to stop them. Town leaders did disavow some of what they saw as the excesses of the mob, but they continued to approve of the destruction of Oliver's house, "as a necessary Declaration of their resolution not to submit to the Stamp Act."[35] In a letter to the Earl of Shelburne, Bernard spent many of his words on James Otis, Jr. who, in his more rational state, took on the mantle of one of the leaders of the Stamp Act protests. Bernard described Otis as "by nature passionate, violent, and desperate," qualities which "sometimes work him up to an absolute frenzy." He was one of the designing men whose end goal was to create a democracy and who had been empowered by the loosing of "the ill humours of the common people" after the passage of the Stamp Act. Like the others described in this chapter, Bernard's political world view was shaped by his medical understandings and, like the unbalanced humors in a sick person, the Stamp Act had unbalanced the humors in the body politic, starting in the most troublesome group, "the common people." Despite Bernard's pleas for rationality to the town's leaders, he found himself powerless to effect change.

In London, Parliament debated what to do in response to the colonial-wide protests. The American champion, William Pitt, no longer a member of Parliament, returned to speak to that body in his role as elder statesman. He spoke eloquently for the rights of American colonists to tax themselves, and blamed Parliament for the disturbances in the colonies. He was opposed in this view by George Grenville who believed that the protesters "border on open rebellion." Grenville stated his fears that if they were allowed to continue, "The government over them being dissolved, a revolution will take place in America."[36] In other words, it was time to confine them or to contain the madness they exhibited. When Grenville finished speaking, Pitt rose to speak again in the midst of a clamor of voices. The speaker called the body to order and Pitt began to speak temporarily interrupted by Lord Strange. Pitt again continued, putting himself squarely on the side of America and on the side of the protesters. Americans may had lost their minds, but "They have been driven to madness by injustice." He then asked, "Will you punish them for the madness you have occasioned?"[37] Pitt, as political doctor, believed it would be good medicine to diagnose the causes of the illness properly. In his mind, the mental illness of the colonists was caused by the actions of Parliament and, therefore, it would be well to change course and restore both the colonies and the empire to health. Pitt called for the total and immediate repeal of the Stamp Act as the best course of medicine.

In the end, Parliament did repeal the Stamp Act, likely hoping that this action would cure the madness of the colonists. Secretary of State for the Southern Department, Henry Conway, who had been one of the chief voices for the repeal, likely breathed a sigh of relief and then reached out to governors of the American colonies asking them to help craft "a dutiful and affectionate return to such peculiar proofs of indulgence and affection."[38] Parliament had done the right thing and Conway hoped that order and good health could be restored and that the relationship between the metropole and the colonies would once again become mutually beneficial. He feared that if the colonists did not cure themselves of their ill humor, that members of Parliament would become enraged, the road to reconciliation would be rocky, and the possibility for further illness in the body politic would remain. Parliament had repealed the loathsome law. The King wished to forgive and forget as well but would not be able to do so unless the colonists showed their good faith. The best way to do this was to provide compensation for the people who had property destroyed during the Stamp Act protests.

Conway wrote variations on his letter based on the ways subjects in the different colonies had responded to the Stamp Act. To the governors of colonies where there had been destruction of property, he asked the governors to work with their colonial assemblies to make compensations to those injured "from the madness of the people."[39] Some of the governors responded that they felt sure of compliance and thus the return of tranquility. But Massachusetts Governor Bernard found that he could not convince the Massachusetts assembly to take this step. While the members of that colony's House of Representatives claimed "the greatest abhorrence of the madness and barbarity" of those who harmed others, they also claimed that their goal was to bring the perpetrators into the legal system for any other step exceeded the bounds of their power.[40] When Bernard urged their compliance with the request in order to prove their good feelings toward King and Parliament, the House was unmoved. It was not that they did not believe that the King and Parliament were good but the members of the House insisted that the charge exceeded the bounds of power of the Massachusetts House of Representatives.

While the repeal tamped down the worst of the madness that had shown itself in mob action, the colonists' desires to check the excesses of government power remained in place. London merchants feared that the colonists would display an excess of pride and passion in the wake of the repeal and gloat over their victory, further angering Parliament. They published a letter directed to their American counterparts asking them "to express filial duty and gratitude to your parent country."[41] They should not celebrate the repeal, but rather get on with the business of business. Their tone of parental chiding and correction did not go over well in all quarters. In Virginia, George Mason responded stating, "There is a passion natural to the mind of man, especially a free man, which renders him impatient of restraint." Just as men and women unjustly confined for madness took every measure to win their freedom so would American colonists unjustly fettered by laws. This stance was not the ravings of a madman, but of a man "who looks upon Jacobitism as the most absurd infatuation, the wildest chimera that ever entered into the head of man." The majority of American colonists were just like him, he insisted, and should no longer be "treated as rebels and outlaws" to be punished or restrained.[42]

Mason and his fellow colonists were impatient of restraint and wary of the fact that simultaneous with their repeal of the Stamp Act, Parliament passed the Declaratory Act. This act claimed Parliament had the "full power and authority to make laws and statutes of sufficient force and validity to bind the colonies and people of America . . . in all cases whatsoever," and it was not long before Parliament tested this theory. In 1767, Parliament passed the first of the laws that comprised the Townshend Acts, a Revenue Act that set taxes on imported British goods. This was not passed in a fit of pique or madness but in response to a particular reading of the situation. After all, when testifying about the colonial reaction to the Stamp Act, Benjamin Franklin had insisted that colonists opposed that act because it was an *internal* tax, designed to tax the business of everyday life in the colonies and that he believed there would be no opposition to an *external* tax, or a tax on imports. Franklin, removed from the colonies although tied through correspondence, had misread the tenor of the anti-tax protest on the ground in North America. Almost immediately in response to the Revenue Act, towns held meetings, passed non-importation resolutions, and then enforced their resolutions, publishing the names of merchants who refused to comply.

In Boston, when Theophilus Lillie refused to sign the non-importation agreement, his name (alongside others) was printed on a handbill where he was declared an enemy to his country. Coercion worked in Lillie's case. He met with the merchant supporters of non-importation and signed the agreement. However he did not do so of his own free will. "But it was no more my own act than if I had been in prison, or upon the rack," he wrote in a long piece published in *The Boston New-Letter*. He felt unjustly punished for following his own conscience, stating that "it always seemed strange ... that People who contend so much for civil and religious Liberty should be so ready to deprive others of their natural Liberty."[43] In language very similar to John Macpherson's discussed in chapter 1, he asked if liberty could exist when an extra-legal body could deprive others of it. He had not given his consent to the non-importation agreement except under threat of losing everything. He had become unfree not due the passage of laws of Parliament but because of the tyranny of the few in Boston who ruled without a mandate and with no legal authority. Similarly, Peter Oliver, still steaming over the destruction of his brother's house during the Stamp Act protests, believed those leading the non-importation movement led ordinary people into mass delusion, that he again had to endure government by a mad mob instead of the reasonable and rational government with Parliament at its head.

Even those in opposition to the new laws by Parliament could object to the tactics of coercion. Writing as a Farmer, lawyer John Dickinson opposed the laws that comprised the Townshend Acts as oppressive, reaffirming the earlier Stamp Act cries that Parliament could not pass tax laws over the colonies because colonists were not represented in Parliament. However, Dickinson asked that his fellow Americans act with restraint, to resist being drawn into madness, and to resist those who wished them to draw them in irrational directions. Using a medical metaphor, he urged his fellow Americans to proceed with caution in order to avoid allowing political differences to "be enlarged to an incurable rage."[44] If they reached that point, reason flew out the window "and a blind fury governs, or rather confounds all things." Americans should be indignant at Parliament's attempts to take away American liberties but colonial leaders should act with rational restraint, boycotting and petitioning but resisting mad and mobbish behavior. Instead of succumbing to passions that opened the door to lunacy, colonists needed to remain committed but calm.

Colonial women weighed in as well. Quaker Hannah Griffitts supported the boycotts and insisted women needed to step up to help enforce them, manufacturing alternatives to imported items to fill local needs. Women could also administer medicine, Griffitts insisted in her poem, "The Female Patriots." While a male doctor would make the final diagnosis of the illness in the body politic, "Woman by honest Invention,/ Might give this State

Doctor a Dose of Prevention."[45] Nineteen-year-old Charity Clarke joined in with other women in home manufacturing, writing to a cousin in London that she saw the actions taken by her fellow colonists not as irrational or unpatriotic but reasonable.[46] Most telling, Sarah Gill wrote to the English historian Catharine Macaulay that while there may be "Madness and Faction" in the actions of the colonists, it was a "Generous Madness, and a truly Loyall Faction."[47] For those fettered against their will by the laws of Parliament, it was not unlikely that they go mad. Just like the iniquity of being put in a madhouse when one was sane thus to be driven mad by the barbaric practices therein, the iniquitous Stamp Act could drive rational men and women insane. In this case, however, their madness freed them from restraint and led them to defend their liberty even more ardently, standing against the tyrants who attempted to take away rights from American colonists.

While boycotting, spinning, weaving, and knitting might not unsettle the rational mind of the body politic, the tactics of attacking customs officers' bodies and properties did just that according to Ann Hulton. For Hulton, the Sons of Liberty went beyond an embrace of liberty and descended into madness and became, in her styling, the "Sons of Voilence" [sic], who enforced their anarchist and leveling principles on society as a whole. The minds of the people had been "inflamed by designing men," causing them to act in erratic, dangerous, and irrational ways.[48] Christian Barnes called the Marlborough Massachusetts Sons of Liberty, "the Sons of Rapin[e]" who sowed discord among the "Poor deluded people with whom we have lived so long in Peice & harmony."[49] For Hulton and Barnes the lawless authority of the so-called Sons of Liberty presented danger to the body politic but also the physical body of men and women. For Barnes, the Sons of Liberty were no better than rapists, criminals who forced themselves on the colonists against their will.

The continued discord in the colonies was enough to convince the British government that harsher measures were needed to act as a cure to the growing madness in the body politic. When Massachusetts sent a circular letter to other colonial assemblies asking them to join together as they had in protest of the Stamp Act, the Colonial Secretary Lord Hillsborough instructed American governors to dissolve their assemblies if they responded. Under Hillsborough's orders, Governor Bernard instructed the Massachusetts House to rescind the circular letter, the House refused by a vote of 92-17, and Bernard dissolved the legislature. With this step, he attempted to revoke membership in the body politic for both the elected officials and the people they represented in the same way a diagnosis of insanity revoked membership in the body politic. However, the leaders resisted the revocation of their membership and in the wake of this move by the governor, the legislature simply moved across the river to Cambridge and continued to meet in defiance of his orders. With clear evidence of colonial intractability and the leaders' tendency toward madness, Hillsborough determined troops were needed in Boston and other colonies to maintain order and to enforce obedience to Parliament's laws. This confirmed the fears of those in Boston that Britain would use any means, including a standing army in times of peace, to divorce colonists from their rights and try to force them to submit to tyranny.

By the time the decision was made to send troops to Boston, the New York General Assembly had already taken measures to express its displeasure over paying for a standing army in times of peace. While they would house and supply soldiers gladly in times of war, absent war, armies were symbols of tyranny and disorder. Without a war to fight, commanders might become mad with power and, as Benjamin Franklin wrote, an army could "put it in the Power of the Captain General to oppress the Province."[50] In December 1766, the New York General Assembly petitioned the royal governor claiming duty and loyalty to Crown and Parliament while also protesting that the cost of quartering troops was too much to bear, that "this Expense would become ruinous and insupportable."[51] There was no need for an army in New York City and therefore no reason to requisition funds for their maintenance.

For those already suspicious of the Americans' intentions, the New York Assembly's action confirmed their belief that the rebellions in the colonies had not come to an end and that the colonists' true intention was independence. Just as confinement for madness became proof of madness, resistance to Parliament's laws became proof of a desire for independence. In response to these fears Parliament passed the New York Restraining Act which threatened to suspend that colony's Assembly if they did not comply. The Assembly caved to Parliament's pressure but provided only a meager £1800 for the soldiers' maintenance. In relationship to these political maneuverings, both colonists and soldiers made their positions known through their actions on the ground.

For the Sons of Liberty, their liberty pole was the symbol of resistance to oppression. That group had erected their first liberty pole in 1765 in response to news of the passage of the Stamp Act. For the soldiers, the liberty pole was the symbol of resistance to the government they represented and, therefore, they cut it down. Several times the Sons of Liberty erected a liberty pole only to see it destroyed by soldiers. Learning a different lesson than the soldiers thought they were teaching them, the Sons of Liberty finally secured their pole with iron bands to make it harder to destroy. On January 13, 1770, angered at the low amount requisitioned for their support by the Assembly, soldiers attempted to cut down or blow up the reinforced pole and threatened citizens who sounded the alarm. Maddened by their failure to destroy the liberty pole, the soldiers entered Montayne's Tavern, threatened patrons with swords and bayonets and then destroyed their surroundings. Thus, the soldiers stationed in the colonies to put down the mobbish behavior of the colonists descended into mobbish behavior. Two nights later, the soldiers finally succeeded in destroying the pole, cutting it up in pieces and throwing it in front of Montayne's.

From here, the disturbance escalated. The Sons of Liberty declared that any off-duty soldier bearing arms "shall be treated as Enemies to the Peace of this City."[52] When two colonists came upon soldiers posting a handbill that mocked the Sons of Liberty, they brought the offenders to the mayor's house to lodge a complaint. When a unit came in arms to free their fellow soldiers, a Captain ordered them to return to their barracks, an order they initially obeyed. As they began their return to their quarters, a group of colonists walked closely behind them. At the top of Golden Hill, the soldiers and their followers were met by another British unit that formed behind the trailing colonists. The soldiers who had been following orders now turned and one of them described as dressed "in Silk Stockings and neat Buckskin Breeches (who is suspected to have been an Officer in Disguise)" ordered them to cut through the crowd with their bayonets.[53] The colonists initially defended themselves with rungs they had pulled off a sleigh near the mayor's house but were forced into retreat. A later account said the soldiers "madly attacked every person they could reach."[54] In New York City, the soldiers' only apparent enemies were fellow Britons, unruly and liberty mad, but no real threat to the empire. Nonetheless, an enemy was an enemy, and the body of soldiers seemed to express little hesitation at using violence against the colonists and the symbols of what they considered the colonists' intransigence. Their behavior against the colonists who were residents of New York City certainly supported an argument that a standing army was a tyrannical threat to British liberties. It was not the colonists' passions that had gotten the better of them, but the soldiers' and they channeled their rage through violent actions in response to real and perceived slights.

In Boston, the arc of resistance followed a similar path. While Samuel Adams called on his fellow colonists to oppose the entry of British troops into the town of Boston in 1768, the delegates from ninety-six towns who assembled to craft a response would not go that far but did reiterate their aversion to "an unnecessary Standing Army, which they look upon as dangerous to their Civil Liberty."[55] Because of this decision by the convention, the troops who had been sent to put down a rebellion and force obedience to Parliamentary laws found no rebellion and no overt resistance to the laws. As this was the case, there was no way to paint the army in Boston as anything but a body used to threaten a peaceable people and take away their liberty.[56] The Massachusetts House repeated the refrain that military power used to enforce laws was both unnecessary and in opposition to the very nature of the government that usually kept Britons free; it was "a power without any check here; and therefore so far absolute."[57] Bostonians had not consented to submit to the arbitrary rule of the sword or to any restraint on their birthright liberty.

Like James Horrocks, with whom this chapter began, Lieutenant Governor Thomas Hutchinson worried that Bostonians had breached the barrier of true liberty by allowing their inflamed brains drive them into madness. In letters he wrote to Thomas Cushing in London in 1769, he feared that if Parliament did not do something more decisive than pass a Declaratory Act that the colonies would descend into anarchy. "There must be an Abridgment of what are called English Liberties," Hutchinson wrote, in order to keep good government and guide colonists away from the natural liberty that would break the bonds between the mother country and the colonies.[58] Liberty needed restraint to keep health in the body politic.

As in New York City, in Boston the year and a half of a tense but relative truce between the troops and the residents of that town, exploded into violent expressions of passion in early 1770. In February, a group of boys first picketed the store of a merchant who refused to comply with the boycott of British goods and then proceeded to the house of the tax collector, Ebenezer Richardson. What did Richardson see when he looked out his window? Did he see unruly boys gone amadding and refusing to give him the deference he was due? Did he believe in the contagious properties of madness, that they began with written petitions and ended with boys threatening order? Whatever he saw, Richardson made the decision to shoot at the crowd from his window and in doing so, he fatally wounded eleven-year-old Christopher Seider. Perhaps Richardson saw it as a just and rational response, but a piece published in the *Boston Gazette* called his actions "a barbarous Murder," and Richardson "an execrable Villain . . . who could not bear to see the Enemies of America made the *Ridicule of Boys.*"[59] Those opposed to the British military presence and the Townshend Acts turned Seider's funeral into a political affair. According to the *Boston News-Letter*, several hundred school boys led the procession, followed by family members, then more than 1300 women and men on foot, closing with "about thirty chariots, chaises, etc."[60] The newspaper assured its readers that everyone behaved rationally and in good order. The mourners were also protesters, sorrowed by the death of Seider, but also bitter because of the behavior of British officials and royal appointees.

A week later, on March 5, that bitterness exploded in a confrontation between civilians and soldiers. It began like a number of previous incidents with an exchange of insults between a two young apprentices and Hugh White who served that night on guard duty at the Boston Custom House. The men verbally jousted and then White struck one of the apprentices, Edward Garrick, in the head with his musket. These actions drew notice from other townspeople and in responsesomeone started ringing the church bells. As this was the usual signal for a fire, it brought a crowd to the Customs House where White's sentry position had been reinforced by Captain Thomas Preston and six privates. The crowd hurled objects and insults at the British soldiers. In the midst of confusion and chaos, soldiers fired into the crowd, killing three instantly, fatally wounding two more, and injuring three additional men before order was restored and the soldiers and their commander arrested. As Bostonian John Rowe noted in his journal that night, "the Inhabitants are greatly enraged and not without Reason." The next day he noted that, "Most all the Town in Uproar & Confusion."[61] In the midst of the chaos that followed this incident, Bostonians met at Faneuil Hall and asked for the immediate removal of the troops to Castle Island.

The soldiers involved were arrested and the trial postponed until November to give the mad fury that followed what Paul Revere and others took to calling the Boston Massacre time to abate. In the trial, Robert Treat Paine argued for a conviction of murder and painted a picture of bedlam created not by unruly inhabitants, but by "the Riotous barbarous ungoverned and ungovernable Behaviour" of the soldiers.[62] While there was a lot of confusion on the night of March 5, none of the confusion should have been met with brute force, according to Paine. For the defense, John Adams also painted a picture of madness, but one that should exonerate the soldiers or at least soften their sentence to manslaughter. He asked the court to imagine, "the multitude . . . shouting and huzzaing, and threatning life, the bells all ringing, the mob whistle screaming and rending like an Indian yell, the people from all quarters throwing every species of rubbish they could pick up in the street."[63] Adams described the soldiers' reactions as a *furor brevis* or a temporary madness, and reminded the jury that the law existed to bring order to tumultuous times. In his closing, Adams quoted the British patriot Algernon Sidney that "no passion can disturb" the law, that the law stands against passions or even madness and brings rationality to "flights of enthusiasm."[64] True liberty did brook some restraint; for liberty to flourish, law and order had to be maintained. Adams's arguments won the day; the jury acquitted six of the eight soldiers, and found two guilty of manslaughter. Bostonians revived the memory of the Boston Massacre every year on March 5, but the trial and its outcome briefly calmed the furor in that town.

Parliamentary politics and soldiers on the ground were not the only scenes of potential madness in the North American colonies. In some regions, colonists calling themselves regulators rose up against other colonists holding power. Like the Sons of Liberty, the regulators believed that governmental practices shackled them, denying them "the glorious liberty of free-born subjects."[65] In this case, however, it was not the government across the sea but more local colonial governments run by aristocratic men corrupted by power and the policies they enacted to benefit themselves that were the maddening agents.

If the protesters were right and the doctors wrong, and if oppression made men mad, then the members of North Carolina's Sandy Creek Association had plenty to worry about. In North Carolina in August 1766, the Association published an advertisement making a parallel between the oppression attempted by Parliament under the Stamp Act and the machinations of the leaders in Orange County, North Carolina. They called for a meeting on the question of "whether the free men of this Country labor under any abuses of power."[66] If men did not stand up against the corruption of their local government, the advertisement claimed, the honest people of Orange County would continue to feel the weight of oppression. Although the Sandy Creek Association was not able to oust the men in power in 1766 through election, the regulator movement grew, calling for lower taxes and government accountability. Even though one of the founding members of the Association, Quaker leader Herman Husband, worried that men "too hot and rash, and in some Things not legal," had taken over the Regulator movement by 1768, he remained involved, continuing to call on his fellow North Carolina colonists to resist a government that did not serve the people.[67] For Husband, the potential insanity of the regulators was better than the self-interested and measurable insanity of the men in power. In 1770, he worried that voters would be swayed by bribes of money and strong drink, that they would become "slaves to their lusts." He asked his fellow voters to shun the men coming with bribes "as you would the pestilence" and to vote their consciences instead.[68] Allowing the disease of flattery and bribery to work made voters insensible rather than rational, made people madly vote against their own interests.

Although Husband preferred the tactic of electoral politics, other regulators, like the Stamp Act rioters in 1765, used both legal and extra-legal tactics to assert themselves. By 1769, when the legal tactics continued to fail, regulators tapped into their passions and used force to keep courts from sitting. To those on the other side, those passions the regulators called on made the protesters into madmen. On September 29, 1770, Judge Richard Henderson published an "Account of Mob Violence Witnessed in the Courts of New Bern." To Henderson, the regulation was an insult to good government "perpetrated with such . . . Madness, as (I believe) scarcely has been equaled at any Time." He described the growing mob that filled his courthouse armed with clubs, whips, and switches seeking redress for their grievances. Henderson stated he tried "to soften and turn away the Fury of this mad People." At first he believed he had succeeded, but then the crowd turned on Colonel Edmund Fanning whom they believed guilty of embezzlement and abuse of tax collection. The regulators pulled Fanning out of the courthouse; Henderson was sure Fanning would be killed by the "Rage and Madness" of the mob, but Fanning managed to escape.[69] His house however, did not. The regulators first destroyed his belongings and drank his liquor and then pulled down Fanning's house. Continuing in their rage, they put a rotted body of an executed enslaved person at "the lawyer's bar and filled the Judge's seat with human excrement."[70]

Absent other means to overturn a system that worked against them, they resorted to violence against person and property and grisly and grotesque symbolic gestures of derision. Beyond revulsion, what did the protesters want to achieve with this particular action? For people protesting the absence of their own liberty, what did they see in the symbolism of using the body of a dead chattel slave? It is unlikely they thought deeply about the inherent hypocrisy of using a body of an enslaved person to protest for their own liberty and the utter disregard of black bodily autonomy in life and death under slavery while they demanded their own autonomy be recognized. While white regulators claimed they had been made into slaves by the legal and governmental system in North Carolina, they were not slaves in the way that their desecrated body would then be used for political fodder. I do not know the identity of the man or woman they placed at the bar, nor what he or she had been executed for—disobedience, potential for revolt, theft, or something else—but men in New Bern had decided on and carried out a death sentence for that slave. Those in power would not question the execution of a slave, but the use of the rotted body certainly made them think that the actions of the regulators were the actions of men gone mad.

A few months later, in January 1771, the North Carolina General Assembly passed a riot act that gave power to prosecute those "unlawfully, tumultuously and riotously assembled together." If the rioters did not appear within 60 days of being summoned by the court, their property would be seized by the government and they could be killed with impunity. The forces of law and order would not tolerate the madness of the people to tear down what they saw as good government. While the regulators continued to resist, Royal Governor William Tryon mustered a militia of approximately 1,000 men and marched to Orange County. On the morning of May 16, 1771, Tryon sent a proclamation to the regulators demanding that they lay down their arms and surrender but all attempts to negotiate peace failed. The regulators relied on guerilla tactics but as they ran out of ammunition many of them fled the battle. In the end, Tryon's forces prevailed. With this victory, government forces won the initial battle to diagnose the problem, that it was the madness of liberty run amok rather than the problem of corrupt government and corrupt officials that ailed the body politic. With their defeat, the regulators' political movement against high taxation and government misconduct died down and those who had escaped hid out for another year or moved into new territory where they would be outside the bounds of North Carolina law.

While the North Carolina government may have believed they had correctly diagnosed the illness in the body politic in the immediate aftermath of the crisis, as the news spread others contested that diagnosis. Virginian Richard Henry Lee did not like the regulators' tactics, but understood that they had been driven mad "by repeated injuries" by lawyers and judges.[71] As the news filtered into Boston where the people were in conflict with British authority figures, the Boston newspapers expressed sympathy with the regulators who, as the *Boston Gazette* opined, had "been intolerably oppressed" by a government that resorted to military force instead of reasonable attention to North Carolinians' grievances. If the regulators were madmen, they had been driven mad by their oppressors just as all colonists had been driven mad by the Stamp Act or Bostonians had been driven mad by military occupation.

The actions of Parliament and other ruling elites brought Americans to ask themselves who should be entrusted with liberty and under what circumstances. Throughout the 1760s and early 1770s, men and women put in place local and colony-wide mechanisms that ranged from mob action to written resolutions. These mechanisms began to build foundations for a relatively-shared American understanding of the answers to the questions about liberty. Many disagreed with the language of the Declaratory Act that stated Parliament could make laws to bind the colonies in all cases whatsoever and instead became more insistent that Parliament had no right to pass laws without representation from the colonies. Protesting Americans described these laws as shackles and themselves as people made into slaves. They believed any attempt by Parliament to pass laws, particularly tax laws, without their consent violated both their rights as British subjects and the rights laid out in colonial charters. While not all colonists agreed with this assessment, it became a powerful tool of continued protest and eventually of nation building.

When Parliament passed the Tea Act in 1773, colonists called on this shared understanding in ways that continued to affect the body politic and lead to what some saw as continued delusion but others saw as a cure. The Tea Act was an effort by Parliament to shore up the British East India Company. This law allowed the British East India Company to ship directly to America while requiring a small import tax on that tea. As Mercy Otis Warren later wrote in her 1805 *History of the Rise, Progress, and Termination of the American Revolution*, "The people throughout the continent, apprized of the design . . . summoned meetings in all the capital towns, and unanimously resolved to resist the dangerous project by every legal opposition, before they proceeded to any extremities."[72] In other words, Otis believed that colonists had acted rationally in their response, first using the laws within the colonies until they were pushed to act in less rational ways by the continued oppression by Crown and Parliament.

The first step taken by colonial leaders was to pass resolutions reaffirming their commitment to resist any tax laws passed without their consent. The citizens of Philadelphia additionally stated that the Tea Act was an attempt "to introduce arbitrary Government and Slavery" into the colonies. Unlike the members of the 1765 Virginia House of Burgesses, leading Philadelphians in 1773 had no qualms about labeling as enemies supporters of Parliament's laws, writing that "whoever shall, directly or indirectly, countenance this attempt . . . is an enemy to his country."[73] After all, as citizens in Plymouth, Massachusetts declared, the new law was "an affront to the common sense and understanding of mankind." In their assessment, the Tea Act was not a rational law passed to benefit British subjects, but was an irrational and alarming effort that was "evidently repugnant to every principle of our constitution" and "dangerous to the liberty and commerce of this country."[74] In localities throughout the colonies, men met and resolved to resist the Tea Act and to brand those who did not agree with their interpretation of the relationship between colonies and empire as enemies to "this country."

Others challenged the interpretation of the resolutions. The Plymouth document read that their resolutions had been passed unanimously by the town. However, forty men from Plymouth objected publicly to the resolution. While it might have passed unanimously, it only did so because leaders in that town had not only "attempted to delude an innocent and loyal people," but they had succeeded in their attempt. Temporarily brought to madness by the local furor over the Tea Act, voting members in the town had signed onto the resolution, but in a clearer and saner moment had realized they had done so in error. Away from the madness of the town meeting, these men had come to their senses and resolved to resist efforts to force compliance with an illegal protest. Barnabas Hedge, in an additional retraction printed in *Rivington's New-York Gazetteer*, wrote that he had acted with "precipitation and folly."[75] A man writing under the pen-name Poplicola added his voice to the dissent, writing that those who objected to the Tea Act were not lovers of liberty, but had their private interests at heart and attempted to impose "a tyranny of so high a nature as not to permit a fellow citizen even to think differently from them without danger." The "cabal," as Poplicola called it, would happily take away liberty from the colonists and fan the flames of unrest.[76] Like John Macpherson, like Theophilus Lillie, and like others, these dissenters found it extremely troubling that men claiming liberty seemed bent on taking liberty away from those who disagreed with them. Who was empowered to define liberty and who was empowered to take liberty away from others? Americans answered those questions differently depending on their political worldview and pushed their political leaders to respond to their answers.

In some locations, the remonstrances and resistance of those against the Tea Act had an effect as governors decided to store the tea or send it back until a resolution could be reached. However, the Massachusetts governor, Thomas Hutchinson, decided to enforce the rule of law. He insisted that the tea be landed, unloaded, and that the tax be paid. This did not surprise those opposed to the Tea Act for earlier that year Hutchinson's private correspondence had been published in a pamphlet. They would have read his assertion that "what are called English liberties" needed to be abridged in the colonies "rather than the connexion with the parent state should be broken."[77] It became clear to Bostonians that their town meetings, resolutions, and ultimatums to merchants had no effect on Hutchinson's actions, thus they turned to large-scale destruction.

On December 16, 1773, a group of men boarded the three ships in Boston Harbor and destroyed 342 chests of tea. For these men and their supporters, this was a rational action taken to counter the irrationality of the Tea Act and those who supported it. Even some generally uncomfortable with mob action saw the destruction of tea as a needed remedy to the unbalanced humors in imperial relations. John Adams mused in his diary that this action was necessary to assert the principle of resisting taxation made without colonial representation. It was a blow against tyranny in the persons of Thomas Hutchinson and the customs officers who were "hardened and abandoned" to "the distresses of the People." After all it was "but an Attack upon Property" rather than an attack on the people.[78] Adams praised the actions taken the previous night but also worried about what measures Parliament would take, anticipating the Coercive Acts that punished Bostonians.

Incensed by what came to be known as the Boston Tea Party, Parliament passed four laws they called the Coercive Acts to try to force compliance to British law in Boston and Massachusetts Bay Colony. They closed Boston Harbor until the colonists paid for the destroyed tea, took away the Massachusetts charter and put the colony directly under the rule of the British, removed trials of royal officials to be moved elsewhere in the empire, and allowed soldiers to be placed in private homes. What came next did little to check the growing colonial protest. Parliament found itself unable to tamp down madness and instead inflamed colonists to action. Their actions increased division in the colonies and opened the door to further violence. It started on local and individual levels but eventually rose to the level of a war for independence.

NOTES

1. Thomas Barnard, *A Sermon Preached before His Excellency Francis Bernard, Esq; Governor and Commander in Chief, the Honourable His Majesty's Council, and the Honourable House of Representatives, of the Province of the Massachusetts-Bay in New-England, May 25th 1763. Being the Anniversary for the Election of His Majesty's Council for Said Province* (Boston: Richard Draper, 1763), 44, Evans Early American Imprint Collection.

2. James Horrocks, *Upon the Peace. A Sermon. Preach'd at the Church of Petsworth, in the County of Gloucester, on August the 25th, the Day Appointed by Authority for the Observation of that Solemnity* (Williamsburg: Joseph Royle, 1763), 8, Evans Early American Imprint Collection.

3. East Apthorp, *The Felicity of the Times. A Sermon Preached at Christ-Church, Cambridge, on Thursday, XI August, MDCCLXIII. Being a Day of Thanksgiving for the General Peace* (Boston: Green and Russell, 1763), 8, Evans Early American Imprint Collection.

4. Quoted in C. Hale Sipe, *The Indian Wars of Pennsylvania: An Account of the Indian Events, in Pennsylvania, of the French and Indian War, Pontiac's War, Lord Dunmore's War, the Revolutionary War and the Indian Uprising from 1789 to 1795* (Harrisburg: The Telegraph Press, 1929), 466, https://archive.org/details/indianwarsofpenn00sipe.

5. In John R. Dunbar, ed., *The Paxton Papers* (The Hague: Martinus Nijhoff, 1957), 62.

6. "Petition by the Inhabitants of Lancaster County," *Digital Paxton: Digital Collection, critical Edition, and Teaching Platform,* http://digitalpaxton.org/works/digital-paxton/petition-by-the-inhabitants-of-lancaster-county.

7. In Samuel Hazard, ed., *Hazard's Register of Pennsylvania, Devoted to the Preservation of Facts and Documents, and Every Kind of Useful Information Respecting the State of Pennsylvania,* Vol. XII (Philadelphia: William F. Gedes), 12, https://books.google.com/books?id=t30UAAAAYAAJ&ppis.

8. *A Serious Address, to Such of the Inhabitants of Pennsylvania, As Have Connived at, or Do Approve of, the Late Massacre of the Indians at Lancaster; or the Design of Killing Those Who are Now in the Barracks at Philadelphia* in Dunbar, ed., *The Paxton Papers,* 93.

9. *A Dialogue, Containing Some Reflections on the Late Declaration and Remonstrance, Of the Back-Inhabitants of the Province of Pennsylvania,* in Dunbar, ed. *Paxton Papers,* 118.

10. *The Conduct of the Paxton Men, Impartially Represented* (Philadelphia: Andrew Steuart, 1764) at http://digitalpaxton.org/works/digital-paxton/the-conduct-of-the-paxton-men-impartially-represented.

11. "Remonstrance and Petition of the South Carolina Back Country" in Merrill Jensen, ed., *English Historical Documents: American Colonial Documents to 1776* (New York: Oxford University Press, 1964), 592.

12. In Edmund S. Morgan, ed., *Prologue to Revolution: Sources and Documents on the Stamp Act Crisis, 1764–1766* (Chapel Hill: University of North Carolina Press, 1959), 13.

13. Edmund S. Morgan and Helen M. Morgan, *The Stamp Act Crisis: Prologue to Revolution* (Chapel Hill: University of North Carolina Press, 1953).

14. Morgan, *Prologue to Revolution,* 24.

15. Charles Garth to the Committee of Correspondence of the South Carolina Assembly, 5 June 1764, in Morgan, *Prologue to Revolution,* 27–28.

16. John Haslam, *Illustrations of Madness,* ed. Roy Porter (London: Routledge, 1988), 15.

17. Jasper Mauduit, 9 February 1765, in Alden Bradford, ed., *Speeches of the Governors of Massachusetts, 1765–1775. The Answers of the House of Representatives Thereto with Their Resolutions and Addresses for that Period* (New York: Da Capo Press, 1971), 30.

18. "The French Traveller's Account" in Morgan, *Prologue*, 46–47.

19. "Governor Fauquier's Account," in Morgan, *Prologue*, 47.

20. Benjamin Grosvenor, *Health: An Essay on Its Nature, Value, Uncertainty, Preservation and Best Improvement* (Boston: D. and J. Kneeland, 1761), 193.

21. Quoted in Richard M. Ketchum, *Divided Loyalties: How the American Revolution Came to New York* (New York: Henry Holt and Company, 2002), 119.

22. "The Declarations of the Stamp Act Congress" in Morgan, *Prologue*, 63.

23. "A Letter from a Plain Yeoman," in Morgan, *Prologue*, 75–77.

24. "John Dickinson Appeals to William Pitt," in Morgan, *Prologue*, 119.

25. Edward Channing, *A History of the United States*, Vol. III (New York: Macmillan Company, 1912), 60–61.

26. "Newport, November 11," *The Coming of the Revolution*, https://www.mashist.org/revolution.

27. Alfred F. Young, "Ebenezer Mackintosh: Boston's Captain General of the Liberty Tree," in Alfred F. Young, Gary B. Nash, and Ray Raphael, eds, *Revolutionary Founders: Rebels, Radicals, and Reformers in the Making of the Nation* (New York: Vintage Books, 2001), 24.

28. John Hughes to Benjamin Franklin, in *The History of the War in America, between Great Britain and Her Colonies, from the Commencement to the End of Year 1778*, Vol. II (Dublin: The Company of Booksellers, 1789), 84–86, https://google.com/books/edition/The_History_ofthe_War_in_America_Betwee.

29. Joseph Galloway to Benjamin Franklin, in *History of the War in America*, 86.

30. Deborah Franklin to Benjamin Franklin in Louise V. North, Janet M. Wedge, and Landa M. Freeman, eds, *In the Words of Women: The Revolutionary War and the Birth of the Nation, 1765–1799* (Lanham: Lexington Books, 2011), 5.

31. Buchan, *Domestic Medicine*, 93.

32. Duane, William, ed., *Letters to Benjamin Franklin, from His Family and Friends, 1751–1790* (New York: C. Benjamin Richardson, 1859), 21, https://catalog.hathitrust.org/Record/006255147.

33. In Douglass Adair and John A. Schutz, eds, *Peter Oliver's Origin & Progress of the American Rebellion* (Stanford: Stanford University Press, 1961), 53.

34. Governor Bernard to Lord Barrington, 23 November 1765, in Edward Channing and Archibald Cary Coolidge, eds, *The Barrington-Bernard Correspondence and Illustrative Matter, 1760–1770. Drawn from the "Papers of Sir Francis Bernard" (Sometime Governor of Massachusetts-Bay)* (Cambridge: Oxford University Press, 1912), 94–95.

35. In *The Parliamentary History of England, from the Earliest Period to the Year 1803*, Vol. XVI (London: T. C. Hansard, 1813), 131.

36. *History of the War in America*, 91.

37. "The Role of William Pitt," in Morgan, *Prologue to Revolution*, 141.

38. Henry Seymour Conway to William Tryon, 31 March 1766, *Documenting the American South*, https://docsouth.unc.edu/csr/index.php/document/csr07-0094.

39. Henry Conway to Francis Bernard, quoted in, *The Acts and Resolves, Public and Private, of the Province of the Massachusetts Bay*, Vol. IV (Boston: Wright & Potter, 1890), 934, catalog.hathitrust/org/Record/008374362.

40. Massachusetts House of Representatives to Francis Barnard, 25 June 1766, in Alden, ed. *Speeches of the Governors of Massachusetts*, 94.

41. Letter of the London Merchants to the American Merchants," 28 February 1766, in Morgan, *Prologue*, 158.

42. George Mason to the Committee of London Merchants, 6 June 1766, in Morgan, *Prologue*, 162–163.

43. Quoted in Andrew Stephen Walmsley, *Thomas Hutchinson and the Origins of the American Revolution* (New York: New York University Press, 1999), 112.

44. John Dickinson, *Letters from an American Farmer* in *Memoirs of the Historical Society of Pennsylvania*, Vol. XIV (Philadelphia: Historical Society of Pennsylvania, 1895), 327.

45. Hannah Griffitts, "The Female Patriots," in Louise V. North, Janet M. Wedge, and Linda M. Freeman, *In the Words of Women: The Revolutionary War and the Birth of the Nation, 1765-1799* (New York: Lexington Books, 2011), 7.

46. North et al., *In the Words of Women*, 9–10.

47. Sarah Gill to Catharine Macaulay, 8 December 1769 in North et al., eds, *In the Words of Women*, 18.

48. Ann Hulton in North et al., eds, *In the Words of Women*, 11.

49. Christian Arbuthnot Barnes in North et al., eds, *In the Words of Women*, 15.

50. "From Benjamin Franklin to Lord Kames, 25 February 1767," *Founders Online*, National Archives, accessed September 29, 2019, https://founders.archives.gov/documents/Franklin/01-14-02-0032.

51. Quoted in William Griffith, ed., *Historical Notes of the American Colonies and Revolution, from 1754–1775* (Burlington, NJ: Joseph L. Powell, 1843), 28, https://www.google.com/books/edition/Historical_Notes_of_the_American_Colonie.

52. *Historical Magazine, and Notes and Queries, Concerning the Antiquities, History and Biography of America*, Vol. 5 (Morrisania, NY: Henry B. Dawson, 1869), 15, https://archive.org/details/historicalmagazi1869morr/page/n19.

53. *Historical Magazine*, 17.

54. *Historical Magazine*, 26.

55. Massachusetts House of Representatives to D. DeBerdt, Esq. Agent for the Province, In England," 12 January 1768, in Bradford, ed., *Speeches of the Governors of Massachusetts*, 130.

56. Edmund S. Morgan, *The Birth of the Republic, 1763–89* (Chicago: University of Chicago Press, 1977), rev. ed., 45–46.

57. *Speeches of the Governors of Massachusetts*, 171.

58. Quoted in Ray Raphael, *Founders: The People Who Brought You a Nation* (New York: The New Press, 2009), 116.

59. Quoted in Robert A. Ferguson, *The American Enlightenment, 1750–1820* (Cambridge: Harvard University Press, 1994), 9.

60. Quoted in J. L. Bell, "The Funeral of Christopher Seider," *Boston 1775*, http://boston1775.blogspot.com/2007/02/funeral-of-christopher-seider.html.

61. Edward L. Pierce, *The Diary of John Rowe, A Boston Merchant, 1764–1779,* (Cambridge: John Wilson and Son, 1895), 73, https://catalog.hathitrust.org/Record/001262059.

62. *The Trial of the British Soldiers, of the 29th Regiment of Foot, for the Murder of Crispus Attucks, Samuel Gray, Samuel Maverick, James Calwell, and Patrick Carr, on Monday Evening, March 5, 1770, Before the Honorable Benjmain Lynde, John Cushing, Peter Oliver, and Edmund Trowbridge, Esquires* (Boston: William Emmons, 1824), 121, https://www.loc.gov/law/help/rare-books/pdf/john_adams_1824_version.pdf.

63. *Trial of the British Soldiers*, 99.

64. *Trial of the British Soldiers*, 116–117.

65. "Remonstrance and Petition of the South Carolina Back Country," in Jensen, ed., *English Historical Documents*, 596.

66. Quoted in Elizabeth A. Fenn and Peter Wood, *Natives and Newcomers: The Way We Lived in North Carolina before 1770* (Chapel Hill: University of North Carolina Press, 1983), 83.

67. Fenn and Wood, *Natives and Newcomers*, 88.

68. In William Edward Fitch, *Some Neglected History of North Carolina, Being an Account of the Revolution of the regulators and of the battle of Alamance, the First Battle of the American Revolution* (New York, 1914), 113–114. https://archive.org/details/someneglectedhis00fitcuoft/page/n9.

69. Richard Henderson, *An Account of Mob Violence Witnessed in the Courts of New Bern.* Adams Matthews Colonial America Database.

70. James P. Whittenburg, "Planters, Merchants, and Lawyers: Social Change and the Origins of the North Carolina Regulation," *William and Mary Quarterly* 34, no. 2 (April 1977): 237.

71. Whittenburg, "Planters, Merchants, and Lawyers," 238.

72. Lester H. Cohen, ed., *History of the Rise, Progress and Termination of the American Revolution by Mrs. Mercy Otis Warren*, Vol. I (Indianapolis: Liberty Fund, 1994), 58.

73. "The Philadelphia Resolutions" 16 October 1773, *The Avalon Project* https://avalon.law.yale.edu/18th_century/phil_res_1773.asp.

74. "Citizens of Plymouth, Massachusetts," *America in Class* https://americainclass.org/sources/makingrevolution/crisis/text6/teaactresponse.pdf.

75. "Citizens of Plymouth."

76. "Poplicola," New York Gazetteer, 12 November 1773, https://americainclass.org/sources/makingrevolution/crisis/text6/teaactresponse.pdf.

77. *Copy of Letters Sent to Great-Britain, by His Excellency Thomas Hutchinson, the Hon. Andrew Oliver, and Several Other Persons, Born and Educated among Us. Which Original Letters Have Been Returned to America, and Laid before the Honorble [sic] House of Representatives of This Province* (Boston: Edes and Gill, 1773), 16, Evans Early American Imprint Collection.

78. John Adams diary 19, 16 December 1772–18 December 1773 [electronic edition]. Adams Family Papers: An Electronic Archive. Courtesy of the Massachusetts Historical Society. /www.masshist.org/digitaladams/.

Chapter 3

Impolitic Madmen
Dividing into Enemy and Friend

The growing confusion and conflict deepened by 1774. Men and women proclaimed liberty, equality, and rational government but also violated those principles regularly. Passions, and often angry passions, overrode rational principles.[1] It was easy to play to passions and bypass rationality because conflict hardened existing divisions or created new ones. This chapter examines the ways passion overruled reason as ordinary people made decisions about whether family members or neighbors were friends or enemies. It asks a variation on John Macpherson's question: "[W]here will then be the liberty we pretend to contend for, when the hands of doctors and divinity and physic, are the only persons entrusted with it?" More broadly, what happens to liberty when individuals or groups of individuals could enact what they saw as justice against those who thought, believed, or acted in ways that violated the community norms that changed rapidly and were nowhere clearly defined? Who got to claim the word *patriot?* Not everyone who opposed the acts of Parliament embraced extralegal action but few who urged caution remained unscathed by the growing divisions. Those who called themselves patriots could point to the violence and irrationality of their opponents at the same time as they engaged in violent and irrational behavior. Increasingly, a powerful minority of colonists moved the thirteen colonies into conflict with Great Britain and those who remained loyal to the British system.

For Joseph Galloway, a man who had been a Pennsylvania delegate to the First Continental Congress and a close friend to Benjamin Franklin, the colonies, "where Freedom, Peace and Order have always equally triumphed over those Enemies to human Happiness, Oppression and Licentiousness," had become "governed by the barbarian Rule of ambitious Fools and impolitic Madmen."[2] He was not entirely wrong. The history of extralegal violence in this era meant reason and civilization were not always (or even often) triumphant. Instead, impolitic madmen and women brought to a frenzy by anger performed barbaric acts of cruelty on people who were not strangers or soldiers but were neighbors, family members, or former friends. Galloway likely used the word *madmen* simply as a way to characterize what he saw as unreason in his opponents, but his use of the word invoked the physicians of the ancient world. Eighteenth-century mad doctors read and referenced the ancient texts. Consciously or unconsciously, Galloway did as well, echoing the interpretation of the second century Greek physician Aretaeus of Cappadocia. Aretaeus had observed that furious madmen "see exactly as they ought, but do not judge of objects as they ought to judge."[3] Galloway believed the "impolitic Madmen" in North America deluded themselves in seeing danger everywhere they looked, even where it did not exist, and in taking it upon themselves to enforce compliance to their delusions.

The determination that someone was an enemy has a long history but this chapter begins in 1774. After Parliament passed the Coercive Acts to punish Massachusetts Bay for the destruction of East India Tea, men from twelve North American colonies gathered in what they called the Continental Congress in Philadelphia to craft a reasoned and sane response to grievances they believed "threaten[ed] destruction to the lives, liberty, and property of his majesty's subjects." In the document they created, the Continental Association, they called on fellow colonists to cease importing, exporting, and consuming goods and to create local Committees of Safety as an enforcement mechanism. Like their fellow colonists, these men had been "affected with the deepest anxiety, and the most alarming apprehensions," ones that might unsettle the mind of the body politic absent a measured response. The Association gave instructions that the names of those breaking the non-importation, non-exportation, and non-consumption agreement would be published and "universally contemned as the enemies of American liberty." Once someone was determined to be an enemy, friends to liberty needed to "break off all dealings with him or her."[4]

Although the men who crafted the Association believed they were acting rationally, the document alarmed a significant minority of the colonists. Prominent men like Samuel Seabury responded to the Association in print (albeit anonymously). He believed the resolutions by Congress were a series of "mad schemes" and in his pamphlet, he spun out a nightmare scenario caused by those mad schemes. The adoption of the Association would immediately result in unemployment for all those working in the shipping trade followed by the oddly specific "twenty mobs and riots in our own country."[5] The chaos and financial hardship that followed would result in hunger which in turn "will make these people mad." Hungry men and women would then "come in troops upon our farms, and take that by force which they have not money to purchase."[6] Seabury and others believed that this action by Congress had the potential to overturn a rational, stable, and relatively prosperous society and lead to violence and anarchy. The delegates had deluded the people into believing they were defenders of liberty, but that was just the babble of men mad for power.

In fact, the Association did result in mob actions and a whole lot of chaos. Although the language of the Association was relatively mild, exacting embarrassment and economic sanctions, the practice of policing so-called enemies could become anything but mild. Peter Stretch, a Philadelphia Merchant, wrote to William Neate "that man's property would be destroy'd & perhaps his Life Sacrifiz'd into the Bargain if he Dar'd to Contradict" the Association.[7] Like others who opposed the Association, Stretch knew that resistance to Congress's measure put people into harm's way. In a memoir published the year the war officially ended, James Moody described the tenor of 1774. He wrote that the popular leaders, "were able to throw the whole continent into a ferment" that year, "and maddened almost every part of the country with Associations, Committees, and Liberty-poles, and all the preliminary apparatus necessary to a Revolt." The Continental Association, in Moody's mind, was a conduit for disease. Absent law and order, the disease would spread rapidly and the colonies would revert to a state of nature with little to no protection from irrational actors. At first, Moody tried to remain safe from infection by dissembling, but, "The general cry was *Join or die!*" He found that staying silent was not an option because, "Some infatuated associations were very near consigning him to the latter of these alternatives."[8] If he were to diagnose them, he might say that he leaders were furiously mad, ready "to imbrue their hands in human blood."[9]

While in some regions the words were a rhetorical flourish more than anything else, the most ardent supporters of the Association really did speak the language of this stark and brutal choice: join us or we will harm or kill you. The written record has left us clear evidence that sometimes the men and women who cried, "Join or die," really meant it. Their tactic was to terrify their political opponents in order to make it clear that people were either on the side of the Associators or they were not. And if they were not, their person or property could be attacked regardless of age, sex, or social standing. In order to escape the mob, those who resisted the Association or were suspected to resist the Association needed to carve out a third option for their own survival and sanity because both their physical and mental health was at risk. In many regions, this meant physically leaving homes and family. By 1777, Moody made common cause with the loyalists in order to preserve what little liberty was left him.

Like Moody, others sought for an alternative. From the pulpit, Isaac Smith, Jr. continued to preach obedience to law, fearful of the changes that some of his neighbors and friends embraced, changes he believed had the potential to do great harm. A century before Smith stood in front of a Massachusetts congregation, Roger Williams had worried about "the madness of the *Children of Man*," and asked, "Into what furious *Extremes* do we leap and run into?"[10] Smith, too, worried about the extremes that led to mad and impolitic behavior. Like the Virginian James Horrocks had eleven years earlier, Smith argued that liberty needed to be checked by legal constraints to keep good order and prevent a descent into madness and anarchy. Smith tried to counter the madness of extremes, put limits on unchecked liberty, and steer a middle course.

His cousin, Mary Cranch, cautioned him against his continued preaching in the manner he had been. She wrote, "Orthodoxy in Politicks is full as necessary a quallification for Settling a minister at the present Day as orthodoxy in divinity was formely, and tho you should preach like an angel if the People suppose you unfriendly to the country and constitution and a difender of the unjust, cruil and arbitary measures that have been taken by the ministry against us, you will be like to do very little good." Her letter did not simply lay out a hypothetical situation. She had heard gossip about him, had "been told by several in two meetings houses in this town within these Six weeks" that they would rather leave the meeting than listen to him preach. She worried because "the spirit of the People runs so high." She assured him of her love and support but thought that maybe he had not fully considered the consequences not just for himself but for his parents as well as he preached himself onto the side of those considered enemies to the people. His father's business would suffer "for it will be said and I know it has been said 'If the son is a Tory the father is so to be sure.'" If that were not enough guilt to bear, he should also remember that, "You will grieve your mother beyond description."[11] Cranch not only disagreed with her cousin's politics, she hated the fact that he publicly aired those politics from the pulpit making himself and his family a target.

Smith's reply to his cousin tells us a great deal about resistance to the measures of both the Continental Congress and more local governments. He replied politely and with real affection to his cousin, but also let her know that he disagreed with her. He was not an enemy, but a friend to his country and felt it was his duty to preach order and caution. He asked, "Into what times are we fallen, when the least degree of moderation, the least inclination to peace and order, the remotest apprehension for the public welfare and security is accounted a crime?" Like others, he had disagreed with the policies passed by Parliament, but the British government was his government and he worried about transferring power from legitimate bodies that might sometimes err to illegitimate bodies that could break down the sinews that kept society functioning. While Cranch argued that the resistance to Parliament was in good hands, Smith asked, "is it not also in bad ones?"

When he looked at the protesters, he did not see heroes; instead he saw "the conduct of a few bad men" who had "already done infinite mischief." He asked, "And may not the violence and temerity of such men precipitate us into measures, which the united efforts of the good cannot prevent?" The good men who resisted could not control the madness of the people. "I must freely own, that I had rather calmly acquiesce in these, and an hundred other acts, proceeding from a British Legislature, (tho' we need not even do this,) than be subject to the capricious, unlimited despotism of a few of my own countrymen, or behold the soil, which gave me birth, made a scene of mutual carnage and desolation."[12] He could see no good end to the actions taken by colonists. In 1775, he left North America, spending the war years as a minister in England before returning to the new United States after the war was over.

Others also feared potential consequences that might come from disobedience to law and the move away from order. In 1774, William Hooper, Sr. wrote to his wife from New York that he was worried about her, "lest the present confused state of Boston should tend to impair your health." He worried that there was nowhere in the colonies that would be safe for, "the Spirit of Contention hath gone forth & I know no people or Province which is not infected with it." For Hooper, the resistance to Parliament's action was an infectious disease that had spread far and wide. He acknowledged that he had a different view of the troubles than his friends in Boston and that this difference of opinion had made him an enemy to them, that "they will readily condemn me for a contrary conduct." Like Smith, when he looked around he did not see rational actors engaged in working toward liberty, he saw madness and danger. From where he stood, he saw, "A Government subverted & for what—for the intemperate folly of a rabble. Deluded men!"[13] Again and again, those worried about extralegal forms of government saw delusion in the protests that shook society to the foundation. Liberty was worth defending, but unleashed, liberty led to insanity.

His son, William Hooper, Jr., had experienced the intemperate folly of a rabble in North Carolina in 1771. Hooper, Jr. had supported British policies. As a result, a mob dragged him through the streets and destroyed his house. Perhaps his father had that in his mind when he wrote to his wife. Unlike his father, however, Hooper, Jr. moved toward support for the American cause. In April 1774, Hooper, Jr. wrote to his friend James Iredell, "The Colonies are striding fast to independence, and ere long will build an empire upon the ruins of Great Britain; will adopt its Constitution, purged of its impurities, and from an experience of its defects, will guard against those evils which have wasted its vigor."[14] Like his father, he saw chaos, but instead of delusion and madness, he believed that a better, healthier, and more rational political system was to come from the growing rebellion.

For the colonists who continued to worry about unchecked liberty, as the Association was put into practice, they calculated that acts of resistance to the restrictions imposed by Congress were possible. Resistance meant operating within the existing British legal system, something that certainly still seemed a viable option. How could temporary governments operating outside of the sanction of the British empire get away with punishing those who broke no existing law? Surely law and order would win out over anarchy and confusion. Throughout the colonies, many made just this argument. In Hollis, New Hampshire, members of the Town Meeting voted unanimously to pass a series of resolves aimed at following British law rather than the dictates of the Continental Congress. Why? They saw the Association as "unlawful proceedings of unjust men, congregating together to . . . very outrageously trample under foot the very law of liberty, and madly destroy that jewel." Excess liberty had, indeed, led to madness, just as the medical doctors feared. The members of the Hollis Town Meeting saw anyone trying to enforce the Association as operating only under "the authority of a mobbish company of disorderly men, unlawfully assembled to commit riots and unlawful actions."[15] The Coercive Acts were bad, but anarchy was worse. Rationality dictated that they follow British law for, after all, liberty needed constraint.

Ridgefield, Connecticut took a similar approach, voting to reject the Association. When men in nearby Wethersfield heard two Ridgefield men bragging about this at a tavern, they decided to treat them in the same way they treated "strolling ideots, lunatics, &c." These two dissenting men were considered as dangerous to the good order in Wethersfield as the furiously mad were. A crowd forced them out of town with "hisses, groans" and the music of a funeral march, a threat of violence if not actual violence enacted on their bodies.[16] The town government further resolved no one opposing the Association would be allowed to stay within their town limits. When delegates from other Connecticut counties met together in a Provincial Congress, they passed what can only be called coercive acts against the towns of Ridgefield and Newtown which had also protested the Association. This meeting voted to "withdraw and withhold all commerce, dealings, and connection from all the inhabitants of those two Towns," cutting them off from government and trade, as Parliament's Coercive Acts had done for Massachusetts Bay.[17] The local governments turned to measures like those they had deemed oppressive when enacted by Parliament, taking away the British liberties of those who refused to protest with them. These governments did not think of mad houses and straightjackets when they passed these measures, but nonetheless they denied the liberty of conscious of rational actors, constraining them against their will.

Despite actions by local and colonial governments against those who refused to participate in the boycotts, some colonists continued to articulate their opposition to the Association. In James Rivington's *New York Gazetteer*, A Freeholder of Essex complained that the resolves were not "*wise* and *prudent*," but rather "rude, insolent, and absurd . . . calculated to answer no end but to stir up strife, and increase confusion among us." This writer called out what he saw the hypocrisy of those in Congress and elsewhere. He had been told Congress met to do something to "secure our liberties, and make up the breach with the mother country." Instead, "by this Congress the liberty we had is taken from us, and the breach widened." He likened Congress to the Spanish Inquisition, a force that operated through intimidation and violence. If he submitted to this inquisition, "I shall not dare to think or act, but I shall be in danger of being held up as an enemy to my country, and tarring and feathering is the least I am to expect." He then turned patriot claims on their head. It was not the acts of Parliament but instead the acts of Congress that attempted to make him a slave. The Association was in clear violation of the British constitution and its purpose in his mind was nothing more than to allow those in Congress "to be clothed with power to revenge themselves upon their neighbours, without control, and the poor victim of their mad zeal, malice, or wrath, is to be exposed to infamy and disgrace, unheard, without the form of a trial, and against the laws of his country."[18] The madness of Congress was that they claimed liberty, but stripped liberty from men who dissented and did away with the rule of law. American politicians had become worse than their British oppressors, maddened by a drive for personal power and operating outside constraint. Their wild passions led them down a dangerous path.

Other writers penned similar responses to the Association. In Rye, New York, eighty-three men testified in a letter to their "dislike to many hot and furious proceedings . . . which we think are more likely to ruin this once happy country, than remove grievances."[19] In Massachusetts, those who opposed the restrictions handed down to them from the Continental Congress signed variations of a covenant that laid out their resistance. In their protest, they stated that they would "not acknowledge, or submit to the pretended authority of any Congresses, committees of correspondence, or other unconstitutional assemblies of men." And if, inevitably this put them in harm's way, then they would "at the risk of our lives, if need be, oppose the forcible exercise of all such authority."[20] Over and over, these writers and covenanters repeated the language of those protesting British policies back to them, pointing out the hypocrisy of Americans who complained about their lack of liberty while they actively engaged in interfering with the liberties of others. These men and women, called Tories by their enemies, did not have to look far for examples. John Connolly wrote to a friend that the protesting Americans were "infatuated people." In his mind, there was only one explanation, for "nothing but madness could operate upon a man" willing "to form unwarrantable associations with enthusiasts."[21]

The infatuated people directed their enthusiasm at forcing compliance through violence or the threat of violence. If the Associators could not find a person to threaten directly, they found other means to intimidate their opponents. For example, when local enforcement committees could not discover the identities of pamphlet or letter writers that opposed the Association, they destroyed the publications instead, thereby actively interfering with the free flow of information. In Hanover, New Jersey, Associators tarred and feathered "Free Thoughts on the Resolves of the Congress" and then nailed it to a pillory. They did not know the author was Samuel Seabury so they could not use direct intimidation of violence against him. Instead they threatened him and others with similar opinions obliquely, harming the pamphlet in lieu the author. In Ulster County, New York, a meeting determined to burn that same pamphlet and, if discovered, the author and others like him should "be henceforth deemed the enemies of their country."

For many bent on obeying the Association destroying pamphlets and other publications was not enough as committees went after the sympathetic readers of those publications. In a letter of protest, Ulster County residents expressed their alarm that they had been threatened, "merely for reading and communicating . . . such publications."[22] Thomas Bradbury Chandler, in an anonymously published pamphlet called, "What Think Ye of the *Congress* Now?" warned his readers that if they discovered the names of people like him, "there is reason to believe, that the *writers* and their *writings* would both be consumed together in the same fire."[23] If rationality was held dear as a key to liberty, should not rational people read all the publications, debate them, and use the power of reason to come to a conclusion rather than be madly pushed into a false consensus? In their madness for liberty, committeemen became tyrants. Their tactics worked as can be seen when fifteen of the eighty-three men who had protested against the Association in Rye publicly recanted, writing to "utterly disclaim every part thereof, except our expressions of loyalty to the King, and obedience to the constitutional law of the Realm."[24] It is not hard to imagine that their minds had not been changed, but that they chose to join rather than to die or be otherwise harmed.

Like a contagious disease, violence spread along the pathways carved by the committees of enforcement. In a letter that started, "To the Americans," the writer expressed his horror at the "arbitrary and unlimited power" of the committees. Against every principle of British liberty, these committee men "may judge by appearances, and condemn unseen and unheard; they are under no check, there is no appeal to another Court, they are not accountable to any power."[25] Liberty had meant, among other things, having access to trial by jury and having the power to face one's accusers in a court of law. The committee men took that all away without evidence and without a trial; they determined who was guilty and inflicted punishments that ran the gamut from intimidation to property damage to physical harm. Those who faced intimidation or harm had no mechanism for appeal or redress, they were debarred from the social compact as effectively as if they were furiously mad and institutionalized.

In Massachusetts, the men who affixed their signatures to what was sometimes called the Loyalist Association or Ruggles Covenant were among those who were marked for punishment without trial. The language of the Association became more than words on a page as crowds took it into their own hands to exact justice with no trial or no legal protections for those they deemed guilty. The Massachusetts Provincial Congress sanctioned this violence. In session, they decreed that the covenant signers' "names may be published to the world," and that "their persons treated with that neglect, and their memories transmitted to posterity with that ignominy, which such unnatural conduct must deserve."[26] Their use of the words "unnatural conduct" is interesting. English common law emphasized natural justice when defining the duties of children to their parents, considering it unnatural for children to refuse to support their parents in times of need. If this was the construction they referenced, they had already substituted the Continental Congress in place of Crown and Parliament as the metaphorical parent. In *Blackstone's Commentaries*, the law of nations meant that natural law was dependent on "compacts, treaties, leagues, and agreements" among communities. If this were the reference then the Association superseded British common law and was less an agreement and more of a demand. Were they associating the behavior of covenanters with "crimes against nature," or sodomy, or with monstrous births "brought forth contrary to the common decree and the order of nature"?[27] Although it is unlikely they thought this much about those two words, *unnatural* suggests revulsion and that irrational reactions to the conduct of their opponents were merited.

For colonists already enraged by the acts of Parliament and looking for vengeance, the Ruggles covenanters made easy targets. For loyalist Ann Hulton, the actions of the colonists against anyone who dared to protest against new forms of government were signs of "the licentiousness & barbarism of the times." Government regulations had ceased to function, she wrote. "There's no Majestrate that dare or will act to suppress the outrages" perpetuated on so-called Tories. "No person is secure[,] there are many Objects pointed at . . . & when once mark'd out for Vengence, their ruin is certain."[28] For Hulton it was as if the madmen had become jailers, roaming the city in which she lived with the intent to harm. The colonists were not harmless lunatics but were the furiously mad who interfered with the peace and safety of good people.

Timothy Ruggles, for whom the anti-Association covenant was named, suffered assault on his person and property. This was not just because he opposed the Association but also because he had become a mandamus councilor. According to the Massachusetts Government Act, the representatives in the upper house of the Massachusetts legislature became appointed by royal writs of mandamus. Previously those serving in the upper house had been elected by incoming members of the House of Representatives and outgoing members of the Council. Men like Ruggles, however, were put in place to do the will of Parliament and the King rather than to act as representatives of the people of Massachusetts Bay. Because he accepted this position, Ruggles was warned out of his Dartmouth home by "the People assembled there." Once warned out, he agreed he would leave in the morning but angry colonists decided not to wait until he was gone. Resorting to violence on his property, they cut off his horse's mane and tail, covering it with paint, and maimed and poisoned his cattle. Where was liberty when left in the hands of men willing to engage in this sort of behavior against their peaceable neighbors? Ruggles found temporary safety in Boston under the protection of Thomas Gage, but he was not able to return home. Two other councilors, Timothy Paine and Abijah Willard, resigned from their positions. Willard had been arrested by citizens in the neighboring colony of Connecticut where, according to one account, a crowd of 500 people then made sure he was brought over the line into Massachusetts. After that, he signed a statement that asked forgiveness for taking the oath of office and promising that he would "not sit or act in the said Council, nor in any other that shall be appointed in such manner and form."

In response to these and other acts of threat and intimidation, Daniel Leonard responded in a series of letters signed Massachusettensis, urging calm resistance to the disease of anarchy that ran rampant through the colonies. This anarchy had led to "hatred and wild uproar," for the crime of a man who "acts, speaks or is suspected of thinking different from the prevailing sentiment of the time." For Leonard this was the "height of madness!" or "a despotism cruelly carried into execution by mobs and riots."[29] Liberty was not at stake; reason, rationality, and order were. In Massachusetts, the covenanters had written, "That we will, upon all occasions, mutually support each other in the free exercise and enjoyment of our undoubted right to liberty, in eating, drinking, buying, selling, communing and acting, what, with whom, and as we please, consistent with the laws of God, and of the King."[30] In New York, a writer who went by the pen-name Grotius, felt that the Association was "a savage invasion of private right and private property, which neither the laws of God or man could warrant or countenance."[31] These loyalists were not going to allow those who rebelled undisputed claim over rights language. They also had unalienable rights as Britons that came from God, man, and the King. Local forms of government did not override the government and laws already in place.

Despite the fact that many believed local committees were put in place by an "impolitic, absurd and mad association," mad Associators acted as if they had just and legal authority.[32] Their assertion of control in unsettled times came without all the mechanisms in place to reinforce that control. This meant that the people out of doors had a freer rein than usual to act beyond the limits of authority. We see one case of this in Philadelphia in August 1775. The case involved linen that might have been obtained outside of the rules set by Congress's Association, but more so, it involved the actions of a lawyer, Isaac Hunt, who did not cooperate with the committee's inquiries. Hunt believed the restrictions were unjust interferences with the liberty of commerce and thus, he would not abide by them. When the committee did not take vigorous enough action to punish Isaac Hunt and others for their lack of compliance, "several of the freemen of the City, men of prudence and discretion," took the matter into their own hands. These freemen decided that Hunt, as an enemy to the people, "ought to receive an American coat of tar and feathers, laid on with decency, without further injury to his person, and then to be expelled from the province forever." They gathered at his house and asked Hunt to recant. He not only refused to do so, he threatened the crowd with a pistol. The crowd put Hunt on a cart but as more people gathered threateningly the men ostensibly in charge decided that leaving Hunt at the mercy of a growing mob would put his life in danger. After parading him around, the men who initially argued for tarring and feathering deposited him back into his house. At that point, the crowd, "fell to, with the utmost violence, and broke his windows and doors with stones and brickbats."[33]

This clearly lay outside of any legal proceedings, whether British or American. The "freemen" had determined that the committee had proceeded too cautiously and therefore took the law into their own hands. Luckily, while Hunt was humiliated he was not physically harmed. While the leaders of this action protected his person, they were unable to protect his property, however. A long letter in the *Pennsylvania Journal* detailed the action that followed. This letter claimed that those who planned the action were "gentlemen," neither "mobbish or mobbishly inclined." For their part, they acted "with sobriety, decency and decorum." While the sober and rational gentlemen did what they could to mitigate the situation, they did not have full control over the crowd. The letter blamed the damage to Hunt's property on "a number of hearty jolly tars, market people, and others out of the crowd, who were enraged that he escaped from them without tarring and feathering." Even the "others out of the crowd," however, should not be held accountable. They may have been temporarily mad but they had been driven to madness because "no magistrate is commissioned to act against those who attempt to destroy the Continental Association, or any other law of the Congress, but our Committees." This language is telling as the letter writer acknowledged that the people had acted extralegally. However, the letter insisted that there was no shame in the actions, only an object lesson that, "Transgressors against" the Association "shall be brought before the publick." The blame for any violence lay squarely with Hunt or men like him who flaunted the Continental Congress's resolutions, the danger Hunt faced "arose from his own madness and folly." They reminded their readers of the war in New England (discussed in chapter 4) and while sympathy could be extended to Hunt's wife and children, that same sympathy was needed for the wives and children of the men slain in Massachusetts.[34]

In each of the colonies, as actions like these against so-called Tories increased in number, royal governors worked to gain control although this became more difficult as colonists either used existing governmental frameworks or set up alternative ones to resist actions by Parliament and the King. Men in power who wished to continue obedience to Crown and Parliament used every means to persuade colonists to stay the course under British law. In Georgia, Governor James Wright reminded the colonists of their precarious borderlands position. "We are in a very different situation and on a very different footing from other Colonies," he wrote in a letter to the assembly.[35] Wright specifically referenced the ongoing conflict in that colony with the Creek Indians. He did not need to add that they also shared a contentious and ill-defined border with Spanish America or that slaves were potential enemies in their midst. The upper house of the assembly replied to this plea praising the governor for his "real and friendly concern," and to the King for providing troops to protect white colonists against the Creeks. They confirmed that they "disapprove[d] of all violent and intemperate measures" taken in other colonies.[36] The lower house did not respond with praise, however. Even in relation to the ongoing conflict with the Creeks, they did not believe the Governor or King had done enough and wrote, "we cannot, but with horror, reflect on the dreadful crisis to which this Province must have been reduced, had we experienced no other recourse than those dilatory succours which the administration meant conditionally to afford us."[37] These members of the lower house saw a world that was stacked against them, where men with more power than they had were slow to act. It was not hard for them to make common cause with the colonists in Massachusetts Bay although their circumstances were very different. When they looked at the actions of those enforcing the Association, they did not see madmen acting outside of the law, but rational actors pushing against unjust restraints.

Taking matters into their own hands, Noble Jones, Archibald Bulloch, John Houstoun, and John Walton placed a notice in the *Georgia Gazette* on July 20, 1774 calling on "all persons within the limits of this Province" to attend a meeting in Savannah to consider the "arbitrary and alarming imposition of the late acts of the British Parliament respecting the town of Boston," as well as the tax laws passed by Parliament. The meeting was originally set for July 27 and then postponed until August 10 to give men in the further reaches of Georgia time to travel to attend.[38] In the August 10 meeting, those sitting passed a series of resolutions, *nemine contradicente*, or unanimously, that claimed allegiance to the Crown, but also made common cause with the other colonies in resisting the Coercive Acts. While the men who attended could claim the resolves were passed unanimously, the records tell a different story, one that shows coercion rather than consensus.

Was the meeting truly open to all people in the colony of Georgia? Those who opposed the growing rebellion claimed that, "when several gentlemen attempted to join" the meeting, "the tavern-keeper, who stood at the door with a list in his hand, refused them admittance, because their names were not mentioned in that list." Behind those closed doors, the men might have reached consensus, but that was only because they had schemed to keep out anyone who might dissent. This was not the reasonable action of the whole people nor was it conducted with "truth and decency;" rather was the treasonable action of a few. The dissenters tried to highlight the hypocrisy of these actions, calling the attendants of the meeting "pretended advocates for the liberties of America."[39] For colonists who claimed there could be no curtailment of liberty without consent, shutting the doors of the tavern went was hypocritical. What about representation and the consent of the governed? For supporters of Parliament and Crown it signaled that those clamoring for liberty were disingenuous, that there was something more sinister behind their claims.

When Governor Wright looked at the colonial world he had helped to create, he despaired. He believed that there was a "licentious spirit" abroad throughout the colonies, and conflict had reached such a head that there was little that could be done to stop it. He believed that "neither coercive nor lenient measures will settle matters, and restore any tolerable degree of cordiality and harmony with the Mother country."[40] No rational action could counter the work of frenzied and irrational protesters. In a letter to Lord Dartmouth he wrote that the colonies had increased in size and wealth more than those remaining in England could imagine, and had become so large and wealthy that he believed that the relationship between colonies and mother country could only be saved if Parliament entirely abandoned the principle of taxation in regards to the colonies. Anything less could only be a temporary fix, for "the flame will only be smothered for a time and break out again at some future day with more violence." He put his despair on the page in this letter. He had invested so much of his life and energy into building a good colony, but at this moment, "everything [was] unhinged and running into confusion, so that in short a man hardly knows what to do or how to act; and it's a most disagreeable state to one who wishes to support law, government and good order, and to discharge his duty with honor and integrity."[41] The body politic, in Georgia and elsewhere, was subject to confusion and disorder, to a mental illness without a good remedy. The licentious spirit furthered divisions between colonists.

Crowd actions made people change course, claim error, and resign from political posts, but one of the ways that madness could work was through deception. Madness could deceive a person into believing he or she was royalty or that Air Looms were channeling their thoughts. A madman or woman could also deceive their acquaintances. It was hard to know if people were what they seemed at the best of times. In the midst of political turmoil, there was madness in trying to guess whether conversion of principles was genuine or not, particularly if it had come through coercion. Joseph Scott's story was one case in point, highlighting the folly and madness of a changing political landscape. Scott had sold military stores to General Gage in Boston, but when he realized how high public opinion was against him, he closed and locked the cellar that housed the stores. Determined to get needed war material, Gage sent 100 soldiers to break into the cellar and carry cannon and other supplies to their ships. Despite the fact that Scott had changed his allegiance and acted accordingly, the Selectmen and Committee of Correspondence brought him in front of their body and "told him he deserved immediate death for selling warlike stores to the enemy."[42] Hearing this news, Gage offered Scott military protection but Scott was told (it is unclear by whom) that this would incite the people to even further violence. While Scott managed to escape death, incensed townspeople attacked his home. According to John Andrews, "Sometime last night they gave Scott a Hillsborough treat, and not content with disfiguring the outside of his shop, they by help of a ladder opened his chamber window and emptied several buckets full into it."[43] The Hillsborough treat was a mixture of mud and excrement—either animal, human, or both—that was routinely used to show displeasure for opponents. According to other sources, the Selectmen stepped in to stop the damage to Scott's home, but Scott was treated as an enemy rather than a friend.

People's words, and sometimes even their actions, could mask deception which was a gateway to disordered thinking and potential madness. For those colonists who believed it was their duty to root out this deception in order to properly police adherence to the Association, this could add additional layers of suspicion and paranoia to their everyday transactions. Could they trust someone who began acting or speaking in a different manner? Was that person dissembling or had he or she descended into madness? The artist who created the 1774 satirical print, "Liberty Triumphant, or the Downfall of Oppression," showed one group of men who lied about their desire for landing tea in order to save their reputations "with the People who are easily deceived (see figure 3.1). The print is a scene of mad confusion as

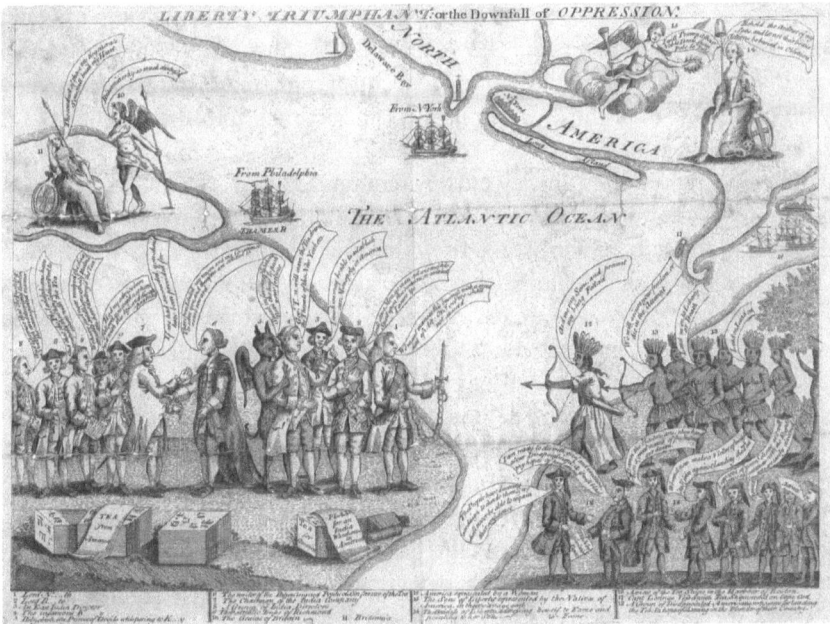

Figure 3.1 "Liberty Triumphant, or the Downfall of Oppression" (Philadelphia: Henry Dawkins, 1774), Courtesy of the William L. Clements Library, University of Michigan.

ministers negotiate with East India representatives and the devil on the left side of the print. On the bottom right is a group of men labeled, "A Group of Disappointed Americans, who were for landing the Tea." These men did not care about violations of British liberty, they cared only for their own gain. The man on the left of this group despairs that their plans had been discovered by the "People," and that "we shall never be able to regain their confidence." Yet the others are not so sure that all hope is lost. One man pipes up, "We must now make a Virtue of necessity & join against landing the Tea." He argues that they must appear to be on the side of the protesters in order to retain the faith of the people. One of his fellow merchants agrees for this act "will save appearances with the People who are easily deceived." These designing individuals believed that the colonists' brains were weak and therefore they could be led into the twisted paths of confusion and madness. The merchants hoped that, with their powers of delusion, they could continue to profit off of the tyrannical policies of Great Britain. However, the print's artist was not deceived; his message was that, despite the confusion, the people are clear-headed rather than disillusioned fools or madmen. They will unmask the perfidy of the merchants, aid the cause of liberty, and fight if they need to in order to prevent America, pictured as an Indian woman, from "being Fetter'd." They resisted straightjackets or chains. If the default assumption among the protectors of the Association was that others were lying in order to betray them, however, that assumption also allowed them to curtail others' liberty without evidence of wrongdoing. In this sense, they were not better than those who put men and women into the madhouse for their own purposes.

As they guarded their liberty closely, committee men not only watched for violations of non-importation, non-exportation, and non-consumption, but also violations in behavior, some of which were easier to police than others. The Association had declared that Americans should "discountenance and discourage every species of extravagance and dissipation," including one of the main forms of entertainment among better-off colonials: the ball. This restriction brought women solidly into the political sphere. Women were often the organizing forces behind the balls and active consumers of that entertainment. In some locales, before the Association went into effect colonists threw one last extravaganza while they could. In North Carolina, Janet Schaw noted, "We have an invitation to a ball in Wilmington, and will go down to it someday soon. This is the last that is to be given, as the congress has forbid every kind of diversion, even card-playing."[44]

Once the Association was in effect, local committees of safety did not balk at shutting down popular forms of entertainment. The Wilmington Committee of Safety sent a letter to Mrs. Austin on March 1, 1775 that read, "The committee appointed to see the resolves of the Continental Congress put in execution, in this town, acquaint you, that the Ball intended to be given at your house, this evening, is contrary to the said resolves; we therefore warn you to decline it, and acquaint the parties concerned, that your house cannot be at their service, consistent with the good of your country."[45] If Mrs. Austin held the ball in opposition to this directive, she would have been labeled an enemy and actions taken against her. As the committee labeled the house as hers, she was presumably a widow and therefore outside of the restrictions of coverture. This meant, too, that she was solely responsible for her own actions and therefore also a potential target for coercive actions against her and her property.

Mrs. Austin likely did not hold her ball. The members of Congress made it clear that they believed both men and women were capable of proper or improper action when they wrote that refusing the terms of the Association meant that other Americans would "break off all dealings with him or her." The historical record also makes it clear that women as well as men were targets of attack for crossing the line into what others deemed extravagance and dissipation. In Plymouth, Massachusetts, townswomen had met at the assembly hall "to divert themselves." If there were only women there, this diversion was unlikely a ball but, offended, a mob gathered, threw stones at the windows of the hall and forced the women to flee. As they fled, the women faced a barrage of rocks and verbal abuse. When the same group of women then determined to ride together as a substitute for their gathering they, again, "were followed by a mob, pelted and abused with the most indecent Billingsgate language."[46] Was it the social ride that other townspeople found so offensive, or was it that these particular women had already been marked by them as enemies to liberty? Had the women who were threatened and abused believed their wealth, position, or gender exempted them or did they actively resist the edict? Regardless of the answers to those questions, the Association created space for extralegal actions with few checks from old or new systems of government.

From the distance of time and with the lack of supporting records, it is often difficult to determine what was resistance in men and women and what was simply obnoxiousness, laziness, or indifference. It can be inferred that some of the actions taken were forms of passive resistance, that people did what they could to support the British system while trying not to draw too much attention to themselves or to actively take up arms. In Queens, 600 residents turned weapons over to American troops; however, on inspection, the weapons they had relinquished were largely non-functioning.[47] In the same county, Thomas Wooley refused to muster. A committee determined that he was "dangerous to the liberties of America," and he was sent to jail. After serving some time there, Wooley petitioned the Provincial Congress for release, acknowledging that he appeared obnoxious, but claiming he was "a friend to his native country (a greater love for which no man can have)." This, of course, could be read in a number of different ways. It could have been a sincere statement of attachment to the American rebellion. It equally could have been a sincere statement of attachment to the British government. Or it could have been deliberately duplicitous: Wooley, like the Americans mocked in the satirical print discussed above, could have simply worked to use the right language to win release.

In these ways and many others, the Association compelled colonists to choose a side, to mark their allegiance through their actions and words. By the 1775 Battles of Lexington and Concord, careful neutrality became increasingly difficult. Like many of his neighbors, Pennsylvanian James Allen opposed Parliament's tax laws, believing them to be unconstitutional and unjust. By his own account he had "zeal for the great cause," but he found the actions of his fellow colonists troubling, writing, "I frequently cry out—Dreadful times!" He worried that his neighbors and other Pennsylvanians did not want remedy or regulation but only independence. In October 1775, he mustered with his local militia, writing in his diary, "My Inducement principally to join them is; that a man is suspected who does not; & I chuse to have a Musket on my shoulders, to be on a par with them."[48] He also hoped that his presence would help to inject some logic and reason into a body of armed men who were averse to following orders and were quick to act on impulse. In many ways, it was a disguise for Allen. In 1775, he did not identify as a loyalist but found little common ground with other Philadelphians working for liberty. A musket on his shoulder as he stood in formation with his neighbors allowed him, temporarily, to blend in. By spring 1776, he despaired because those like him were not speaking out and the mobility now had the reins of power. "I love the Cause of liberty," he wrote. However, madness had taken hold of the people, transforming what had been a just resistance into a frightening movement toward independence. "The madness of the multitude is but one degree better than submission to the Tea-Act."[49] Allen continued to try to act in both private and public to sway fellow colonists away from independence and temper the madness of the multitude.

If men like Allen tried to figure out how to remain neutral in the midst of the frenzy of protest in 1774 and battles and war preparation in 1775, it became increasingly difficult when Congress declared "that all political connection between them and the State of Great Britain, is and ought to be totally dissolved." In the Declaration of Independence, Congress sold their war to the world as a just war, a war for liberty and equality, for rational government based on the consent of the governed. The language of the Declaration was exultant and grand, promising much. But just as they had before declaring independence, American men and women afterwards violated the principles of liberty, equality, and rational government regularly.

After Congress signed and published the Declaration of Independence, Allen still tried to stay on a middle course. Like some others, he said that he would not fight for independence but he also would not stand in the way of those who did. If the revolutionaries believed in liberty of conscience, they should respect this choice. He would not serve the British in any way, he would abide by the new government in Pennsylvania and pay his taxes, but he would put down his musket and sit out the military conflict. For Americans ablaze with the cause of independence, this choice made him suspect. The militiamen who called themselves Associators and seized control of the government in and around Philadelphia saw the world in the stark terms later laid out by James Moody and discussed above: join or die. Anyone not actively participating in the conflict was undoubtedly an enemy. Like the mobs that had come before them, they took matters into their own hands when they believed legislative bodies did not act quickly or decisively enough. The Associators saw their actions as a rational response to the loss of liberty but for their victims, their actions were anything but rational.

In December 1776, Allen's home was surrounded by Associators who arrested him and brought him to Philadelphia. When his accusers gave Allen the opportunity to speak, he reminded them that he opposed independence from the beginning but that he "had not interfered in publick matters," and wished to remain out of the conflict. Although his accusers found this answer unsatisfying, Allen was allowed to return to his home. He returned to a home where the surroundings were familiar, but where the geography had changed. When he looked at the world the new government and the Associators had created, he did not see liberty triumphant. To Allen, Pennsylvania could now be divided into two groups. These groups were not patriots and loyalists, but, "Those that plunder and those that are plundered." Whereas the Associators believed they helped to create a new and better world, to Allen their credo was that "To oppress one's countrymen is a love of Liberty." By 1777, Allen was convinced, "This civil war has rendered the minds of our Governors desperate & savage: they not only trample on the most express laws of their own Government, but those of natural Justice & humanity."[50] As one of the leaders of the initial opposition to acts of Parliament, he saw a new government that loudly trumpeted liberty but did nothing to protect it. The war had disordered the minds of the men who held positions of power. As one loyalist imprisoned in Boston wrote in a song, Americans "rav'd through the land," for "Their madness was boundless."[51] No longer rational and civilized, they had become desperate and savage.

Those whose religious principles required them to remain unentangled in war found their situations no better than Allen's. Each of the doctrines of the peace churches varied slightly, and within each of the churches individuals chose which tenets to follow and which to ignore. However, when members of these denominations felt that it was their religious duty to refrain from participating in measures of war, they put themselves at risk of physical harm or imprisonment at the hands of Americans proclaiming a different kind of duty. Like the men and women in chapter 1 who claimed to be sane but were confined against their will for being lunatics, men and women who claimed to be neutral were confined against their will or forced from their property for being loyalists.

The Moravians comprised one such denomination. The Moravian immigrants to North America had settled primarily in North Carolina and Pennsylvania. Their settlements were admired by many of the men and women in colonial America for being models of efficiency and order. Several Moravian leaders had developed what they believed to be long-standing and abiding friendships with their non-Moravian neighbors. The Bishop Nathaniel Seidel in Bethlehem, Pennsylvania had considered Benjamin Franklin a friend and therefore he called on that friendship in the summer of 1775. By the time of his writing, he told Franklin, that "some good inoffensive Persons have been already ill-treated" by their refusal to take part in military exercises, and that others had been threatened with the destruction of their property and livelihood. Seidel told Franklin that they knew "how to excuse this vehement Heat," after all, their religion taught them how to turn the other cheek. Using every argument available to him, Seidel continued that while they, as true followers of Christ, would endure, the bad treatment of Moravians or others who followed a doctrine of nonviolence created difficulties for the cause Franklin and others espoused. He assured Franklin that neither he nor any of the brethren would act against the American cause and asked that Franklin, from his seat of power, take some action to help them against the committees or the self-appointed guardians of patriotic fervor and work to provide protection for his brethren and others. Making good use of the language of liberty to which Franklin was attached, Seidel prodded, "[We] should think ourselves extremely unhappy if in the Struggle for common Liberty, we should lose our Liberty of Conscience."[52] Seidel claimed a common cause with other liberty-seekers but to him and his brethren, violence could not be used to achieve that cause.

Franklin's reply must have frustrated Seidel. Although Franklin did assure Seidel that he was "persuaded that the Congress will give no Encouragement to any to molest your People on Account of their Religious Principles," there was little he could do to stop the people from acting. In addition, Franklin opined that his understanding of Moravian doctrine was that the brethren were allowed to arm themselves for defensive wars. Moravians had done so, Franklin reminded Seidel, in the Seven Years' War. Therefore, Franklin concluded that Seidel and other leaders should allow men who were so inclined to arm themselves and to exercise with the militia. This might make their neighbors less suspicious. In addition, being armed was the best protection against dangerous neighbors. Whether Franklin willfully or genuinely misunderstood the Moravian doctrine of peace, he assured Seidel that, "having Arms in Readiness for all who may be able and willing to use them, will be a general Means of Protection against Enemies of all kinds." He advised, "a Declaration of your Society, that tho' they cannot in conscience compel their young Men to learn the use of Arms, yet they do not restrain such as are so disposed, will operate in the Minds of People very greatly in your Favour."[53] He did not respond at all to Seidel's liberty arguments, nor could this letter have provided much reassurance for Seidel or other Moravians who found themselves threatened or harmed by neighbors who found their pacifism to be a clear sign of loyalism.

Men and women in Moravian communities faced danger from American patriots. In December 1776, American General Charles Lee believed Bethlehem harbored a nest of loyalists and threatened "that in a few hours he would make an end" of the community. As soldiers flooded into Bethlehem, another American general, Horatio Gates, set up bodyguards at the dwelling of the Moravian Sisters to protect them from rape or other forms of violence. In the midst of the madness of war, two generals on the same side of the conflict saw the Moravians in Bethlehem in polar opposite ways. For Gates, the people he observed made up a hard-working and admirable community, one that did not take up arms, but paid their taxes and ministered to wounded soldiers. For Lee, they were savage enemies who deserved to be attacked. In the end, the more rational head of Gates prevailed but the Moravians remained under suspicion.

Pennsylvania passed the Test Act in 1777, requiring men to sign an oath of loyalty to the American government. Joseph Ettwein, one of the Moravian leaders in Bethlehem, called out the men who passed the act for having "tread exactly in the Steps of the [British] Ministry." Like Seidel, Ettwein pointed out the uncoupling of patriots' language with their action.[54] While lawmakers adopted exemptions for conscientious objectors on paper, men who refused to sign were threatened and sometimes seized and torn from their homes. By September, the Moravians in Gnadenhutten were accused of being loyalists. When a Colonel came to examine the accusations he found no evidence for this, blaming the accusation on "evil disposed neighbors." In that same community, brothers Nathan and Daniel Warner were forced to cut wood for the soldiers in Allentown when they refused to serve in the militia and could not pay the fine.[55] In Lititz, Pennsylvania, troops seized fourteen men and placed them in prison for their refusal to sign the loyalty oath. The men were eventually returned to their community, but only after their fellow Americans brought abuse and terror down upon them. The state government did try to intervene, but as John Bayard, the speaker of Pennsylvania's assembly stated, "we have made a sharp Weapon" with the Test Act, "and mad men have got it into their Hands."[56] The uncertainty of government in time of war meant that men bent on destruction, fueled by irrational desires or anger, acted on impulse, made mad by the circumstances.

While the Moravians did not attract much attention outside of Pennsylvania, the Quakers received national attention throughout the war. As delegates arrived for the Second Continental Congress in 1775, many of them commented on Quaker behavior in their letters. Delegates were impressed by the men sometimes known as "fighting Quakers," that is Quakers who chose to take up arms to fight for the American cause. Richard Caswell wrote home that several of the militia companies were made up fully of Quakers, "and many of them beside enrolled in Other Companies promiscuously." Joseph Hewes commented to Samuel Johnston that, "All the Quakers except a few of the old Rigid ones have taken up arms, there is not one Company without several of these people in it, and I am told one or two of the Companies are composed entirely of Quakers."[57]

Quakers, too, noticed that not all the members of their communities conformed to their religious teachings. From Philadelphia, Joshua Fisher wrote to a friend in England about his fears that so many "young Friends and some

Elder" decided to take up arms or otherwise support the war effort. Fisher believed these Quakers did not have the "stillness patience and resignation of Mind to gain Strength to stand in the trying hours which seems Dayly to threaten like a Storm over our heads."[58] Delegates celebrated the same impatience of the fighting Quakers that concerned Fisher. However delegates' initial admiration did not last long. Many Quakers, both young and old, remained "rigid," or rather, remained true to their pacifism.

Leaders of the Quakers continued to embrace pacifism and worked to enforce their religious rules within their communities, disowning members who supported the war when it began. In January 1775, Quakers from Pennsylvania and New Jersey met in Philadelphia to reaffirm their commitment to nonviolence. In their meeting, they urged their members to remember the teaching of Jesus Christ and to remain steadfast in their faith. In doing so, they used the same language as the Americans who protested against acts of Parliament. Like the colonists who claimed that they simply contended for their liberties, the Quakers claimed that they had "an upright impartial desire to prevent the slavery and oppression of our fellow men, and to restore them to their natural right, to true christian liberty."[59] With this language they painted themselves not as mad loyalists, but, like their fellow colonists, rational Enlightenment thinkers who wanted only their birthright liberty.

As Quaker leaders determined to maintain their religious practices and remain neutral, American patriots looked at Quakers' behavior and saw a country "invaded by open enemies" rather than a principled, moral stance.[60] The members of the emerging American government were particularly angered by Quakers' refusal to accept or use the new continental currency or bills of credit because these both were "money emitted for the purpose of war." In February 1776, a committee determined that Thomas Rogers and Joseph Sermon were "enemies to their country" for refusing continental currency, despite their religious beliefs. This committee believed their refusal did not stem from religious belief for both Rogers and Sermon sometimes accepted bills of credit. Instead, the committee believed these men were duplicitous. Accepting bills of credit sometimes was hypocritical and therefore a sign of disloyalty. The committee barred these men from further trade or intercourse within the colonies.

By 1777, Thomas Paine railed against the Quakers in the second of his number of the "American Crisis." He condemned them for "harping on the great sin of our bearing arms," while they said nothing as "the King of Britain may lay waste the world in blood and famine." Although Paine acknowledged that there were exceptions to this rule, he believed the Quakers were undeniably loyalists, undeniably traitors to the cause. In the third "American Crisis," Paine came back to his anger at the Quakers, calling them "ye fallen, cringing, priest, and Pemberton-ridden people" and faulting them for not supporting the Revolution. After all, Paine claimed, with independence the Americans would create a government "that shall hereafter exist without wars" which was certainly what the Quakers claimed to want. These suspicions that the Quakers were loyalists seemed to be confirmed when General John Sullivan reported finding papers in baggage taken on Staten Island, entitled, "Yearly Meeting at Spank Town." These papers, that reputedly had come from a Quaker meeting, included specific questions about the movement about the Continental Army and answers to those questions: "Where is Washington?" was answered with, "Washington lays in Pennsylvania, about twelve miles from Coryell's Ferry." Although these papers were clearly forged, for Americans already bent on persecuting Quaker men and women for their non-participation, they provided all the evidence needed.

On August 28, 1777, the Continental Congress determined that they had enough testimony that "a number of persons of considerable wealth, who profess themselves to belong to the society of people commonly called Quakers, render it certain and notorious, that those persons are, with much rancour and bitterness, disaffected to the American cause." Among other things, Congress claimed, Quakers communicated with the enemy and worked to harm Americans. The Congress then resolved to arrest fourteen Quaker men, confiscate any of their papers that "may be of a political nature," and guarantee that they be barred from correspondence or connection with others "of the same persuasion."[61] There was no specific evidence against these men; nevertheless, a general warrant was served against them, and they were imprisoned in the Masonic Hall. As Sarah Logan Fisher wrote about the arrest of her husband, Thomas, "About 11 o'clock our new-made council sent some of their deputies to many of the inhabitants whom they suspected of Toryism, & without any regular warrant or any written paper mentioning their crime, or telling them of it in any way, committed them to the confinement."[62] The men arrested asked to see the warrant, which they were not allowed to do.

The arrested men believed they still had access to legal protections and took a number of different courses to restore themselves to liberty. They were told they would not be exiled if they signed a statement promising not to leave their houses, be available for questioning at any time, and to not do anything to harm the American cause, but most refused to sign this statement because they felt it infringed on their liberty. As they put it in the long pamphlet they published to defend their liberty and call on their rights, they "refused to become voluntary prisoners." Like John Macpherson who claimed he had been imprisoned against his will for insanity, these men claimed they had been imprisoned against their will from "intemperate zeal, and personal animosities," or simply at the whim of those in power. They refused the stain on their reputations that signing the statement would make.

If they were going to lose their liberty, it was going to have to be taken from them. They asked how base a government must be that took liberty away without just cause.

In their pamphlet, they called on the same writers the revolutionaries did, using the same language as their adversaries to support their claims for liberty. They wrote that, "no man can lawfully be deprived of his Liberty, without a warrant from some persons having competent authority, specifying in offence against the laws of the land, supported by oath or affirmation of the accuser, and limiting the time of his imprisonment until he is heard, or legally discharged, unless the party be found in the actual perpetration of a crime." Without these protections, without any accusation of a crime, without being able to face their accusers, their arrests could be nothing more than a sign of power exerted under a tyrannical government; it was not justice, but rather the "over-turning every security that men can rely on." Any knowledgeable reader would hear echoes of the list of the King's crimes in the Declaration of Independence that included being robbed of the benefit of trial by jury. Who were the enemies here? If it were wrong for Parliament to pass laws without representation from the colonists or for the King to abolish trial by jury in some cases, this act was "far more dangerous in its tendency, and a more flagrant violation of every right which is dear to Freemen." If under the social contract, no rights could be taken away without the consent of the governed, then they would not "endanger PUBLIC HAPPINESS AND FREEDOM by a voluntary surrender of those Rights which we have never forfeited." Like the men fighting the war, they would not be reduced "to a tame acquiescence with your arbitrary proceedings."[63] They printed fifty-two pages of objections and resolutions. Like the revolutionaries, they formed a government based on the social contract within the confines of the Masonic hall, to speak and act out against measures they felt were unjust. Unlike the revolutionaries, their pacifist doctrine would not allow them to take up arms against their enemies.

These men also applied to the Chief Justice of Pennsylvania, Thomas McKean, for writs of habeas corpus. McKean originally issued these, and like the Quakers, he felt it was their due to be treated within the bounds of the law. In a letter to John Adams, McKean cited cases of American prisoners who were granted this right and even "the Ministry despotic as they were, did not complain of it." Should not the Americans also extend this right to men suspected, but not convicted of crimes? "*Fiat justitia, ruat coelum,*" he wrote, or let justice be done though the heavens should fall. In the madness created by a culture of suspicion, as men in power claimed war exigencies, initially no non-Quakers came to argue for the rights of these men. Despite McKean's plea for justice, and despite his attempts to follow both the letter and the spirit of the law, in the end, the Pennsylvania government forced most of the men who had been imprisoned into exile in Winchester, Virginia where they were forced to pay for their room and board.

From Winchester, in January 1778, exile Thomas Wharton wrote to his cousin who had issued the general warrant that allowed Wharton and others to be seized and imprisoned without trial. He asked his cousin how he could "in the Cool Hour of Reflection rest Contented, seeing thou had so great a share in Afflicting & sorely distressing the Wives & Innocent Children of so great a Number of fellow Citizens"? The younger cousin may have felt justified when he looked at the new governments created by the war and hoped for a better future, but the Quaker exiles and their families were not going to remain quietly in a world where men claiming to be fighting for liberty did not live up to their principles and instead acted as intemperate madmen.

The exiles, their family members, and their supporters continued to pressure the wartime governments to reverse their decision. The pressure apparently worked, for Congress ordered the Board of War to allow the exiles to return home on March 16, 1778.[64] Even after the exiles returned home, however, their lives remained difficult because of their religious principles. After the news of Cornwallis's defeat at Yorktown reached Philadelphia in late October 1781, celebrating Americans illuminated their houses. Because of the Quaker stance on war, they did not participate in this ritual, and because they did not participate, once again they were deemed enemies whose property and bodies were open to attack. In Philadelphia, Anna Rawle described a night of terror as a mob surrounded her home, breaking windows. When she and the other women in the house went into the yard to hide, two of their neighbors came over the wall and put lights in their windows to stave off further damage. Rawle was not the only one, she wrote, "Even the firm Uncle F was obliged to submit to have his windows illuminated, for they had pickaxes and iron bars with which they had done considerable injury to his house." The next day she concluded that "Philadelphia will no longer be that happy asylum for the quakers that it once was."[65]

These examples and others provide answers to the question asked at the beginning of this chapter. What happens to liberty when it is in the hands of the people and outside the checks offered by the legal system, when individuals or groups of individuals can enact what they see as justice against those who think, believe, or act in ways that violate community norms, norms that changed rapidly and were nowhere clearly defined? Clearly, liberty-loving Americans could become maddened. Their goals, first of overturning oppressive laws and then of winning liberty, sometimes became more important than the principles they espoused. Pitched battle on the field pitted friend against enemy, but those divisions existed before anyone even reached the plains of war. Long-standing ideological differences and the creation of enemies led to violent and irrational behavior that was often unchecked by the new forms of government that arose.

NOTES

1. For in-depth analysis of passion and the coming of the American Revolution: Eustace, *Passion Is the Gale*.
2. Joseph Galloway to Samuel Verplanck? December 30, 1774. In Paul H. Smith, ed., *Letters of Delegates to Congress: 1774–1789*. August 1774–August 1775 (Washington: Library of Congress, 1976), 283.
3. John Monro's translation which appears in *Remarks on Dr. Battie's* Treatise on Madness (London: John Clarke, 1768), 4, catalog.hathitrust.org/Record/009290937.
4. Articles of Confederation. https://avalon.law.yale.edu/18th_century/contcong_10-20-74.asp.
5. Samuel Seabury, *Free Thoughts, on the Proceedings of the Continental Congress, Held at Philadelphia Sept. 5, 1774*, Project Canterbury, http://anglican history.org/usa/seabury/farmer/01.html.
6. Samuel Seabury, *A View of the Controversy between Great-Britain and her Colonies: Including a Mode of Determining Their Present Disputes, Finally and Effecually [sic]; and of Preventing All Future Contentions* (New York: James Rivington, 1774), http://anglicanhistory.org/usa/seabury/farmer/03.html.
7. Francis Hazley Lee, ed., "Early Revolutionary Letters of Peter Stretch, a Philadelphia Whig Merchant," *Pennsylvania Magazine of History and Biography* 36 (1912): 327, https://www.jstor.org/stable/20085604.
8. James Moody, *Lieut. James Moody's Narrative of His Exertions and Sufferings in the Cause of Government, Since the Year 1776; Authenticated by Proper Certificates*. 2nd ed. (London: Richardson and Urquhart, 1783), 5.
9. Spurzheim, *Observations on the Deranged Manifestations of the Mind*, 2.
10. In Perry Miller, ed., *The Complete Writings of Roger Williams*, Vol. 7 (New York: Russel & Russell, Inc., 1963), 245.
11. "Mary Smith Cranch to Isaac Smith Jr., 15 October 1774," *The Adams Papers, Adams Family Correspondence*, Vol. 1, ed. Lyman H. Butterfield (Cambridge, MA: Harvard University Press, 1963), 171–172.
12. "Isaac Smith Jr. to Mary Smith Cranch, 20 October 1774," in Butterfield, ed., *Adams Papers*, 174–176.
13. William Hooper, New York, to Mary Hooper, 7 November 1774. James Murray Robinson Papers. Massachusetts Historical Society.
14. Quoted in Jeff Broadwater, "Declaring Independence: William Hooper, Joseph Hewes, and John Penn," in Jeff Braodwater and Troy L. Kickler, eds. *North Carolina's Revolutionary Founders* (Chapel Hill: University of North Carolina Press, 2019), 47.
15. Hollis, New Hampshire. Town Meeting Resolves. 7 November 1774. In *American Archives: Consisting of a Collection of Authentick Records, State Papers,*

Debates, and Letters and Other Notices of Public Affairs, the Whole Forming a Documentary History of the Origin and Progress of the North American Colonies; of the Causes and Accomplishment of the American Revolution; and of the Constitution of Government for the United States, to the Final Ratification Thereof, Vol. 1 (Washington: M. St. Clair Clarke and Peter Force, 1833), 1229, https://books.google.com/books/about/American_Archives.html.

16. *American Archives*, 1236.
17. *American Archives*, 1237.
18. Letter, 5 June 1775, *New York Gazetteer*, 5 January 1775. Reprinted in *American Archives*, 1094–1096.
19. "We the Subscribers," 24 September 1774 in *American Archives*, 802.
20. "Ruggles Covenant," in William Lincoln, ed., *The Journals of Each Provincial Congress of Massachusetts in 1774 and 1775, and of the Committee of Safety* (Boston: Dutton and Wentworth, 1838), 68, https://google.com/books/edition/The_Journals_of_Each_Provincial_Congress.
21. *American Archives,* 72.
22. Ulster County, New York. 11 February 1775 in *American Archives*, 1280.
23. Thomas Bradbury Chandler, *What Think Ye of the Congress Now? or, An Inquiry, How Far Americans are Bound to Abide by and Execute the Decisions of, the Late Congress?* (New-York: James Rivington, 1775). Evans Early American Imprint Collection.
24. 17 October 1774 in *American Archives*, 803.
25. "To the Americans," 4 February 1775 in *American Archives*, 1212.
26. Lincoln, ed., *Journals of Each Provincial Congress,* 69.
27. Ambroise Parré quoted in Paromita Chakravarti, "Natural Fools and the Historiography of Renaissance Folly," *Renaissance Studies* 25, no. 2 (April 2011): 215, https://doi.org/10.1111/j.1477-4658.2010.00674.x.
28. Ann Hulton, *Letter of a Loyalist Lady: Being the Letters of Ann Hulton, Sister of Henry Hulton, Commissioner of Customs in Boston, 1767–1776* (Cambridge: Harvard University Press, 1927), 72.
29. Daniel Leonard, "Massachusettensis" (Boston: Mills and Hicks, 1775) http://oll.libertyfund.org/titles/leonard-massachusettensis.
30. Ruggles Covenant.
31. Grotius, *Pills for the Delegates: Or the Chairman Chastised, in a Series of Letters, Addressed to Peyton Randolph, Esq.; On hi Conduct, as President of the General Congress: Held at the City of Philadelphia, September 5, 1774* (New York: James Rivington, 1775), 8, Evans Early American Imprint Collection.
32. Grotius, *Pills for the Delegates,* 27.
33. *American Archives,* 174.
34. Letter published in Peter Force, ed., *American Archives,* 175–176.
35. *American Archives,* 1153.
36. *American Archives,* 1154.
37. *American Archives,* 1155.
38. George White, ed., *Historical Collections of Georgia: Containing the Most Interesting Facts, Traditions, Biographical Sketches . . . Compiled from Original*

Records and Official Documents (New York: Pudney & Russell, 1855), 44, https://bo oks.google.com/books?id=oWIGNjgAlpkC.

39. White, *Historical Collections of Georgia*, 48.

40. Hezekiah Niles, ed., *Republication of the Principles and Acts of the Revolution in America* (New York: A.S. Barnes & Co, 1876), 390, https://books.google.com/books?isbn=5881459903.

41. James Wright to Lord Dunmore, August 24, 1774. In Hezekiah Niles, ed. *Republication of the Principles and Acts of the Revolution in America* (New York: A.S. Barnes and Company, 1876), 390.

42. Boston, 27 September 1774 in *American Archives*.

43. Journals of the Continental Congress, 56. "Mooning and Hillsborough Treats as the Revolution Comes to a Boil," at http://www.newenglandhistoricalsociety.com/mooning-hillsborough-treats-revolution-comes-boil/.

44. Janet Schaw, *Journal of a Lady of Quality; Being the Narrative of a Journey from Scotland to the West Indies, North Carolina, and Portugal, in the Years 1774 to 1776*, ed. Evangeline Walker Andrews (New Haven: Yale University Press, 1921), 149, Documenting the American South, https://docsouth.unc.edu/nc/schaw/schaw.html.

45. Thomas Loring, ed., *Proceedings of the Safety Committee: for the Town of Wilmington, NC from 1774 to 1776—Printed from the Original Record* (Raleigh, 1844), 20, https://books.google.com/books?id=gHItAAAAYAAJ.

46. Frank Moore, ed., *The Diary of the Revolution: A Centennial Volume Embracing the Current Events in Our Country's History from 1775 to 1781 as Described by American, British, and Tory Contemporaries, Compiled from the Journals, Documents, Private Records, Correspondence, etc. of that Period, Forming an Interesting, Impartial, and Valuable Collection of Revolutionary Literature* (Hartford: J.B. Burr Publishing Company, 1876), 42, https://books.google.com/books?id=UWIFAAAAQAAJ.

47. Joseph S. Tiedemann, "A Revolution Foiled: Queens County, New York, 1775–1776," *Journal of American History*, 429.

48. October 14, 1775. In "Diary of James Allen, Esq., of Philadelphia, Counsellor-at-Law, 1770-1778, *Pennsylvania Magazine of History and Biography* 9 (July 1885): 186.

49. March 6, 1776, "Diary of James Allen," 186.

50. October 1, 1777, "Diary of James Allen," 293.

51. "A New Song Composed by a Prisoner in Boston Jail," in *Philadelphia Evening Post*, 4 December 1777.

52. Nathaniel Seidel to Benjamin Franklin, in *The Pennsylvania Magazine of History and Biography* 29 no. 2 (1905): 246.

53. Benjamin Franklin to Nathaniel Seidel, 2 June 1775 in *Pennsylvania Magazine of History and Biography*, 246.

54. Quoted in Scott Paul Gordon, "Patriots and Neighbors: Pennsylvania Moravians in the American Revolution," *Journal of Moravian History* 12 (2012): 113, https://www.jstor.org/stable/10.325/jmorahist.12.2.0111.

55. John R. Weinlick, "The Moravians and the American Revolution: An Overview," *Transactions of the Moravian Historical Society* 23 (1977): 5.

56. Quoted in Gordon, "Patriots and Neighbors," 125.

57. In *Letters of Delegates to Congress,* http://memory.loc.gov/ll/lldg/001/lldg00 1.sgm.

58. Joshua Fisher, Philadelphia, to Robert Walker, Gilderson, England, 8 September 1775. Joseph Francis Fisher Papers. Historical Society of Pennsylvania.

59. Society of Friends, *The Testimony of the People Called Quakers, Given Forth by a Meeting . . . Held at Philadelphia the Twenty-Fourth Day of the First Month, and Subsequent Documents, 1776 to 1777* (Philadelphia: John Dunlap, 1777), https://www.loc.gov/item/2006566657/.

60. *Pennsylvania Packet,* 15 September 1778, quoted in Peter C. Messer, "'A Species of Treason & Not the Least Dangerous Kind': The Treason Trials of Abraham Carlisle and John Roberts," *Pennsylvania Magazine of History and Biography* 123 (1999): 318, https://www.jstor.org/stable/20093317.

61. "Observations on the Charges Contained in Several Resolves of Congress against the Society of People Called Quakers in General, and Some Members of that Society in Particular," in *Exiles in Virginia: With Observations on the Conduct of the Society of Friends during the Revolutionary War, Comprising the Official Papers of the Government Relating to that Period.* (Philadelphia, 1848), 239–246.

62. Quoted in Robert F. Oaks, "Philadelphians in Exile: The Problem of Loyalty during the American Revolution," *Pennsylvania Magazine of History and Biography* 96 (1792): 304, https://www.jstor.org/stable/20090650.

63. Quoted in *Exiles in Virginia: With Observations on the Conduct of the Society of Friends during the Revolutionary War, Comprising the Official Papers of the Government Relating to that Period, 1777–1778* (Philadelphia, 1848), 101, https:/lccn.loc.gov/06042550.

64. Paige L. Whidbee, "The Quaker Exiles: 'The Cause of Every Inhabitant.'"*Pennsylvania History: A Journal of Mid-Atlantic Studies* 83, no. 1 (2016): 28–57. https://www.muse.jhu.edu/article/606388.

65. Diary of Anna Rawle, Shoemaker Family Papers, Historical Society of Pennsylvania.

Chapter 4

The Folly and Madness of War, 1775–1783

Sitting in Boston early in April 1775, General Thomas Gage acknowledged a letter he had received from a fellow governor, Josiah Martin. Martin had expressed optimism that the people in North Carolina had begun to reject the "arbitrary power of the Continental Congress and of their Committees" and move back to due obedience of law. If this were true, Gage was jealous. He responded to Martin that in Massachusetts Bay, leaders of the opposition "by their arts and artifices, still keep up that seditious and licentious spirit, that has led them on all occasions to oppose Government, and even to acts of rebellion."[1] When he wrote this letter, Gage still believed there were measures he could take to halt the spread of that spirit. Gage was intelligent but, like any human being, his understanding of the situation around him was limited by his own worldview and by the company he kept. Operating within the British empire, ultimately under others' command, and surrounded by like-minded people, Gage believed that the rebellion could be contained and that the majority of Americans opposed the actions taken against imperial policy. Ironically, Gage's own actions to contain the rebellion closed doors to alternative possibilities and led to increasingly violent opposition to British authority first in Massachusetts Bay and then in other colonies.

Gage was not an outlier. He held the same view of many Britons on both sides of the Atlantic. They shared a stubborn belief that acts of rebellion in the colonies had been started by a few bad apples, by rabble rousers who held temporary power but could easily lose support. Many of those who thought this way believed a show of force would bring rebelling colonists to heel. In England, George Cressener wrote to his friend William Knox: "I look on the Bostonians as Men in a high fever, bleeding will bring them to their senses." While he used a medical metaphor, his bleeding was far from metaphorical. He believed that the British regulars should move to crush the rebelling colonists, literally making them bleed even to the point of death. In his mind, a quick and decisive military action would scare the majority of the colonists back to mental health. This bleeding could force "the better sort" of New Englanders, sick and tired of "being governed by the rabble" to realize how dangerous the situation had become and join in to restore law and order.[2] Cressener, like so many others of his time, did not or could not understand the depth of the unease (or disease) that ran throughout the colonies that stemmed not from a delusion brought about by a few power-hungry colonial leaders, but by a deep-seated mistrust of the acts of Parliament and the motivation behind those acts.

For ten years, colonists had organized resistance against laws or actions that signaled tyranny. In cities like Boston, they had grown used to, but never reconciled with, a standing army; people in towns without a standing army followed the news of occupied cities closely. Men and women organized, raised liberty poles, worked on home manufacturing, wrote petitions, developed intelligence networks, mustered militia, and engaged in other actions. Many were independent and perhaps even *independence*-minded, quick to take offense at threats to liberty and quick to act in liberty's defense. When the British placed an embargo on military stores, colonists began an arms race, stockpiling weapons and powder. In Worcester, Massachusetts the newly formed American Political Society declared that each member of their society be well armed. One of their organizers, Timothy Bigelow, also worked to supply the society's members with weapons. They even launched a successful raid in Boston, smuggling four cannons out from under British watch.[3]

The colonists were not the only ones to develop impressive networks. Thomas Gage employed an intelligence network that watched colonists' movements closely and mapped out the roads around Boston. In hopes of ending stockpiling and destabilizing the resistance in his colony, on April 18, 1775 Gage gave the order to his troops to confiscate weapons at Concord and to capture John Hancock and Samuel Adams who were reported to be at Lexington. He sent "an improvised brigade" of about 800 men, each carrying only "one day's ration but no knapsack."[4] A British soldier recorded that they crossed the Cambridge Marsh at about 11:00 p.m. and then waited until 2:00 a.m. for additional provisions to be brought over on crossing boats. This writer later concluded that "from beginning to end [it] was an ill planned and ill executed" expedition.[5] Weary, soaked through, and anxious, some of the British regulars must have wondered if they were playing out a madman's dream. If they allowed themselves to think about or question their orders, they may have wondered about the mental health of those issuing them.

As the British mobilized, Americans watched and acted. Understanding Gage's intent, Paul Revere and William Dawes rode to carry the news to the colonial populations along the routes the British might take. On his way to Lexington, Revere crossed paths with British scouts. Although they saw him, Revere managed to escape capture and find Hancock and Adams in Lexington. He convinced the two men to flee for their own safety. Although Revere and Dawes had proceeded as quietly as possible, in their wake the news they carried became accompanied by the cacophony of alarm as people tolled bells and fired guns to alert others, signaling danger and heightening fear and excitement. Men and women rose from their beds to observe or participate, gathered weapons, and kept fires burning. Instead of a night of rest before the next day's tasks, it was an unsettled night that must have worked on the nerves of all who were there whether they were ardent friends to the government of Great Britain or supporters of the American resistance.

In Lexington, about seventy militiamen mustered on the Common near midnight. When it became clear that the British forces had not yet approached, the men returned to their beds or to Buckman's Tavern for whatever sleep they could wrest from the night. At about 4:00 a.m., certainly crazed from too little sleep and too much adrenaline, these same men and a number of observers heard the drum beat of warning followed by shots and the tolling of the meetinghouse bell. They roused themselves to return to the Common as the British forces approached. The sun would not rise for another hour and according to most observers it was a typically misty spring morning.

We have many accounts of what happened when the British regulars encountered the American militia. Depositions and other accounts each tell a kind of truth although they all must be approached with caution. The men telling their stories certainly swore to relay only facts, but each of the storytellers had a purpose. Even if they felt morally obliged to tell the truth, memory is problematic particularly when joined by the trauma of battle and death. The accounts agree on some things. One of the British commanders cried, "Disperse, ye rebels!" There was deafening noise as the British soldiers shouted and huzzahed, likely both to give themselves courage and to frighten the militia in front of them. There was a gun fired, but whether it was a pistol or musket and who fired first was up for debate. In a heightened atmosphere of fear and anxiety, British soldiers then opened fire on the assembled militia who broke and ran. This brief altercation left eight Americans dead and one wounded.

At that moment, no one understood the significance of the event they had witnessed. In American social memory, this moment has become freighted with meaning as we write and rewrite our past to fit our nationalist purposes. It later became the "shot heard 'round the world," but at that moment the first shot and those that followed were not heard by the world but only by those in and immediately around Lexington Common. It was not as if a voice whispered in the participants' ears, "This will change everything." (That would have been truly mad.) Those there understood it was a dangerous moment that required a response. For the participants, the present and not the future called to them. What did they need to do right then to keep or shift the tide in their favor? British officers' first task was not to fight a war to crush an insurgency or maintain an empire but was to regain order in troops maddened by the lack of sleep and the experience of armed conflict. As one British officer later wrote, "the men were so wild they could hear no orders."[6] For Americans, their task was to get the news out to the nearby towns and to regroup in continued resistance, making it as hard as possible for the soldiers to complete their tasks.

The fact that British officers could not bring their men immediately under control gave Americans time to reform militia, bring in reinforcements, and set themselves in advantageous positions. As British troops approached Concord they found that "the country people had occupied a hill." The British Light Infantry attacked the country people on the hill, but "the Yankies quitted it without firing, which they did likewise for one or two more successively."[7] All of this chase and retreat worked to further delay British progress toward Concord and further tire the already exhausted troops, allowing Americans time to move some weapons and to gain defensive positions. In Concord, the British captured or destroyed what military stores they could find, burning cannon carriages. The smoke made the "Yankies" believe that the British had set fire to Concord and prompted their advance on the North Bridge. Faced with large numbers of armed Americans, the British at the North Bridge opted for a strategy of retreat, pulling up planks from the bridge as they did so in order to delay the American approach. In the ensuing confusion of shouts, orders obeyed and ignored, one British soldier fired and then others followed suit. The Americans managed to gather and fire over each other's heads, driving the British more rapidly into retreat.

The confusion did not end there. On the British return to Boston, Americans ambushed them from all sides "but mostly from the rear, where people had hid themselves in houses till [they] had passed and then fired."[8] British soldiers broke into these houses to protect themselves by routing, capturing, or killing those who shot at them but also to plunder "notwithstanding the efforts of the officers to prevent it."[9] This long night and day of military conflict was not army against army but British forces against country people, some but not all formed into militia units. And, they were a country *people* meaning that women as well as men fired at the British forces.

To the British, the fact that American men *and women* placed their bodies on the line was evidence that they were not in their right minds nor would they act reasonably. Captain W. G. Evelyn of the King's Own Troops denounced the Americans as "the most absolute cowards on the face of the earth," who were "just now worked up to such a degree of enthusiasm and madness that they are easily persuaded the Lord is to assist them in whatever they undertake."[10] In one house, John Crozier later wrote, "8 resolute fellows" tried to hold off the British Grenadiers. Even after seven of them had been killed at close range by bayonet, "the 8th continued to abuse" the soldiers "with all the moat like [rage] of a true Cromwellian," going to his death with "such epithets as I must leave unmentioned."[11] Other writers falsely reported that the Americans scalped and otherwise mutilated the bodies of the British wounded, leaving them to die. The evidence of American madness, and perhaps religious madness, gave pause to some Britons. The bleeding that came with military action could not act as a cure for madness, for men and women beyond reason. If he were paying attention, the British mad doctor William Battie (then in the last year of his life) would not have been surprised by this. While some mad doctors believed that bleeding could help alleviate madness, Battie wrote that it was "however no more the adequate and constant cure of Madness, than it is of fever." Instead the lancet "when applied to a feeble and convulsed Lunatic" was no "less destructive than a sword."[12] If the colonists were insane, these battles had just increased their insanity.

The British strategists had to deal with an enraged population that defied their understanding. John Crozier lamented that Gage had "a difficult and unpleasant task" and concluded that military force could do nothing to damp down the people's "enthusiastic zeal." Gage, of course, never did come up with a formula for quashing the zeal of those he called "the infatuated multitude."[13] Instead, *rage militaire* spread beyond the boundaries of Massachusetts Bay, infecting Americans in all of the colonies. Broadsides appeared like the one printed in Virginia by Alexander Purdie, announcing that it was "full time for us all to be on our guard, and to prepare ourselves against every contingency." After all, the broadside continued, "The *sword is now drawn*, and god knows when it will be sheathed."[14] The letting of blood, far from acting as a corrective, acted as an infecting agent for resolve, continued resistance, and a resort to an armed and defensive posture.

The country people in and around Lexington and Concord immediately felt the effects of April 19 in one way or another. Experience Wight Richardson sat down to write on the day of the battles that "not only our minnet men but almost all of our men took up their arms." She feared that two men from her town of Sudbury had been killed. Two days later her only son joined others to keep "our Enemies" hemmed into Boston. Less than a month later she noted that she was "much sunk in my spirits for the civil war that is in our Land."[15] Richardson and her son supported the actions of the Massachusetts Provincial Council that managed the everyday workings of the war that had come, but that did not prevent their lives from being unsettled by the civil war that ensued. Richardson, like so many others near the scenes of fighting, experienced this moment not only as a fearful observer and mourner of the dead, but also as a recorder of the destruction of peacetime calm and the movement of madness from the battlefields into the homes and lives of civilians.

Across the ocean, Britons initially felt the reverberations of war less strongly than their American counterparts. The British responses to the opening battles of the war and to the military and political conflict that followed were mixed. Several prominent men placed their sympathy fully with the North American colonists. Other Britons demonstrated deep misunderstandings of the nature of the conflict and vastly underestimated the determination of the American people to resist what they saw as clear violations of their rights and liberties. British men and women who remained at home as well as those who were stationed in or traveled to North America had difficulty translating both the words and actions of the Americans, often misreading in ways that deepened the divides and made reconciliation increasingly difficult. These men and women wondered how the American people could be so deluded as to believe that just exertion of imperial power over colonies were part of an evil design with an end goal of enslaving a multitude.

Many of the documents from this point of view repeat certain words that show how similar the language of politics was to the language of medicine. According to these writers, the vast majority of the people in America made up an "ignorant multitude" whose reasoning was weak. It was therefore possible for a few men to mislead the people, convincing them to follow in their mad schemes. Henry Ellis's language was typical. From his post in Marseilles, he wrote about "the infatuation with which wicked and designing Men had found means to infect the minds of the ignorant multitude."[16] The disease with which the ignorant multitude was infected was a madness that allowed them to throw reason to the wind and engage in acts of violent treason. The frequency with which these words were repeated in almost identical fashion from the pens of different writers in different parts of the empire reveal that this analysis had traction. Those who believed that the majority of the people in North America were friends to the British system of government and only needed guidance from more reasonable men overlooked any and all evidence that contradicted this view. These believers could not see or hear the eloquence of the words of articulate and rational writers who argued the case against British policy, nor could they read the actions of those who did not write but instead picked up a weapon to join in the fray.

Some Britons who did understand these words and actions tried to translate them. In the House of Lords, the Earl of Shelburne asked, "How comes it that the Colonies are charged with planning independency"? This claim, he said, was "contrary to fact, contrary to evidence, [and] notorious to the whole world."[17] For George Johnstone, New Englanders surpassed all others "for wisdom, courage, temperance, fortitude, and all those qualities that can command the admiration of noble minds." Their fellow subjects in North

America were not mentally ill and therefore were not writing or acting the way they did because they were a deluded multitude. Rather they presented a rational response to what they believed were irrational policies or actions. In this view, it was not the liberty-loving colonists who were a threat to rational order, but rather the ministers. In a response to a speech by the King to Parliament where George III called resisting Americans "the unhappy and deluded multitude," nineteen members of the House of Lords argued that it was the ministers who had "proved themselves unequal to the task, and in every degree unworthy of publick trust."[18] According to these dissenters, when faced with policies that worked to destroy traditional British liberties, the colonists responded only as thinking, liberty-loving people, not as madmen and women.

Resisting Americans celebrated and reprinted the words of their supporters. Earlier in the year, they had celebrated William Pitt's January 1775 call for Parliament to vote to remove Gage's troops from Boston, a measure he and his supporters lost by an overwhelming vote of 68-18. Despite his inability to sway Parliament, Pitt's words took hold in North America. When a printer published news about the Battles of Lexington and Concord in Williamsburg, Virginia on April 29, he prefaced the report with an excerpt from Pitt's speech, reminding Americans that Pitt had told Parliament, "the very first drop of blood that is spilled will not be a wound easily skinned over." Instead, he said, "it will be . . . a wound of that rancorous and festering kind, that, in all probability, will mortify the whole body."[19] Pitt had tried to provide a method to heal the body politic by removing the infecting factor of British troops in Boston. Instead, as he predicted, the troops and the actions of those troops led to a festering wound with fewer and fewer antidotes possible.

Pitt and others who advocated for the American cause made no headway in 1775. John Wilkes might have sworn and shouted that the war was fatal and ruinous to Great Britain, but the majority in Parliament continued to support military and other coercive measures against the North American colonists and they were bolstered by other prominent men in England. For example, university leaders at Oxford and Cambridge agreed with the majority of the members of Parliament that the Americans were deluded. The Chancellor, Masters and Scholars of the University of Cambridge issued a statement that the Americans brought the misery of war upon themselves. "We pity their infatuation," they wrote, conveying their belief that resisting Americans were not in their right minds.[20] Samuel Johnson raged that it was the Americans who had "inflamed this pernicious contest," and called on his "insulted nation" to "pour out its vengeance."[21] Support from prominent public figures gave the majority in Parliament the confidence they needed to continue to outvote the opponents of increased military conflict at every turn.

It is not surprising that men in power, who were separated from North America by an ocean, prejudice, conflicting intelligence, and false reports could misread the situation and believe that it was only a matter of time before the majority of Americans abandoned their leaders and were restored to their right minds. What is surprising is that Britons on the ground in North America could also grossly misread the situation. Perhaps their worldview acted as blinders to what was going on in front of them, perhaps they gave too much credence to their supporters, or perhaps they hoped their deliberate misreading of the situation would, in the end, force their desire for a continued British empire in North America into being.

Henry Strachey is a good case in point. He owned a plantation in Florida but lived in England. In 1776 and 1777, he was in North America serving as secretary to Lord Richard Howe. He accompanied Howe to New York for a peace commission, carrying a declaration of reconciliation. Delays meant that Congress had already declared independence from Great Britain before Howe sought an audience, but still Howe and Strachey were confident that they would get a hearing and, perhaps, start down the road to peace rather than continued war. Howe's declaration guaranteed pardons for all who would "aid and assist in restoring the publick tranquillity" in order to bring about "the establishment of legal government and peace." Instead of receiving an audience at Washington's headquarters, however, Howe found himself turned away by American Colonel Joseph Reed because the letter was addressed to "Mr. Washington" instead of "General Washington." According to Colonel Henry Knox's version of the story, Washington also sent word that the British had come to the wrong place with their offers of pardon as "the American had not offended, therefore they needed no pardon."[22] The rejection frustrated both Howe and Strachey who continued to believe that reconciliation was possible.

Congress had declared for independence (discussed further in chapter 5) and Washington had rejected Howe's peace commission, but Strachey wrote home to his wife Jane that he did not believe the American people agreed with this move. Instead it was only that "the violent Members of Congress" had already riled up the people with "the intoxicating Arguments for Freedom and Independency."[23] Because these madmen with their pretended government had led some people astray, Washington felt empowered to reject the healing medicine offered by Howe's declaration. None of this made sense to Strachey and he wondered how to turn Americans' attention back to their rational duty. Despite Strachey's close proximity to the rebelling colonists, he existed in a bubble that distorted his view of the situation on the ground. In his reading, declaring independence was an act of the overheated imaginations of a small handful of powerful Americans. The idea that some were so deluded as to believe they could successfully wage war for independence against the powerful British empire could only be a fevered dream. Surrounded by British military personnel and in contact with colonists who supported Crown and Parliament, Strachey overestimated British strength and loyalist commitment and underestimated the will of Congress, American military commanders, and their supporters.

Perhaps if Strachey had been a soldier rather than a noncombatant his view of the rebelling colonists would have shifted. Instead, in the summer of 1776 he remained optimistic about the British war effort, writing home that it was only a matter of time before Americans were led "back to their Duty." He was mistaken in his optimism and more accurate in his worry that "the infatuated Expectations, and Perseverance of the present Rulers of America, appear so much beyond Reason, and Nature, that no common Powers of Penetration can determine the Effect of even the completest Victory." He tempered his initial rosy analysis of British strength with concern that madness had taken such a complete hold on American minds that they would continue to fight even when faced with clear evidence that they could not win. Like the British observers of the conflict in Massachusetts he wondered what to do to remove the American people from the thrall of Congress and to restore them to sanity.

On August 27, 1776, two weeks after Henry Strachey suggested that American rulers were beyond reason and nature, his theory would be put to a test at the Battle of Long Island. On the American side, George Washington sent out a general order on the eve of the battle that reminded the soldiers that they were freemen fighting for a just cause, and asking them to "Be cool, but determined; do not fire at a distance, but wait for orders from your officers." Washington appealed to the best angels of their natures, but also the worst, as he also emphasized that if they hid or ran without orders, they would be shot on the spot: a carrot (acknowledgment for the bravery of freemen) and a stick (death to those who disobeyed). Despite Washington's speech, not every freeman was brave although many fought even when terrified. Before battle, Joseph Plumb Martin wrote that he "saw a lieutenant who appeared to have feelings not very enviable." The lieutenant was "snivelling and blubbering," among his men and "praying each one if he fought against him, or if *he* had injured any one, that they would forgive him." Martin concluded, "I would have then suffered anything short of death rather than have made such an exhibition of myself."[24] The brutal nature of war tested the mental health of those who witnessed it, although military culture and the eighteenth-century construction of bravery, virtue, patriotism, and manhood worked to suppress outward shows of terror. In the end, it did not matter whether Americans exhibited bravery in addition to cowardice that day; their forces were crushed as Americans blundered and miscalculated and the British forces took full advantage. In the wake of such a decisive British victory, many believed that "the affair will be over this campaign."[25] For Strachey, the victory must have bolstered his confidence in the outcome he predicted.

Instead, having defeated the American forces, General William Howe did not press his advantage and therefore did not crush the American forces. Using the window of opportunity to escape offered to him, Washington orchestrated a night-time retreat over the East River protected by a timely fog that hid the last of the retreating forces at dawn. Washington's move saved the remaining troops and kept the possibility of military engagement alive but he understood that he had a supremely difficult task ahead of him. His men had experienced the confusion and madness of a battle with large numbers of casualties. They experienced exhaustion even in their retreat. On August 31, Washington wrote Congress that he had been so tired he could not write them immediately on gaining safety. In his first report, Washington painted as optimistic picture as was possible, praising the soldiers for their orderly retreat. His optimism did not last, however, for only two days later he wrote again, this time about how defeat had "dispirited too great a proportion of our Troops and filled their minds with apprehension and despair." Instead of mentally tough and battle-ready troops, Washington had spooked troops. He did not know how to remedy it, particularly as he was still so dependent on militias rather than regular Continental troops. For Washington, operating with militia posed an insurmountable problem for, in his mind, the men who served in that capacity would never be properly subordinate to military command. Without a more regular army, he believed that the American cause could be doomed. Whatever advantage he gained from the additional numbers that the militias provided was "nearly counterbalanced by the disorder, irregularity and confusion they Occasion."[26] It was impossible to avoid the madness of battle, but he did not want to add to that madness and confusion with undisciplined and sometimes recalcitrant troops.

As Henry Strachey witnessed the British victory from on board the *Eagle*, he knew, or at least guessed at, the despair of the American commanders and their troops. The conditions the American soldiers faced had been the stuff of nightmares, complete with death, destruction, and seemingly utter defeat. He had seen that not even surrender saved American soldiers in every instance. As one British officer wrote, "We took care to tell the Hessians that the Rebels had resolved to give no quarters to them in particular, which made them fight desperately and put all to death who fell into their hands. You know all stratagems are lawful in war."[27] This officer had described and justified Hessians bayoneting Americans who thought they could save themselves by throwing themselves at the mercy of the enemy only to find there was no mercy.

Despite the nightmare of death even in surrender, of retreat and high rates of desertion, Americans seemed set on fighting an unwinnable war. To

Strachey they proved themselves "beyond Nature as well as Reason." On September 3, Henry wrote to Jane, "I shall ever hereafter think it possible that a Phrenzy may seize a whole Nation as well as an Individual." By the end of the same month, he wrote her again, "I begin to think it possible, that a whole Country as well as an Individual may be struck with Lunacy."[28] With these remarks, Strachey signaled his growing belief that the war would not end in the near future and that reconciliation was no longer possible. The madness had spread from the inflamed brains of a few individuals to the mind of the body politic. It would be impossible for sane individuals to prevail because it had gone beyond the actions of any one person and had infected the collective. He was not yet reconciled to the idea of an independent nation in North America but he recognized a nation nonetheless. The nation raved and acted irrationally, but it was there, animated by principles with which he disagreed.

Madness cannot explain the American Revolution entirely, of course, but looking at it this way adds to our understanding of an era that is otherwise hard to understand. Americans now believe that the Revolution was a rational solution to oppression, but many immersed in the crisis could make little sense of it. As John Shy tells us, "the American Revolution challenges the historical imagination." Because of this, one explanation is the war was "an extraordinary phenomenon, akin to collective madness," for ordinary people acted in extraordinary ways, up to and including imbruing their hands in human blood.[29] Perhaps Strachey was partly right in his belief that the collective had gone mad. If victory over the British Empire and independence were the fevered dreams of impolitic madmen, enough people dreamed of both to continue fighting.

Strachey not only diagnosed a madness in the body politic, he also suggested a cause. He believed that all the advantages that had accrued from a resource-rich continent tied to a powerful empire had made the colonists overly wealthy. They had "been too happy," he wrote, and their "Prosperity has made them mad."[30] Other Britons offered different causes for the illness of rebellion and war. Charles Inglis, the first consecrated Anglican bishop in North America, preached a long sermon on the Christian soldier's duty before newly raised loyalist troops on September 7, 1777. He praised the soldiers for taking up arms "to defend your Families, your Lives, Liberties and Property" against "usurped Power" which removed Americans from the protection of good government under the British Constitution. Inglis believed that while Americans might prevail temporarily, they could not achieve a lasting independence. In his view, if the colonists defeated the British, America would be in such a weak state that the French or the Spanish, "our inveterate and popish Enemies," would fill the void left by Great Britain. Nothing could explain Americans bent on independence other than "astonishing Infatuation and Madness."[31] Independence-loving Americans were mad and had become mad in a number of different ways. His analysis could have come straight out of medical text. "A wrong Byass of Mind, inordinate Affections and Desires, or an overweening Opinion of ourselves," he said, "frequently produce this unhappy Temper."[32] In his analysis, he concurred with a sermon preached 23 years earlier by Samuel Finley that "Precipitant Conclusions concerning Persons, Things, or Opinions, formed without evidence, and often in Defiance of Demonstration to the contrary, discover a Degree of Madness." All evidence pointed toward the goodness of the British system, but mad Americans had reached other precipitant conclusions that they could not shake. Inglis asked the soldiers to pray for God's intervention to bring about peace "to our distracted Country," and to "remove the Delusion of our misguided Brethren."[33] We do not know how the soldiers heard or interpreted this sermon, but Inglis was clear that the men who were temporarily their enemies were not in their right minds. Like most madmen, however, they could be led back to rationality and therefore be restored to full enjoyment as members in a healthy body politic.

No matter what men like Strachey and Inglis concluded, American soldiers and civilians were (for the most part) not lunatics. If madness did not drive them to put themselves in harm's way, what did? Shy has examined what he calls the "psychic web spun from logic, belief, perception, and emotion that draws people to commit terrible acts and to hazard everything they possess."[34] He concludes that their motivations were likely as many and varied as the men who participated, ranging from anger at the British political and military policies, other forms of ideology, financial need, ideas about manhood, and peer pressure, but not lunacy.

While it remains impossible to untangle the motives for many of the soldiers, what matters for this study is that there was a perception from both American military commanders and other observers that while the soldiers were not lunatics, they did tend toward disorder. Americans with military, political, or economic power worried a lot about the fact that many within the ranks were of the lower sort who had long existed at the margins of society. Shy found that most Continental soldiers were poorer than the average American. While Strachey thought that prosperity had driven the body politic into a frenzy, the majority of the men who fought had not benefited from prosperity. Even before the war began, town leaders and other residents brooded about the danger these poorer sort posed to their communities. They monitored them closely, considered them a threat to the economic stability of their towns, and sometimes demanded they leave. Now these same men formed the base of the fighting forces.

While some of the records left to us are from ordinary soldiers with limited education, more come from men and women who expressed distaste for and unease toward the poor. Shortly after he took to the field in Long Island, Pennsylvanian General Persifor Frazer wrote to his wife Mary about his loathing of the New England men over whom he had command. They were, he wrote, "the strangest mixture of Negroes, Indians, and Whites, with old men and mere children, which together with a nasty lousy appearance make a most shocking spectacle."[35] From Philadelphia, John Adams wrote to Joseph Hawley in Massachusetts worrying that even the commanders coming out of Massachusetts were "awkward, illiterate, [and] ill bred."[36] Adams believed there was a preponderance of illiterate commanders because they were elected rather than appointed. He believed the poorer sort put self-interest above the common good in ways elite members of society did not. It fed into his and others' fears of faction and party, that the divisions that existed between groups of people would be furthered by an ill-informed electorate. Men driven by economic need could be more easily swayed, Adams argued, than men of independent means. His comments reflected his own prejudices against the lower sort: of course, poor men voted in ways that reflected their interests, but wealthy men did as well. The men whom Adams denigrated needed money in a way he did not understand and also in a way that drove them into military service. Acquiring financial means and status was a motivating factor for the poorer sort, just as keeping financial means and status was for the better sort.

Unlike the better sort, the poorer sort also had fewer escape hatches if they did not want to serve in the military. Once states instituted drafts, poor and middling men could not buy their way out of the draft the way their better-off neighbors could. In the slave-holding states plantation owners benefited from exemptions, claiming they needed to keep their enslaved people from running off. The white tenant farmers in Washington's Virginia whose labor was truly needed to keep their families solvent found themselves among the ranks of soldiers, despite petitions claiming that they were "poor men with families that are Incapable of Supporting themselves without Labour."[37] According to George Washington, even when men initially were motivated by ideology, Congress should not expect soldiers to be "influenced by any other principles than those of Interest."[38] While this might have seemed like greed or selfishness to Washington and other wealthy Americans, the fact of the matter was that the soldiers looked down upon for their poverty and lack of education could not live without pay. Even if they had no family to support, they had to support themselves and think about their futures if they managed to survive the war.

Poor men serving as soldiers bore the brunt of the fighting. They were the torso and limbs of a military body politic whose head was often disordered by poor command and political infighting. Later in his life, Joseph Plumb Martin described the British landing at Kip's Bay on the island of Manhattan. The day began with advance fire from the British naval forces. Once the British troops began to move, Americans precipitously retreated with or without the orders of their immediate officers, often discarding everything from weapons to items of clothing as they fled. For the militia, Martin later noted, "the demons of fear and disorder seemed to take full possession." Even among the Continental soldiers, disorder reigned in ways that led to a day that was a nightmare of privation and death with no clear sense of direction or purpose. Washington tried to rally subordinate officers to stand and fight with their troops, but to no avail. According to General George Weedon, Washington physically struck at the officers who fled. Angered, Washington threw his hat on the ground and exclaimed, "Good God, have I got such troops as those!" In his memoir, Martin wrote, "The men were confused, being without officers to command them.... How could the men fight without officers?"[39] Benjamin Trumbull also blamed the disorderly retreat on the officers, writing that they did not "give the men a rational prospect of defence and a safe retreat should they engage the enemy."[40] The retreat had not been honorable, Trumbull acknowledged, but lives had been saved because of it. Without competent officers, there was no one to give orders and therefore impose order on the day. Weedon wrote that Washington temporarily lost his mind, breaking down over this lack of martial spirit and that those around him had to drag him from the field.

While Kip's Bay played out in one particular day of madness and confusion, warfare is never rational even under the best of circumstances. In every region, on every field of conflict, soldiers reported back on their particular experiences. In 1832, Park Holland recollected serving under General Philip Schuyler in 1777. He remembered the fear of knowing there were "foes in every direction." Even in the sparse prose of his memoir, the reader gets a sense of how unsettled Holland was by the uncertainty of what was to come and the danger they were to face. To make it worse, Holland and the men he served with had little confidence in their commander. Geographic prejudice was part of it: the soldiers were young and old New Englanders, many of them both poor and poorly equipped, and Schuyler was an aristocratic New Yorker. After abandoning Fort Ticonderoga because it was indefensible, Schuyler kept his men engaged in making it extremely difficult for the British General Burgoyne to move through the wilderness, cutting down trees to block roads, destroying bridges, and changing the course of the waterways. The toil of unglamorous work may have added to the disenchantment of the men who served under Schuyler. In 1832, Holland apologized for their lack of confidence, writing: "He certainly did everything a man in his situation could do. But the situation of a retreated army is never a very pleasant one, and as often remarked, a commander is blamed for misfortunes over which he could have no control."[41] In his late life, Holland could give Schuyler the benefit of the doubt, but in the heat of the war for New York, the lack of confidence infected the American forces under Schuyler's command.

The military body politic weakened and sickened under the material hardships that accompanied the war. Brigadier General Moses Hazen wrote to Thomas McKean, then sitting in the Continental Congress, "The Reigning Discontent in the Army is a melancholy Distressing Subject." The discontent did not surprise Hazen. He reminded McKean, and therefore Congress, that the soldiers had "suffered the Hardships and fatigues of War, have fought, bled, Defended, and saved these united States from Bondage." Meanwhile, many citizens, "have been accumulating fortunes, and in some Instances Taken the advantage of the Distresses of the army."[42] Playing on Thomas Paine's *American Crisis*, Joseph Plumb Martin wrote that the winter of 1779 and 1780 "not only tried men's souls, but their bodies too," as he described the cold and hunger that ensued.[43] "We were absolutely, literally starved," he wrote, and described men chewing on wood and eating the leather from their shoes in order to survive. Their bodies and therefore the body politic were pushed to the limit. While privation might cure a lunatic under controlled circumstances according to eighteenth-century doctors, it also served to make rational men into lunatics under circumstances beyond their control.

Quartermaster General Nathanael Greene alternately grieved and despaired at the condition of the army fighting for the causes of liberty and self-government. In January 1780, after a severe winter storm, he wrote to Colonel Daniel Hathway begging him to use the officers of the militia and other men to dig out roads in order to get the provisions to the starving army. "The Army is upon the eve of disbanding for want of Provisions," he wrote, "the poor Soldiers having been Several days without." The army would aid in whatever ways they could, but "the Army is stript as naked of Teams as possible, to lessen the consumption of forage." Hathway also needed to convince civilians to supply the army with food and needed materials to lessen the soldiers' reliance of the kinder word for plunder, *forage*. He knew that Hathway should need no reminder of the dangers but then reminded him anyways, explaining that "the surrounding Inhabitants will experience the first melancholy effects of such raging evil."[44] Men willing to starve and freeze and fight would not be willing to keep their hands off the food and clothing of a civilian population if that population did not supply them with some basic necessities. The sight of healthy and well-fed civilians drove them to acts of madness.

From the beginning of the war, Greene had fought tooth and nail with Congress to get the men on the field supplied. He likely understood that the function of a new government would be far from perfect. What he could not stand was when political divisions interfered with the supplying of the Continental Army. It was hard to check the illness in the military body politic when there were not enough resources (medicine) to do so. Finally, unable to take it anymore, he resigned as Quartermaster General in the summer of 1780. He wrote to his wife, Caty that Congress was "so vexed with me that they are about to suspend my command in the line of the Army, as I am informed. Should they take this step and I verily believe they will it will be one of the most high handed and arbitrary measures that ever disgraced the Annals of a free people. Congress have but little power and less influence and seem to take a malignant pleasure in tyrannising over their servants; and in proportion as they sink into contempt their pride and injustice rise."[45] Was this the rational government of a free people? Greene despaired. He believed he had an important role to play in a war whose purpose he believed in. In August 1780, he thought all possibility of playing a part would be taken from him. What surprises us from the distance of more than 200 years is that the language of Greene, a consummate patriot, echoed the language of loyalists who opposed the cause of independence. At this point in the war, Greene saw Congress not as a force for good government but as a force for maddening corruption. Like Strachey or Inglis, he saw American weakness instead of American strength.

The satiric print, "A View in America in 1778" (figure 4.1) speaks to Greene's complaints. Published in London, the print shows freezing, miserable, and ill-clothed soldiers, one bearing a hat that reads, "Death or Liberty."

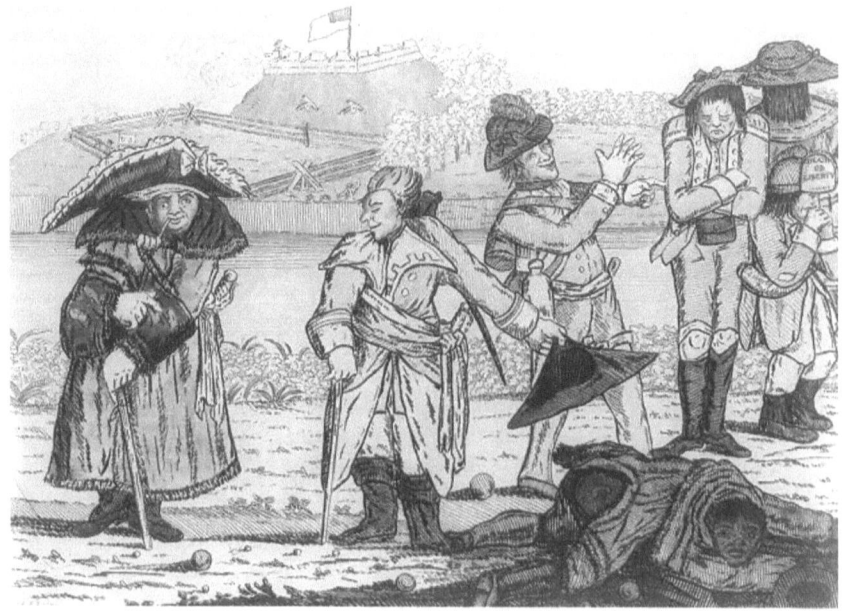

Figure 4.1 "A View in America in 1778" (London: M. Darly, 1778), Courtesy of the Library of Congress.

There is more death than liberty in this print. In the front of the print, a black man lies wounded and neglected giving more lie to the "liberty" half of the "death or liberty" equation. While a well-dressed soldier mocks the other poorly equipped soldiers, an officer with a self-satisfied look on his face, gestures to those behind him while facing an extremely well-dressed civilian. This fur-coat, pipe, and walking-stick attired man represents a number of possibilities. Perhaps he is a civilian profiting off the war or perhaps he is a member of Congress who neglected the plight of the soldier for some other nefarious purpose. Satire plays on concepts of madness, and in this case the print presents a nightmare scenario, a war that followed along disordered pathways, the desire for liberty gone by the wayside.

The hardship of the Continental Army at Washington's winter camp at Valley Forge has been enshrined in our collective memory. The American hardship is often contrasted with a myth of British plenty, but the British army also suffered from material hardship. British and Hessian troops also lacked clothing and food, sometimes because the supplies could not get through or were captured, or sometimes because the administration put in place in North America failed. Clothing for Hessian Troops in Philadelphia arrived in New York in the winter of 1777, but the quartermaster department failed to send them on to those who needed them.[46] And while the British forces never faced the food shortages of their American counterparts, food supply remained a persistent problem as they had to rely on food packaged and sent from Britain rather than local supplies, or, like the Americans, to resort to plunder.[47]

Each one of these stories adds another voice to the thousands of stories of suffering and discontent among the soldiers, and madness and confusion on the battlefield. This madness and confusion spread to the homefront as well. Civilians might be spared the hardships of the battlefield but as war unleashed violence and soldiers needed provisions, civilians faced confusion, injury and the potential for death in their homes or communities. As Nathanael Greene suggested to Colonel Hathway, looting and other depredations were never distant possibilities. From Trenton, Washington forbade plundering, no matter where civilians' loyalty lay. He begged his soldiers to distinguish themselves "from infamous mercenary ravagers."[48] Regardless of this general order, officers did not or could not stop Continental soldiers or militia from destroying property or threatening the safety of civilians, including women, the elderly, and children. In his diary, the Reverend Dr. Henry Muhlenberg recorded the destruction of a church, school, and a number of crops by American forces. Appalled, he turned to a commanding officer, Colonel Alexander Dunlap, to ask if this destruction "was the promised protection to religious and civil freedom"?[49] Muhlenberg's questions led Dunlap and others to call him a Tory and threaten the destruction of his property. It was not safe to be near troops of either side and it was not safe to question the actions of those troops even if the actions contradicted every ideal for which the war was allegedly waged.

British and Hessian soldiers also plundered and physically harmed the civilian population. In December, the American Brigadier General Samuel Parsons wrote Congress describing a British raid on Yonkers a few weeks earlier. About 100 British soldiers had stripped women and children almost naked, turning them out on the street before burning their homes. The troops then led away any captured men with nooses around their necks.[50] Parsons also wrote to the British General William Tryon just a few days after the raid insisting to Tryon that there had been no reason for this grievous behavior. If no actions were taken to remedy the situation, Parsons threatened, American soldiers would retaliate on the civilian property and bodies of those who remained loyal to Great Britain. Tryon dismissed Parsons's indignation, replying that he sanctioned the capture of those disloyal to the King and the destruction of their property. The men he captured were not soldiers, but they were what Tryon called "committee-men," those who had enforced obedience to the Continental Congress and compelled others in North America "to exchange their happy constitution for paper, rags, anarchy and distress."[51] Because the action of these committee-men created disorder and madness, he had no compunction in attacking their person or property.

In a civil war like the American Revolution, considering civilians as non-combatants was madness, Tryon argued, because civilians had led the colonies to ruin. Because of this position, civilians were always in grave danger. In the Carolinas, regular soldiers and militia on both sides engaged in a gruesome war against person and property. In South Carolina, Eliza Wilkinson wrote of the day "the inhuman Britons" came into her house. They took items of clothing, sometimes off the women's bodies. They took earrings from her sister's ears. When one of Wilkinson's friends begged to keep her wedding ring, the British soldiers pointed a pistol at her and threatened to shoot.

Wilkinson described a day of terror from which she and others escaped without physical harm. Other women did not escape, as soldiers raped, brutalized, or killed them. Adam Stephen, serving under Washington's command, wrote to Thomas Jefferson about the barbarity of the British soldiers who "like locusts Sweep the Jerseys with the Besom of destruction." In their destruction, they "Ravish[ed] the fair Sex, from the Age of Ten to Seventy."[52] A New Jersey broadside printed a few months later announced that both British and Hessian troops had captured women, taken them to camp, and raped them. Abigail Palmer, Elizabeth and Sarah Cain, and Mary Phillips had been those captured women and in depositions they told their own stories. British soldiers raped them repeatedly while threatening gruesome death, then dragged them to camp where the soldiers continued to rape the girls and young women before an officer intervened and allowed them to return to the relative safety of their homes. We are left only with speculation about how these girls and women carried the scars of those violent moments with them for the rest of their lives. As reports of these and other rapes circulated widely, bringing the war right into civilian homes, more Americans came to support the war. Whether or not they supported the cause of independence, men joined to help protect their female relatives from harm. The madness these girls and women faced served as propaganda to gain support and participation for the American effort.

The continued madness and folly of war pried open doors that had been shut. After Americans' steady diplomatic efforts to bring the French into the war and the British defeat at the Battles of Saratoga in October 1777, Lord North crafted reconciliation proposals which, if they had gone into place, would have overturned the Tea Act and the hostile position Parliament had assumed toward Massachusetts in 1774. These proposals were carried over by the Carlisle Peace Commission consisting of George Johnstone, Adam Ferguson, Frederick Howard, and William Eden. These men carried with them the possibility of the end to battles and bloodshed, the end of the confusion of war brought into civilian homes, and a resumption of peacetime life. Initially, if these proposals had been more widely known, they might have appealed to a number of Americans, but the Continental Congress refused to consider the proposals and did its best to suppress knowledge of what the Peace Commission offered, or to control and shape what information did leak out.[53]

Despite Congressional efforts to suppress the information, the information moved through the colonies. As the information circulated, Congress had to convince the American people that the British move toward peace was insincere. In a May 9 address to the American people, Congress invoked the travesties of pre-war British policies and the gruesomeness of war on and off the battlefield, reminding readers of the "system of deliberate malice" that included rape and pillage. The address acknowledged that the war had brought economic and other hardships but tried to soothe the readers, proposing remedies to what they called "this dangerous disease." The remedies were rarely adhered-to but persistent calls for cooperation and simplicity.[54] Yes, the epidemic of counterfeiting and devaluation of currency was real, but there was a cure. Fearful that individual states would be seduced to sign on to the British reconciliation proposal, Congress appealed to a social memory of British travesties and to a firmness of purpose among the American people.

This strategy certainly worked among those who championed the cause of independence already. Abigail Adams wrote to her husband, then in France, that the British commissioners had arrived in North America. She assured him they would have no luck in their plot to win Americans' hearts and minds. "We dispise the Nation that can suppose us so nearly assimilated to them, as to renounce treatys, break the publick Faith and tamely give up that Liberty which we have purchased with our Blood," she wrote. These were not friends but enemies "who whilst they are pretending to hold out the olive Branch with one Hand, extend it only to deceive for Blood, Fire, Slaughter and inhumane cruelties are sealed with the other."[55] From her home and hearth, Abigail Adams was one of the Americans who would resist the attempts of the commissioners to deceive and continue to keep the flame alive for independence.

Working to separate American from American or colony from colony was certainly one strategy that commissioners had considered. They were not the only ones. In a long, hand-written manuscript, an unknown writer went into great detail about the problems with the British strategy and suggested that if the British could not annihilate the American insurrection, they could instead work to gain a foothold in the colonies most in need of the empire, notably South Carolina and Georgia. After all, the writer concluded, most had not planned to join a war for independence but had "been drawn in chiefly by misinformation." The British might not be able to reduce all of the colonies to due submission, but they could make life good for "all who are disposed to peace and good order" in a few localities.[56] Then, when people in other colonies still engaged in the madness and folly of war looked southward, they would see a well-off and free people and become jealous. Through good policy and good government, this strategy would work to restore Americans to sanity and, gradually, the British would regain their former colonies by example rather than military force. Whether or not anyone read this manuscript, it reflected an ideology still held that Americans craved the peace and good order of empire but had been led into insanity of war by a few powerful and power-hungry leaders.

Although the ideology that the majority of Americans rejected independence remained, the reality was that the British commissioners could make little or no headway. When the British commissioners realized Congress remained intractable, they wrote what they called a "Manifesto and Proclamation," sending it to loyalist presses in order to make their offer public and thus appealing directly to the American people. In this manifesto they showed they were versant with the forms American government had taken including the dearly held belief in the consent of the governed. Congress had not consulted any of the state assemblies before refusing to consider the offer of reconciliation. They asked if this tactic squared with the liberty for which many Americans claimed to fight. The manifesto proclaimed, too, that far greater martial forces could be brought to bear, claiming that they had "checked the extremes of war" out of benevolence and consanguinity. The mad monster Congress had created was of "unnatural design," and if necessary far greater military forces would follow. Like the 1776 plan of reconciliation, this one carried with it the offer of pardon. The manifesto appealed to the rational minds of those who had never wanted the war and continued to oppose it and to those who had grown tired of the death and destruction that had ensued.

Thomas Paine spat at the commissioners and their manifesto in his sixth issue of the *Crisis*, declaring that the men who had written it were "like madmen biting in the hour of death." It was his first invocation of lunacy in this particular number, but not the last. As Paine did so well, he answered their manifesto measure by measure. In response to the commissioners' call for American soldiers to change sides in order to fight for "their rightful sovereign," Paine exclaimed, "Surely! the union of absurdity with madness was never marked in more distinguishable lines," and remarked that Americans wanted nothing from King George III. Paine had not finished: "Can Bedlam, in concert with Lucifer, form a more mad and devilish request?" he asked. For those who would read his *Crisis*, Paine painted the commissioners as men with diseased brains, more fit for a madhouse than a place at any negotiating table. Paine tried to slam shut the door the commissioners had pried open.

Paine and others opposed to negotiating with England did not manage to slam that door but they did manage to force it closed against continued resistance. As a writer to the *Virginia Gazette* asked the British commissioners, why would Americans have any confidence "in a people who have thirsted after our blood, and sought our utter ruin?" Only "madness" or "pusillanimity" would render a reconciliation possible.[57] The commissioners never did gain an audience with Congress and never swayed enough popular opinion to put pressure on the new American government. Defeated, they returned home where popular opinion began to shift against an expensive and bloody war. With the official entrance of the French into the war on the American side, Great Britain now had another world war on its hands. No longer could they focus solely on the rebellion across the ocean because they had to worry about the enemies across the Channel. The entrance of their long-standing imperial rival spread madness into new corners of the world. For the Americans, the support of their once-hated enemy certainly disconcerted even some of the war's supporters but added needed funds, supplies, naval forces, and soldiers.

Despite the French entrance, the fighting was far from over. Civil war continued to spread attended by rape and torture and all the subsequent madness. Both sides employed Indian tribes putting Anglo-Americans at greater risk particularly in frontier areas.[58] New York loyalist governor, William Tryon wrote to London that he agreed with the strategy of using Indians along the frontier to impose terror against the rebel inhabitants there. When the news reached London of this strategy, the elderly William Pitt stood once more in front of the House of Lords invoking madness and horror in his speech, decrying the use of "the cannibal savage, torturing, murdering, roasting and eating; literally, my lords, *eating* the mangled victims of his barbarous battles!" The practice of allowing Indian soldiers, Pitt argued, made the British no better than the Spanish of the Black Legend and therefore absent morality and not at all deserving of compassion.[59]

On both sides, white and Indian soldiers did engage in a particularly brutal form of warfare. Serving under American General John Sullivan, Erkuries Beatty described coming across the brutalized bodies of two American soldiers. He wrote that they "was both stripped naked and their heads cut off." Lieutenant Boyd had been scalped and his eyes removed. The other soldier's head was missing. They were stabbed repeatedly "and Lt. Boyds privates was nearly cut of[f] and hanging down."[60] The Americans were no better, as Sullivan's forces laid waste to the lands that had been controlled by Seneca, Cayuga, and Onondaga people and scalped and otherwise maimed the bodies of British soldiers. Similarly, American Colonel Daniel Brodhead razed Indian villages and Lieutenant John Harding attacked British-allied Indians with "irresistible fury, tomahawk in hand" forcing the enemy to flee. When Brodhead's forces returned to Fort Pitt, the soldiers proudly displayed the scalps they had taken in the course of the conflict. In her later account of these campaigns, Mercy Otis Warren condemned both the British and the Americans, writing that the spread of "slaughter and bloodshed among innocent and unoffending tribes . . . has no warrant from Heaven."[61] The madness of war had not abated.

In the south, the war was very much a civil war with American military operations often left to still-undisciplined militia. In North Carolina, old wounds festered and rankled as some of the men who had fought against the colonial elite during the regulation now took up arms against the American soldiers. Their enemy was not Parliament across the sea but the men in power more locally. Although Mercy Otis Warren reviled them in her history of the war, she understood that "their aversion to the reigning powers in that state, still rankled in their breasts."[62] The madness of war opened another opportunity to carve a space for themselves, attacking those they considered enemies in a landscape where few people made distinction between soldier and civilian.

Even those who did not join in depredations against civilian populations did not necessarily make common cause with the Americans. One loyalist writing into the *South-Carolina and American General Gazette* in February 1781 sounded a lot like those who in 1774 and 1775 had opposed the Continental Association, arguing for law and order over chaos and confusion. The American leadership had tried to force their opponents to adopt "the most absurd and violent measures" that had no reasonable origin but instead were dreamed up in their "intemperate brains." Even in 1781, this writer characterized the cause of the ongoing conflict as nothing more than "licentiousness and mad ambition ... supported by dissimulation and fraud." For this writer, like Henry Strachey in 1775, it must have seemed as if that madness had spread to the country or nation and was no longer seated only in the addled brains of a few men.

Militarily, as American soldiers and commanders tried to counter the British forces and their allies in the south, they found the same kind of undisciplined fighting men that Washington had worried over early in the conflict. New Englander Benjamin Gilbert complained to his parents that they faced a "melancholy prospect," for trained New England officers "are daily resigning." Gilbert remained to train short-service men, men whose levies lasted only three to six months. "As soon as they are learned their times are out and we must take new ones that makes us perpetual slaves," he wrote.[63] He was despondent at the madness of this situation and further explained that he could not trust the men he trained for they would sleep while on watch and flee in battle. Indeed, serving in Camden, South Carolina, Garret Watts admitted that once the British started firing, "I was amongst the first that fled." He could not remember why except that all the men around him were also fleeing. "It was instantaneous," he wrote. In his retelling, officers made no effort to keep their men in battle but fled as well.[64] Throughout the long years of war, George Washington and his officers were never able to entirely overcome the lack of discipline that had made him temporarily insane at Kip's Bay.

The horrors of battle in the south, and the horrors of attacks on loyalist and patriot civilians were both real but also sometimes exaggerated to make one's enemy look savage. Believing in exaggerated accounts sometimes led men to enact what they believed was justice without orders from commanders or due process for those captured. One example comes to us in the wake of the Battle of Waxhaws. With a mounted British onslaught, Americans under the command of Abraham Buford realized their effort was doomed and some tried to surrender at the same time the British commander, General Banastre Tarleton's horse was killed from under him. His Green Dragoons believed Tarleton dead and began attacking the Americans again as some of the American troops reformed lines and continued in battle. Although this became widely reported as a deliberate slaughter by the British of surrendering American troops it was more likely a confusing moment when it was not clear to anyone who surrendered and who retreated to gain a new position to fight. Nonetheless, the belief that British troops had savagely slaughtered surrendering Americans had serious consequences.

After the battle of Haw River in February 1781, Moses Hall and others went to gawk at captured British soldiers. The idea that these might be the same men who wilfully massacred Americans changed Hall's companions from rational beings to temporary madmen. After yelling, "Remember

Buford!" a number of the Americans hacked the six prisoners to death with broadswords. Hall later wrote, "At first I bore the scene without any emotion, but upon a moment's reflection, I felt such horror as I never did before nor have since." His mind disturbed, Hall returned to his quarters where he replayed what had happened before his eyes. He wrote that he "contemplated the cruelties of war until overcome and unmanned by a distressing gloom." Hall did not become a lunatic, raving across the countryside, but it was clear that the accumulated horrors of war had disturbed him to the point where he felt he had become like a woman, less brave and martial than he should be. Regaining his composure, he marched away from the camp the next morning only to witness further horrors. His regiment came across a suffering boy or young man who had come to watch the British march by earlier in the day. According to Hall, the British believed the boy might act as a spy, bayoneted him, and left him to die. Hall claimed, "The sight of this unoffending boy ... relieved me of my distressful feelings for the slaughter of the Tories." While he had been unsettled by slaughter of prisoners, the cruelty enacted by British soldiers against an innocent bystander made his distressing gloom vanish and allowed him to continue to fight for the cause.

The last major military conflict came at Yorktown, Virginia in October 1781. Here the accumulated madness of six years of regular and irregular warfare played out in siege warfare and the final combined attacks of American and French land and naval forces on the British forces under the command of General Cornwallis. By October 17, the Hessian soldier, Johann Conrad Döhla wrote that the command "could hardly tolerate the enemy bombs, howitzer, and cannonballs any longer." Combined with the lack of food and other supplies, the rational course was surrender, which Cornwallis did on October 19. The surrender was orderly as the British and Hessian troops laid down their weapons as soldiers and civilians watched. In her history, Mercy Otis Warren later remarked on the irony of Cornwallis's capture and imprisonment. She found in ironic because Cornwallis was the Constable of the Tower of London where the American Henry Laurens had been made a prisoner. "By the capitulation, his lordship was reduced to the humiliating condition of a prisoner to the American congress, while [Henry Laurens] remained shut up in the tower, a prisoner to the captured earl."[65] Both became unwilling prisoners, absent their liberty, until a prisoner exchange took place, freeing both men.

Despite the fact that the British surrendered with relative dignity, two weeks later, "An American Soldier" published a letter denouncing Cornwallis for being maddened by desire for gain or "[d]eluded by the splendour of the enterprise."[66] Even as people tried to make sense of the long years of warfare, the only explanation sometimes seemed to be folly, madness, or delusion. On the American side, even in the wake of a decisive victory, people worked to understand the reasons behind such a long and brutal war. And despite the victory, the war was not yet over although the defeat at Yorktown raised a larger chorus of voices in Great Britain against the continued war. If Strachey had been right in 1776 that a whole nation could become mad, that madness had spread and led to a new reality, one in which an American army that had been often defeated, could outlast the trained and disciplined fighting forces of Great Britain and turn the tide of war.

Perhaps what is most remarkable is the fact that throughout the folly and madness of war, the Continental Congress managed to build international alliances and steer a leaky ship of state. By 1781, Congress had finally ratified the Articles of Confederation, the first national government under which Americans functioned. The ignorant multitude, so derided by British who first encountered them on the field of battle, had managed to build institutions on all levels that allowed them to function well enough to see independence, once only whispered softly, published and proclaimed with an increasing chance of success. Independence might have been the dream of a few madmen and women in 1775 and 1776, but it had been dreamed into existence.

NOTES

1. Thomas Gage to Josiah Martin, April 1775, in William L. Saunders, ed. *The Colonial Records of North Carolina*, Vol. IX (Raleigh: Josephus Daniels, 1890), 1220, https://books.google.com/books/about/The_Colonial_Records_of_North_Carolina.html.

2. George Cressener, to William Knox, 30 January 1775, William Knox Papers, Clements Library.

3. Ray Raphael, "Blacksmith Timothy Bigelow and the Massachusetts Revolution of 1774," in Alfred F. Young, Gary B. Nash, and Ray Raphael, eds, *Revolutionary Founders: Rebels, Radicals, and Reformers in the Making of the Nation* (New York: Vintage Books, 2011), 39–40.

4. John Shy, *A People Numerous and Armed: Reflections on the Military Struggle for American Independence* (Ann Arbor: University of Michigan Press, 1976), 109.

5. "From Beginning to End Ill Planned and Ill Executed," in Henry Steele Commager and Richard B. Morris, eds, *The Spirit of Seventy-Six: The Story of The American Revolution as Told by Participants* (New York: Harper & Row, 1958), 74.

6. "From Beginning to End Ill Planned and Ill Executed," *Spirit of Seventy-Six*, 71.

7. "From Beginning to End Ill Planned and Ill Executed," *Spirit of Seventy-Six*, 71.

8. "From Beginning to End Ill Planned and Ill Executed," *Spirit of Seventy-Six*, 71.

9. "From the diary of Lieutenant Frederick Mackenzie," *Spirit of Seventy-Six*, 87.

10. "The Most Absolute Cowards on the Face of the Earth," *Spirit of Seventy-Six*, 89.

11. "The Fatigue Our People Passed through Can Hardly Be Believed," *Spirit of Seventy-Six*, 78.

12. William Battie, *A Treatise on Madness* (London: J. Whiston and b. White, 1773), 94.

13. "Gage Promises to Pardon All Rebels Except Samuel Adams and John Hancock," *Spirit of Seventy-Six*, 96.

14. Alexander Purdie, Broadside, https://cdn.loc.gov/service/pnp/cph/3a40000/3a45000/3a45000/3a45071r.jpg.

15. Elizabeth Wight Richardson, Diary. Massachusetts Historical Society.

16. Henry Ellis, Marseilles, to William Knox, London, 22 March 1774, William Knox Papers, Clements Library.

17. "The Earl of Shelburne Prophesies Ruin, October 26, 1775. *Spirit of Seventy Six*, 256.

18. Reprinted in James E. Thorold Rogers, ed., *A Complete Collection of the Protests of the Lords with Historical Introductions*, Vol. II (Oxford: Clarendon Press, 1875), 162, https://books.google.com/books?id=VPUKAAAAYAAJ.

19. April 29, 1775, https://cdn.loc.gov/service/pnp/cph/3a40000/3a45000/3a45000/3a45070r.jpg.

20. "Oxford and Cambridge Support the King," *Spirit of Seventy-Six*, 243.

21. "Doctor Johnson Has No Patience with American Arguments," *Spirit of Seventy-Six*, 248.

22. Colonel Henry Knox, to Lucy Knox, July 22, 1776, *Spirit of Seventy-Six*, 427.

23. Henry Strachey to Jane Strachey, 11 August 1776, Henry Strachey Papers. Clements Library.

24. "A Common Soldier Has a Snuff of Gunpowder," *Spirit of Seventy-Six*, 442.

25. "Letter from an Officer in General Frazier's Battalion," *Spirit of Seventy-Six*, 443.

26. Washington to President of the Continental Congress, September 2, 1776, http://www.loc.gov/teachers/classroommaterials/presentationsandactivities/presentations/timeline/amrev/contarmy/prestwo.html.

27. "We Have Given the Rebels a D-----d Crush," *Spirit of Seventy-Six*, 443.

28. Henry Strachey, to Jane Strachey, September 3, 1776. Henry Strachey Papers.

29. John Shy, "The American Colonies in War and Revolution, 1748–1783," in P. J. Marshall and Alaine Low, eds, *The Oxford History of the British Empire*, Vol. II *Oxford Scholarship Online*, DOI:10.1093/acprof:oso/9780198205630.003.0014.

30. Everyone should read the excellent forum, "Rethinking Mercantilism," in *William and Mary Quarterly* 69 (January 2012): 3–70.

31. Charles Inglis, *The Christian Soldier's Duty Briefly Delineated: In a Sermon Preached at King's Bridge, September 7, 1777, before the American Corps Newly Raised for His Majesty's Service* (New York: H. Gaine, 1777), 20, Library Company of Philadelphia.

32. Inglis, *Christian Soldier's Duty,* 13–14.

33. Samuel Finley, *The Madness of Mankind, Represented in a Sermon Preached in the New Presbyterian Church in Philadelphia, on the 9th of June 1754,* Library Company of Philadelphia.

34. Shy, *People Numerous and Armed,* 165.

35. July 25, 1776. In "Some Extracts from the Papers of General Persifor Frazer," *Pennsylvania Magazine of History and Biography* 31 (1907): 134, https://www.jstor.org/stable/20085377.

36. John Adams to Joseph Hawley, 25 August 1776 in Richard D. Brown, ed. *Major Problems in the Era of the American Revolution, 1760–1791* (Boston: Houghton Mifflin, 2000), 193.

37. Quoted in Michael A. McDonnell, "'The Spirit of Levelling': James Cleveland, Edward Wright, and the Militiamen's Struggle of Equality in Revolutionary Virginia," in Young, Nash, and Raphael, *Revolutionary Founders,* 139.

38. George Washington to John Hancock, 24 September 1776 in Brown, ed., *Major Problems,* 194.

39. Joseph Plumb Martin, *A Narrative of a Revolutionary Soldier* (New York: Signet Classic, 2001), 37.

40. Journal of Benjamin Trumbull, September 1776, *Spirit of Seventy-Six,* 467.

41. Park Holland, Memoir. Holland Family Papers. Massachusetts Historical Society.

42. Moses Hazen to Thomas McKean, September 29, 1778. Thomas McKean Papers. Historical Society of Pennsylvania.

43. Martin, *Narrative,* 147.

44. Nathanael Greene to Daniel Hatway, January 1780. Nathanael Greene Papers, box 2. Clements Library.

45. Nathanael Greene to Catherine Greene, August 14, 1780, Nathanael Greene Papers, Clements Library.

46. R. Arthur Bowler, *Logistics and the Failure of the British Army in America, 1775–1783* (Princeton: Princeton University Press, 1975), 149.

47. Bowler, *Logistics,* 93.

48. Washington order, 1 January 1777. *Spirit of Seventy-Six,* 525.

49. Journal of Henry Muhlenberg, September 27, 1777. *Spirit of Seventy-Six,* 529.

50. Samuel H. Parsons, Mamoroneck, to Henry Laurens, President of Congress, December 1777. Henry Laurens Papers, Historical Society of Pennsylvania.

51. William Tryon, Kingsbridge Camp to Samuel Parsons, November 23, 1777. Henry Laurens Papers. Historical Society of Pennsylvania.

52. "To Thomas Jefferson from Adam Stephen, [ca. 20] December 1776," *Founders Online,* National Archives, https://founders.archives.gov/documents/Jefferson/01-01-02-0248.

53. Anthony Gregory, "'Formed for Empire': The Continental Congress Responds to the Carlisle Peace Commission," *Journal of the Early Republic* 38, no. 4 (Winter 2018): 643–672.

54. "An address of the Congress to the inhabitants of the United States of America," https://cdn.loc.gov/service/rbc/bdsdcc/04701/04701.pdf.

55. Letter from Abigail Adams to John Adams, June 18, 1778. *Adams Family Papers: An Electronic Archive.* Massachusetts Historical Society. http://www.masshist.org/digitaladams/.

56. *Thoughts on the War between Great Britain & America made in Septr & October 1776 and Thoughts on the Same Subject wrote Feby 1778* handwritten mss., Clements Library.

57. "To the Earl of Carlisle, Sir Henry Clinton, and William Eden, Esq. His Brittanic Majesty's Commissioners" in Thomas Pownall and John Almon, eds, *The Remembrancer; Or, Impartial Repository of Public Events, for the Year 1778, and Beginning of 1779* (London: J. Almon, 1779), 136–137, catalog.hathitrust.org/Record/000641873.

58. John Shy, ed., *Winding Down: The Revolutionary War Letters of Lieutenant Benjamin Gilbert of Massachusetts, 1780–1783 from His Original Manuscript Letterbook in the William L. Clements Library, Ann Arbor, Michigan* (Ann Arbor: The University of Michigan Press, 1989), 9.

59. "Speech of William Pitt, Earl Chatham, Delivered in the House of Lords, November 18, 1777," in *The Spirit of 'Seventy-Six*, 1002–1003.

60. "From the Journal of Erkuries Beatty, Lieutenant with General Sullivan" in *Spirit of Seventy-Six*, 1020.

61. Warren, *History of the Rise, Progress and Termination of the American Revolution*, Vol. II, 285.

62. Warren, *History of the Rise, Progress and Termination of the American Revolution*, Vol. II, 309.

63. Benjamin Gilbert to his parents, 15 October 1780, in Shy, *Winding Down*, 25.

64. Quoted in Matthew H. Spring, *With Zeal and with Bayonets Only: The British Army on Campaign in North America, 1775–1783* (Norman: University of Oklahoma Press, 2010), 232.

65. Warren, *History of the Rise, Progress and Termination of the American Revolution*, Vol. II, 485.

66. "To Earl Cornwallis," *Maryland Gazette*, November 1, 1781.

Chapter 5

"The Whole Country Is Now in a State of Madness"

Life and Government during Wartime

If war on the battlefield created one form of madness, attempts to govern during that war created another. The growing crisis in North America and the outbreak of war in 1775 undermined social and community relations and shook governments on both sides of the Atlantic to their cores. As a large minority of colonists mustered the courage to enter into armed conflict with their mother country and worked to encourage others to do so, they led themselves and others down a path into a brutal and bloody conflict. Even if convinced that war was the answer to the crisis in the relationship between Great Britain and its North American colonies, participants could not help but to see chaos and confusion everywhere they looked. They could hope that the long-term consequences would prove beneficial, but in the short term, they saw that war unleashed folly and madness that needed to be countered. One way to counter this was through the creation of new governments on all levels to try to craft rational responses to an often irrational conflict. This work was so important that even in the regions embroiled in military conflict, Americans engaged in hotly contested debates over the structure and purpose of government.

In 1775, the rebellion that had been building for a decade shifted. While Americans had not known that they were witness to what were the opening battles of the American Revolution on April 19, they did know that the shedding of blood at Lexington and Concord changed the calculus of resistance to imperial policies. Even as the Battles of Lexington and Concord sparked military preparation and conflict, many thought it was madness to oppose the mother country, to even think about new forms of relationships between empire and colonies let alone to consider independence. How could people create rational forms of government in a world where women had muskets and sometimes used them; where apprentices, servants, and enslaved people disobeyed their masters or ran away; where the lower sort organized mob action and took power into their own hands; where sons and daughters did not always obey their parents? It is not surprising that when Americans looked around them they worried about the deleterious effects of the madness of conflict or war on the body politic. Local, colonial, and British governments now had to operate within the reality of war, regardless of what was ultimately decided.

In the official documents published in 1775, colonists still declared for renewed harmony between themselves and Great Britain rather than independence while privately, a committed minority of Americans considered independence the likely and needed outcome of the conflict. For the most part however, they were quiet about this. Even if they could argue rationally about the growing strength of the North American colonies, even if they could convince others that British policies were dangerous to their liberties, working toward independence was fraught with peril. If they failed, their project would be the project of lunatics, an irrational dream rather than a rational contest for home rule. They would be madmen and madwomen in addition to traitors to their country. Even success did not guarantee a rational and sane future because history told them that they could create a system that was far worse than the system under which they existed.[1] There were real possibilities of tyrants rising out of the ruins of the old system, of revenge and bloodshed in the aftermath, of anarchy, or of failed systems. Colonists saw that while some of the members of Parliament were power-mad and corrupt, the British system guaranteed them freedom beyond that of their contemporaries, and their ties to the British empire meant that they could tap into systems that guaranteed some of them economic prosperity.

For years, Americans and Britons leery of the growing confusion in the colonies had suspected that some prominent American leaders were plotting for independence. King George III was not the only one who believed that the New England governments were "in a state of rebellion" by 1775. Massachusetts was the clearest example of rebellion as their Provincial Congress continued to meet and legislate despite the fact that the 1774 Massachusetts Government Act had, on paper, taken that right away. Military governor Thomas Gage derided the Provincial Congress in a letter to North Carolina's governor Josiah Martin. He wrote, "This Province has sometime been, and now is, in the new-fangled Legislature, termed a Provincial Congress, who seemed to have taken the Government into their hands. What they intend to do I cannot pretend to say, but they are much puzzled about how to act."[2] For Gage, the words on the page were more wishful thinking than reality. Members of the Provincial Congress were often puzzled how to act as the world around them changed rapidly, but they still legislated in a relatively organized and united fashion. They erred and stumbled but they also kept an extralegal government functioning better than it probably should have. Thus Gage wrote out of his own fear and puzzlement as he rapidly lost control over the colony he had been charged with keeping under British rule.

Only in Boston had the British kept a tenuous hold on Massachusetts Bay under the command of Gage. He had his supporters throughout the colony, but even in Boston those supporters knew they faced consequences, and sometimes violent ones, for voicing support for Gage or the British government. In January 1774, a mob of men and boys seized the belligerent Tory John Malcom and tarred and feathered him, dragging him through the streets of Boston. Ann Hulton expressed her outrage at this act, writing, "These few instances amongst many serve to shew the abject State of Governm't & the licentiousness & barbarism of the times. There's no Majestrate that dare or will act to suppress the outrages. No person is secure[;] there are many Objects pointed at, at this time & when once mark'd out for Vengence, their ruin is certain."[3] To those who remained loyal to the British government, there were few signs of success in preventing the dissolution of government. For Peter Oliver the violence against those loyal to the British government was telling. He described an attack against Dr. Abner Beebe in the neighboring colony of Connecticut. Beebe "spoke very freely in Favor of Government." Because of this, other colonists attacked Beebe and his property. Oliver's account included descriptions of the physical violence against Beebe. "[H]e was assaulted by a Mob, stripped naked, & hot Pitch was poured upon him, which blistered his Skin. He was then carried to a Hog Sty & rubbed over with Hog's Dung. They threw the Hog's Dung in his Face & rammed some of it down his Throat; & in that Condition exposed to a Company of Women."[4] These were not actions of colonists operating under the rule of law. Their actions signaled growing disorder.

While colonial governments denied that they were in a state of rebellion, colonists increasingly drew lines between friends and enemies and punished those on the opposite side of the lines as discussed earlier in chapter 3. Relating these and other incidents in the appendix to his 1781 *Origin and Progress of the American Revolution*, Oliver pointed out, "All the foregoing Transactions were before the Battle of Lexington, when the Rebels say that the War began." Looking back, Oliver saw a concerted effort for the destruction of British power and independence in the years leading up to military conflict. He was right that, in many ways, the war had begun before April 19, 1775 as colonial governments had already taken actions to block or limit the power of British ministers in North America and colonial Americans used violence against those with whom they politically or ideologically disagreed. Whether the events at Lexington and Concord marked the beginning of conflict or a continuation of an existing war, however, battles in the field did shift and change the nature of a colonial insurgency. When Gage made the decision that seizing weapons stores might stop the insurgency and bring Massachusetts Bay back to rational and good government, he helped bring about that shift and change. In a letter that was reprinted throughout the colonial press, a Roxbury, Massachusetts writer later mused, "What folly could induce Gen. Gage to act a part so fatal to Britain." He continued," I pity the madness which effected their destruction."[5] Gage had tried to get his troops to act with medical precision, attempting to cut out the cancer of stockpiled weapons and steer the body politic back to reason and obedience. Instead, according to this writer, that plan was pitiful madness that led to bloodshed and chaos.

Actual battle on the field meant that governments had to craft responses. Unlike earlier small-scale and unplanned violence like the Boston Massacre, Lexington and Concord resulted from planned network building and the mustering of militia by colonists as measures of resistance to a standing army in Boston. Although the first shots fired may have been accidental, the colonial response was not. The Roxbury letter writer quoted above also proclaimed, *"jacta est alea,"* though what the cast of the die augured was still unclear. Had the battles on April 19 been a mistake? Was there a way to bring Massachusetts Bay back in harmony with the British government or to use enough military force to bring them into submission? The Massachusetts Provincial Congress came immediately out of recess to confront the changed reality of the world and the Second Continental Congress was due to meet again in Philadelphia in less than a month. Levels of government from those in the colonies all the way up to Parliament and King now had to figure into their equation the reality that Americans, both men and women, were willing to fire upon the highly-trained and disciplined British army even at the risk of their own lives.

In the wake of the confusion and bloodshed of April 19, Gage put Boston under siege. The effects were felt immediately. The first Sunday of the siege, Reverend Andrew Elliot noted that it was the most melancholy sabbath of his life, and that all was "hurry and confusion."[6] As Gage attempted to restore sanity and to respond to military conflict, the everyday rituals of Boston became upended. In Sunday meeting, ministers and congregants still gathered in shared faith and worship that helped them make sense of the world but now that work was harder. The relative peace and stability of the previous years had given way to the horrors of bloodshed. Elliot's faith, rooted in Old Testament theology, could survive those horrors in the long term, but in the short term he and others had a sinking feeling that their world had tilted off kilter with no clear path forward.

That hurry and confusion reflected in Gage's decisions. As military governor of all of Massachusetts Bay Colony, could he leverage his fortified position in Boston to keep the dogs of war from slipping their restraints? His decisions reflected the difficulties he labored under and the confusion of ruling in a time of crisis. He understood that the consequences of his decisions could create a form of madness and raise the ire of colonists not just in and around Boston but throughout the British North American world. In an effort to contain the problems he faced and reassert authority and control, he first shut down most travel in and out of Boston and refused to allow residents to leave. He then attempted to act as a conciliator, calling on a committee of the freeholders of Boston to meet.

Gage informed the committee, through the Crown-approved selectmen, that he would not attack citizens in Boston as long as they behaved peaceably toward the British troops but the committee's decisions likely gave him more reason to worry. The document they produced was crafty and sarcastic, assuring Gage that they had no intention of anything but peaceable behavior while also laying the blame for any troubles squarely on Gage's shoulders. The committee's letter responded to Gage's concern that there was an attack against Boston planned by people in the countryside. It claimed no one knew of any planned attack for, after all, "all Communications between the Town & Country has been Interrupted by his Excellencys Order." The committee also emphasized that as long as Boston was closed off from the rest of the colony, residents there would have no access to food, fuel, or other provisions. The letter appealed to Gage as a gentlemen, emphasizing to him that civilized governments did not allow the weakest among them to suffer. His policy as it stood, the committee wrote, would most harm "the Sick & all Invalids."[7] This was not their fault, the men of this committee stated, but came from Gage's orders. The carefully crafted language of the freeholders' meeting was the language of subtle resistance. The men knew better than to directly raise the ire of the governor but they went beyond the initial parameters set out by him and took the opportunity to remind Gage that they suffered because of his actions.

Uncertain, Gage decided Bostonians could leave if they surrendered their weapons and did not travel by carriage or chaise, meaning, out of necessity, any of those departing surrendered many of their household goods. In the midst of this first evacuation, however, other British officials closed the Boston Neck Road—the only way in and out—and ordered the remaining inhabitants back into town. From the safety of Braintree, Abigail Adams wrote to her husband, then sitting in Congress, "The Distresses of the inhabitants of Boston are beyond the power of language to describe. There are but few who are permitted to come out in a day. They delay giving passes, make them wait from hour to hour One day their household furniture is to come out, the next only wearing apparel, and the next Pharaohs heart is hardened, and he refuseth to hearken unto them and will not let the people go."[8] Like the Egyptian Pharaoh, Thomas Gage did not care about the suffering of the people. His government and the government of those around him meant "the whole Town was a prison," as John Leach noted.[9]

In addition to his attempt to work through the local government by appealing to the freeholders, Gage's government also imprisoned suspected enemies, often without concrete evidence. In his diary, 18-year-old Peter Edes detailed his own imprisonment, writing, "No court of enquiry held, So that we are Still held in Suspense. We had been in prison 29 days when we found out by chance from the Serjeant returns, what our crimes were."[10] According to Timothy Newell, some of these men were put into jail "for the most trifling supposed offenses." James Lovell, John Leach, and John Hunt were imprisoned, and "all they know why it is so is they are charged with free speaking on the public measures." Richard Carpenter was arrested for swimming from Boston to Dorchester and back and was sentenced to death, "his Coffin brot into the Gaol-yard, his halter brought & he dressed as criminals are before execution."[11] In the end, Carpenter received a stay and then was pardoned. Mock executions like this, of course, were supposed to serve as examples of government's power to keep transgressors within the bounds of law. The stay and pardon served as a warning but also a signal of mercy to those who came into line. However, in a world so out of the ordinary, operating by different rules from those of rational peace-time life, actions like these instead furthered colonists' anger and led them to more and greater resistance.

Diaries and letters detailing imprisonment and other punitive measures can provide readers in our time of a sense of Gage's failed attempt to gain control over Boston and the rest of Massachusetts Bay. A close reading provides us with other valuable stories as well. The first story is a story of unity. Even from within the prison, men tried to establish forms of government and looked out for one another. Political prisoners organized in an attempt to bring about better conditions for wounded American soldiers alongside whom they were imprisoned. These soldiers had received no medical care and little food. According to John Leach, when the civilians complained that the soldiers were being mistreated and starved, the prison's provost told them that the soldiers "might eat the Nail heads, and knaw the plank and be damn'd."[12] Despite the intractability of the provost, the political prisoners put their heads together in order to try to help the men who suffered more than they did. They shared what little food they had and pushed for better care.

While there are touching stories of unity, however, there are also stories of division. The political prisoners were appalled by the women brought into the jail, women Edes described as "soldier women confin'd for theft," presumably the wives or mistresses of British regulars. According to Edes, these women were placed in close proximity to him and then "acted Such Scenes as was Shocking to nature, and they used language horrible to hear, as if it came from the very Suburbs of Hell."[13] Edes's distaste for these women's behavior should remind us that one aspect of the war that became the American Revolution was that not everyone wanted a world turned upside down, and many were made nervous by the poorer sort who sometimes behaved by different rules. The English rules of decorum remained largely in place. Those with power tended to fret, as New York Magistrate Daniel Horsmanden did, that the poorer sort might "cabal and confederate together and ripen themselves into . . . schools of mischief."[14] Just as John Adams had condemned the lower sort in the 1770 Boston Massacre trial, calling them "the motley rabble of saucy boys, Negroes and mulattoes, Irish teagues, and outlandish jack tars," for the men trying to craft governments in North America, from the level of informal prison government to Continental Congress, rough and shocking women and men threatened to pull their systems toward irrationality and madness.[15] The lower sort invoked Bedlam rather than a social compact.

For Gage, the whole colony seemed like a madhouse and he was the harried keeper of that institution. As Boston life turned on its head during the siege, he continued to try to grab hold of the reins of government and tamp down the insurgency. His attempts had little effect. When Commissioner Henry Hulton looked at the world outside of Boston, he saw that "The whole Country is now is a state of madness, and the distemper may probably run through the Continent." As the distemper spread, so did food and material shortages, but perhaps those shortages could act as a cure. Like others, Hulton turned to the writings of physicians for explanations and solutions. "Perhaps the same treatment as is applied to natural Lunaticks," he wrote, "may be best applied to these political ones; and hunger, and delay, be more effectual than immediate force to reduce them to their senses."[16] Psychology was one tool of analysis applied by Hulton and others. He demonstrated his awareness of the writings of the physicians who believed that lunatics needed to be physically weakened, including by near-starvation diets, before they could be cured. He hoped that the lack of sufficient food would bring the mad colonists' minds back to rationality, away from the fanaticism that drove them to resist British policy.[17]

Sitting governments in other colonies watched the events in Massachusetts closely. The government in neighboring Connecticut drafted a letter to Gage and delivered it to him by way of two of their leading citizens, Samuel Johnson and Oliver Wolcott. The letter asked for an explanation from Gage for the conduct of the British troops and for the siege of Boston. Although the letter claimed horror at the prospect of a civil war, it also stated that colonists in Connecticut were animated by the principle of self-defense and would "defend their rights and privileges to the last extremity . . . [giving] aid to their brethren if any unjustifiable attack is made upon them."[18] They did not want to fight but would take up arms in the face of attempts to further erode their British rights and liberty. From the distance of more than 200 years, this letter reads as a statement of solidarity with Massachusetts Bay. While Hulton held out hope that these Connecticut delegates "may be persuaded that the reports they received before they came here were untrue," he thought it was more probable that their minds were closed against "anything that combats with their prejudices." After all, like their neighbors in Massachusetts, "they are possessed with the notion that Great Britain means to enslave them." Hulton had no faith that the Connecticut delegates were sincere as they too, in his estimation, "mean to try to be independent of Great Britain."[19] Hulton believed the delegates did not mean what they said.

The Massachusetts Provincial Congress also worried that the Connecticut delegates were duplicitous but in a very different way. To Massachusetts leaders, the very seeking out of Gage by Connecticut men made them potential enemies. The Massachusetts Provincial Congress drafted a letter to the Connecticut Congress insisting, in no uncertain terms, that any effort to find common ground with Gage and his government would be seen as nothing less than becoming an instrument of subjugation, slaughter, and desolation. In Massachusetts, the leaders had come to believe that events had moved too far along for anything other than a military solution. They did not yet publicly embrace independence, but they leaned heavily in that direction.

Reactions in New England to the political and military maneuverings in the rest of the colonies were mixed. To some, the Massachusetts insurgents seemed like wild-eyed fanatics who worked to spread the contagion of madness beyond their borders. From North Carolina, Archibald Neilson wrote that the insurgents had engaged in "illiberal wild impolitic and profane violence" when they destroyed the tea in 1773. The participants may have claimed they fought for the cause of liberty, but Neilson saw nothing but "madness and wickedness."[20] In Anson County, North Carolina, loyal British subjects gathered to write that they felt only "disapprobation and abhorrence [for] the many lawless combinations and unwarrantable practices actually carried on by a gross tribe of infatuated anti-Monarchists in the several Colonies in these Dominions." The 227 signers of that loyalty oath held particular contempt for the Massachusetts Provincial Congress, calling them a "profligate and abandoned Republican faction," and condemning their "enthusiastick transgressions" against the British government.[21] Again and again, supporters of the British status quo saw fanaticism, madness, and potential for destruction when they looked at the protests and protesters.

In New Jersey, Governor William Franklin begged the legislature in early 1775 to refuse to act with other colonies in boycotting goods through the Continental Association and, instead, to address their grievances separately to the Crown. He believed that if New Jersey continued to act with the other colonies, they would be led down the road "to Anarchy, Misery, and all the Horrors of a Civil War." He asked them not to listen to "the warm, the rash, and the inconsiderate," but instead to "the moderate, the sober, and the discreet Part of your Constituents."[22] By May, Franklin despaired, writing to Lord Dartmouth, "All legal Authority and government seems to be drawing to an End here." Franklin and other loyal Britons saw new forms of government rising on all sides in contravention to the British government. He reserved his greatest scorn for the protesters, but he also condemned Governor Gage's rashness at moving to capture military stores on April 19. Franklin worried that the consequence of the Battles of Lexington and Concord would be violence "against every Officer of Government in the King's Colonies to the Southward of New England who may refuse to acquiesce" to the proceedings of the Massachusetts Provincial Congress. He then suggested to Lord Dartmouth that every effort be taken to suppress publication of the American grievances that came fast and furiously from the colonies so as not to expose men like himself "to the Resentment of an ungovernable people."[23]

To the agents of Crown and Parliament, large numbers of Americans *had* become ungovernable, wilfully breaking established laws. This was not the rational compact provided by the British constitution, but an irrational and illegitimate tyranny of a few deluded men. These men seemed bent on anarchy, republicanism, and independence. Parliament had believed that the Coercive Acts would contain the contagion of madness before it spread; instead madness appeared everywhere. In opposition to the acts of Parliament, Congress had put the Continental Association in place throughout the colonies and local and colonial governments had created mechanisms to enforce it. When British agents looked south, they saw North Carolinian Richard Henderson signing a treaty with the Cherokees, a treaty that was denounced by the governors in North Carolina and Virginia. When they looked to New York in May of 1775, they saw rogue militia financed by the colonies of Massachusetts and Connecticut seizing the forts and weapons at Ticonderoga and Crown Point. Elsewhere they saw similar examples of colonial governments moving outside of the boundaries set for them under the old systems despite the best efforts of loyal governors to stop them. Perhaps it was true that the colonies had been "seduced by false ideas of liberty and independence, or intoxicated to giddy madness by the pride of opulence and prosperity." If so, British ministers wondered if there was still time to place a check on "the temporary frenzy of her deluded . . . children."[24] By 1775 this seemed increasingly unlikely.

In most colonies, old frameworks of government still held, but the men who operated in those governments became more and more loath to acknowledge ministerial rule. In Massachusetts at the end of May, Samuel Langdon preached a sermon to the Provincial Congress reminding his listeners that the Coercive Acts had taken away their right to the government given in their colonial charter. He marveled that, despite this, "order among the people has been remarkably preserved." He then asked, "But is it proper or safe for the colony to continue much longer in such imperfect order? Must it not appear rational and necessary . . . that the many parts should be properly settled, and every branch of the legislative and executive authority restored to the order and vigour on which the life and health of the body politic depend?"[25] He further explained that it was the duty of the men in the Provincial Congress, with the help of prayer and heavenly guidance, to bring good government back to the people. In eighteenth-century thought, being without government was like existing in a state of nature. While it could work in the short-term, it was not a good long-term solution for without government it would be hard to maintain order and protect property. It was not clear, yet, to Langdon or others what the long-term solutions were. The Massachusetts Provincial Congress did hold out hopes for action from the Continental Congress, that delegates from other colonies would find common cause with Massachusetts and choose to act, as they had with the Association.

As delegates to the Second Continental Congress made their way to Philadelphia for their May 10, 1775 opening session, they traveled along established and known transportation routes and through an unknown political landscape. Even in towns and colonies where government continued to function as usual, more voices clamored for action. As delegates made their way by land and water, the desire for change moved through the veins of the body politic, bringing health or disease depending on one's viewpoint. Men and women need only to pay attention to hear the heart of the body politic beat to a different rhythm than it had before.

One indication of this was that throughout the colonies, men joined militias and women urged men to do so. If any delegate had not seen that martial enthusiasm themselves before they left home, it awaited them when they arrived in Philadelphia. No one had declared war and military conflict had thus far remained small-scale; nonetheless war preparation was everywhere apparent. This struck the North Carolina delegation who wrote home to friends and family members describing the scenes. Richard Caswell, Joseph Hewes, and William Hooper all wrote letters that chronicled companies of militia exercising twice daily on the Common and exclaimed that even Quakers, "except a few rigid ones" had joined. Hooper described what he saw using a disease metaphor: "This City has taken a deep share in the Infection which is so generally diffused thro' the Continent. Men Women & Children feel the patriotick glow."[26] According to Hooper, the infection was a beneficial rather than harmful one, infusing all residents with health and vigor.

In this changed and martial landscape, Congress started the slow process of developing a working colony-wide government on May 11, receiving correspondence and resolving to keep their proceedings secret "until the majority shall direct them to be made public." What was clear to the delegates was that some sort of war had begun. Whether they would be able to shape it, change it, or end it was still up in the air. By May 15, Congress declared the colonies in a state of self-defense and crafted policy for protecting the military stores and calling on additional troops to guard them. They also resolved to keep an exact inventory of all the cannon and stores captured at Ticonderoga so that when harmony was restored between Great Britain and its colonies, an outcome Congress still proclaimed it desired, those items could be returned.

In a city where the militia was highly visible, and in the aftermath of the success of militias at Lexington, Concord, Ticonderoga, and Crown Point, Congress nonetheless remained cautious. Making policy, no matter how carefully crafted in terms of self-defense, raised the ire of Parliament that saw Congress as an illegitimate body but still wished to avoid an all-out war. For his part, Benjamin Franklin worried that the war which had started might last long enough that "the youngest of us may not see the End of" it.[27] He pledged to work to "quench" the war from Philadelphia. Delegate James Duane hoped that Americans would "restrain every emotion of intemperate zeal—every sally of anger and passion." He wrote that he would urge Congress to choose a rational path, to "cooly and deliberately examine and Consider the state of the Colonies."[28] Even in a changed political atmosphere, some of the actors pledged to keep irrationality from triumphing over rationality, to try to check the wilder, more frenetic impulses of some of the American people.

While Hooper had praised the infection of patriotism, to others, so-called patriotism was a disease that rapidly spread with their hopes of containing the contagion fading. John Dickinson made this explicit in his notes for a speech in Congress. Defensive military action might be necessary, he thought, like, "Blisters applied to extract Humours from gross diseased Bodies." He also hoped that only blisters were necessary and that Congress and the American people would not have to resort to more drastic measures: "[A]fter applying Blisters, a prudent Physician will certainly strive to avoid bleeding . . . until the Blisters have been allowed Time to draw." He continued that "during that interval" of time and observation, it was necessary to "keep the Patient in as calm a Temper as may be possible."[29] Dickinson did not oppose the defensive measures agreed upon in Congress but he hoped that Americans would stay calm rather than opening themselves up to a more serious disease in the shape of further military battles. Even John Adams, far less cautious than Franklin, Duane, or Dickinson, declared himself "as fond of reconciliation . . . as any man." He, too, pledged to work toward containing the contagion as long as that could be done without curtailing rights or liberties. Adams feared, however, "that the cancer is too deeply rooted and too far spread to be cured by anything short of cutting it out entire." Adams advocated for a more aggressive approach, but he also worried. After all, the colonists were far from united, and the "continent is a vast, unwieldy machine."[30]

The twelve colonies that were participating in the Continental Congress (Georgia would join later) really were a vast, unwieldy machine and would remain so through the duration of the war. Despite this, parts of that machine functioned, sometimes even well. For those living in the early war zones this was born out of necessity. Household governments reorganized around the absence of men. Militias continued to ready themselves for what came next. Town governments urged men to arms and supplied those men to the best of their abilities. Provincial Congresses continued to legislate. In each locality drawn into the growing war, Americans crafted responses. In New England, a region with a history of resistance to English rule that predated the present conflict and a history of extralegal and brutal warfare against regional Indian nations, perhaps this is not surprising. In regions with a history of obedience, it is. Even the new body of the Congress, for all its faults and weaknesses, functioned well enough.

The Continental Congress could not have functioned without other governments in place. These other governments, however, often made the delegates to the Continental Congress uneasy. Nowhere can this be seen more than in the reactions to military actions taken by local militia or paid for by colonial governments like the raid on Ticonderoga. Almost immediately, delegates to Congress agreed that they must aid in the defense of the colonies but knew they had to proceed with caution. As Congress debated the meaning and outcome of the raid on Ticonderoga, which had occurred on the same day they reconvened as a body, it denied any desire for independence and the existence of a plan to invade Canada, a rumor that had circulated widely. Their June 1 resolve not to invade Canada was translated into French and sent to American forces at Ticonderoga, other military outposts near Canada, and to the inhabitants of Canada. Despite this outwardly cautious policy, some delegates personally expressed unease at what they believed was excessive and bellicose action. In a semi-coded letter to John Dickinson, Thomas Willing wrote that Dickinson needed to be present for the discussion or debate about Canada, writing that he thought what other delegates proposed "must be highly disagreeable to you." He urged Dickinson, "[C]ome to the Congress I beseech you this Morng."[31]

Members of Congress wondered how to keep the colonies functioning in protest without unleashing the full force of the British Empire against them. Where was the line between the stated desire for restoration of peace and the passing of resolutions for military buildup? Congress claimed Americans acted defensively, but the body did nothing to check the actions of the militia in Boston who waged guerilla raids against British stores, killing or wounding British soldiers. The body did nothing, other than to pass a charge to keep a tally of the stores, to check Ethan Allen's Green Mountain Boys as they rampaged and pillaged their way along Lake Champlain. For observers looking for signs that what was said was not what was meant, many of the actions of Congress could easily be seen as masks for a different and more radical purposes.

While Continental Congress did not condemn or check the guerillas, other governmental bodies or agents did as they tried to settle the colonists back to what they considered good government, order, and loyalty. In Parliament, Lord North pushed through the Conciliatory Resolution which, if accepted in the colonies, would allow colonists to tax themselves to raise money for defense. It was also designed to divide the colonies for if it had gone into place, each colony would make separate agreements with Crown and Parliament rather than working through and with Continental Congress. While William Franklin urged men in New Jersey to do just that, in Boston, Gage became convinced that conciliation would not work. In a letter written to Lord North on June 13, he painted a picture of his army hemmed into Boston by numbers that grew every day, numbers that prevented him and his supporters from getting either the goods or intelligence they needed. Massachusetts was not about to agree to be separated from the other colonies for they needed the aid of those other colonies and they opposed what they saw as an occupying army bent on destroying their liberties.

The numbers did grow every day and not just in Massachusetts. In Philadelphia, a woman wrote to a British soldier then stationed in Boston. She informed him that her family "consider you as a public enemy," even though he remained "a private friend." She wrote of her family's zeal in conforming to non-importation and that she had urged her brother to join the American military cause.[32] And, while Gage fretted about his lack of supplies and intelligence, the Continental Congress resolved to form six regiments and unanimously elected George Washington general of this new army. This new army was too late for the Battle of Bunker Hill on June 17, where the American militia fought with "rage and enthousiasm as great as ever people were possessed of," according to Gage, but would start to form and train for what came next.[33]

Governments responded to each of these decisions and conflicts, and each action and response changed the nature of the conflict. Lord North, the Secretary of State for the colonies, came to believe with the Roxbury writer mentioned above that Gage's madness had been the destruction of both effective government and the quashing of the insurgency and therefore issued an order for Gage's removal from North America. By October 11, Gage sailed for England although, strangely, he officially retained the governorship of Massachusetts Bay. In Massachusetts, the Provincial Congress helped to set up hospitals for the wounded and supply doctors to those hospitals. It also continued the business of war, counting soldiers and arms and working in concert with neighboring colonies. On local levels, governments responded to immediate needs. Meanwhile Continental Congress employed different strategies, reflecting the confusion of a still-divided Congress and population.

John Adams perfectly summarized the conflicted nature of Congress in a letter home to his friend James Warren. In a description that mirrored doctors' notes about their mad patients, he wrote that the delegates relied too much on passion and fear rather than "Reason and Evidence." Congress experienced "a Strange Oscillation between Love and Hatred, between War and Peace." This frustrated Adams who believed that only a military option was now viable, but noted that if they did not also continue to petition the King, "Discord and total Disunion would be the certain Effect of a resolute Refusal to petition and negotiate."[34] Thus, on July 5, Congress endorsed and agreed to send the Olive Branch Petition to the King, pledging allegiance to him and asking him to do what he could to stop the loss of life and to repeal the laws that "immediately distress any of your Majesty's colonies." The very next day, Congress endorsed and published their Declaration of the Causes and Necessity of Taking Up Arms.

This, finally, was a declaration of war, one couched entirely in defensive terms. Congress enumerated the colonists' grievances against the policies and actions of Parliament and its ministers. They had tried peaceful routes to resolution, the document claimed, but nothing they had done was able to "stay, or even . . . mitigate the heedless fury with which these accumulated and unexampled outrages were hurried on." They listed the crimes, as they saw them, and reiterated that they refused to submit to "the tyranny of irritated ministers." They had no "ambitious designs of separating from Great-Britain, and establishing independent states" but, because the attacks against them had been unprovoked, they needed to take up arms. Their language of fury and irritation spoke of madness, madness that required the medicine of self-defense to protect the body politic from infection.

John Adams was not displeased with the language. He wrote to William Tudor that this declaration "has Some Mercury in it, and is pretty frank, plain, and clear."[35] In fact, it was so frank, plain, and clear that it alarmed many of the colonists who did not want the military horrors to spread. John Dalrymple, in a pamphlet entitled, *The Rights of Great Britain Asserted against the Claims of America: Being an Answer to the Declaration of the General Congress*, called this Declaration "strange." He felt as if Congress "in a loose, cursory, and superficial manner," had twisted facts to suit its purposes. "But their business is to engage the passions," he stated, "where they can make no impression with their argument." In Dalrymple's opinion, the delegates and their supporters were "madly bent on independence." This was likely more than a turn of phrase as physicians and lay people alike believed that excessive passion led to madness. Because Dalrymple believed that the 1775 declaration reflected a form of madness, he called for Britain to reduce the colonies to a state of dependence for anything else "would be to speak to the winds." Americans had worked themselves up into a "political frenzy," and just like lunatic patients, they had to be put in restraints, at least temporarily, until they regained reason.[36]

While Congress insisted this declaration was not a call for independence, the declaration did by necessity dissolve former governmental systems. Delegate Joseph Hewes called it a manifesto, one that meant, "The powers of Government must soon be superseded and taken into the hands of the People."[37] Others echoed this call for new governments to be formed. If they were to fight a war, even if it were a defensive one, none of the colonies could simply exist in a state of nature, responding to the world around them. They needed systems in place to coordinate efforts, recruit and supply soldiers, retain law and order, among other things. They could no longer rely on the British systems for the British were bent on enslaving them.

By the time Congress passed the Declaration of Causes and Necessity of Taking Up Arms, the colonies separately and together had already created some of these forms of government. Despite this, Americans still hesitated to call for independence. According to Congress, the war was still but an "unhappy and unnatural controversy, in which Britons fight against Britons and the descendants of Britons." On December 1, 1775, Hewes wrote home to North Carolina: "No plan of Separation has been offered, the Colonies will never agree to any till drove to it by dire necessity." Despite fighting in Massachusetts, New York, and Canada, despite the November declaration of martial law in Virginia by Governor Dunmore and his offer to free enslaved people who joined British forces, Hewes did not yet see a dire necessity and continued, "I wish the time may not come too soon." He was not alone in this. While some men and women argued for new forms of government separate from Great Britain's, the risks were great.

If enough Americans moved to support independence, what would happen to well-ordered society and protection of property? In a "Dialogue on Civil Liberty" that took place in Philadelphia in January 1776, one of the speakers rejected independence. He argued that there were, indeed, problems in the British constitution, but that the defects could be remedied. Therefore he "would continue in quiet subjection." For this speaker, while, "[t]here may be sudden occasional groundless tumults in one corner of an empire or government," these were "of no consequence unless the whole body of the people join in them." He then used a Latin phrase, translated as "riots and disturbances often renew support for the government."[38] He urged Americans not to join in the military conflict or the push for independence; if they did, they would only strengthen support for the British system. In other corners of

America, speakers and writers echoed the fears of riots and the possibility of a worse government rising from the ashes of the old.[39]

Even many New Englanders who had been keen to muster to defend their liberties quailed at independence. In New Hampshire, the royal governor, John Wentworth fled for Boston on August 23, 1775 in the face of increased insurgency in that colony. On the recommendation of the Continental Congress, early in January 1776 the New Hampshire Congress adopted a temporary constitution claiming that the departure of Wentworth left them no other choice; they formed a new government, "for the preservation of peace and good order, and for the security of the lives and properties of the inhabitants of this colony."[40] Although they, like the Continental Congress, claimed to have no interest in independence, the wording of their constitution came perilously close to declaring independence. The town of Portsmouth objected to this step, writing to the government sitting in Exeter, "We would . . . have wished to have had the minds of the People fully Taken on such a Momentous Concernment, and to have Known the Plan, before it was Adopted, & carried into Execution."[41] At the same time, a writer using the pseudonym Junius published a letter in the *New Hampshire Gazette* claiming that the New Hampshire representatives had nothing less than independence in mind. He urged his readers to oppose this step. If they did not stand in opposition to independence, "like a neglected wound" their actions could "mortify, and corrupt the whole body."[42] In private letters, John Sparhawk advocated caution. As late as June 1776, he wrote: "it is one thing to Assert Independancy & another to maintain it.—I am afraid the present contest will last many years & nearly ruin both Countries."[43] Even in the most rebellious corners of the colonies, fears of physical and mental illness in the body politic, fears of disruptions to rational systems, meant that Americans hesitated in taking an irrevocable step toward independence.

In the end, other arguments overrode these colonists' fears, at least in the actions taken by the governments in North America. Independence gained traction, helped along by Thomas Paine's timely pamphlet, *Common Sense*, published anonymously on January 10, 1776. As numerous scholars have shown, Paine's language spoke directly to many Americans, leading enough of them to support of independence from Great Britain.[44] He told his readers that, "To talk of friendship with those in whom our reason forbids us to have faith, and our affections wounded through a thousand pores instruct us to detest, is madness and folly." He then proceeded to move their minds away from that madness and folly to a rational and healthy acceptance of what he saw as fact. Paine believed that not only should the colonies declare independence but the new nation that emerged could be a viable one, that the body politic born out of revolution could be free from mental or physical illness and from the disease and corruption of the British system. Paine took the feelings and language that already existed in corners of the colonies and put them on the page in powerful ways for many of his readers or listeners.

While Paine helped move a large minority toward independence, the majority still balked. Some readers found every argument in *Common Sense*, from Paine's title to the last word on the last page, a lie and a potential source of further disease in the body politic. From New York, Charles Inglis fired back in a pamphlet of his own (also anonymously published) entitled, *The True Interest of America Impartially Stated, in Certain Strictures on a Pamphlet Intitled Common Sense.* He believed *Common Sense* was dangerous sedition. In the introduction to *True Interest*, Inglis insisted, "I find no Common Sense in this pamphlet." Instead, there was "much *uncommon* phrenzy." The author must be a lunatic, for the pamphlet was "an insidious attempt to poison [Americans'] minds, and seduce them from their loyalty and truest interest." The words on the page went beyond the illogic of the most furiously mad of men, Inglis wrote. "The principles of government laid down in it, are not only false, but too absurd to have ever entered the head of a crazy politician before." To Inglis, Paine's pamphlet "unites the violence and rage of a republican, with all the enthusiasm and folly of a fanatic." Inglis did not find Paine's argument compelling or logical. Inglis pled for a different approach, one he hoped would bring Americans back to their senses.

Even some who had come to believe that independence was the only solution for their disordered world were discomfited by *Common Sense*. By 1776, the Virginia planter, Landon Carter believed that the colonies had been compelled to independence by necessity, but he was alarmed by what he deemed "Republican distractions," or a mad turn toward unworkable government structures. In his diary he wrote of his dread that "we might fall into a worse situation from internal oppression and commotions." While he reluctantly supported independence, he took a particular exception to *Common Sense*. The pamphlet did not sway him as it had others; he found it illogical and badly argued. In February 1776, Carter deemed the pamphlet "rascally and nonsensical as possible." In April, Carter wrote that Paine "advances new and dangerous doctrines to the peace and happiness of every society." In May he fretted that the republican ideas embedded in calls for independence "do avow a conduct more arbitrary than ever the English constitution in its Purity could admit of."[45] To Carter, perhaps the author was only temporarily mad rather than furiously mad. Either way, calls for a republican form of government could only come from a madman.

For those who did believe that breaking from Great Britain was the only possible path, Paine and Carter represented two points on the spectrum. Paine not only argued that Americans should choose independence, he exalted in the idea. For Paine, it was "infinitely wiser and safer, to form a constitution of our own in a cool and deliberate manner," rather than leaving the potential for future independence or a future nation to chance. He argued independence was the only rational step. Carter, on the other hand, believed he and other Americans did not choose independence but had been forced in that direction. That compulsion came only after the British ministers had become "so mad" that no other solution was possible. While independence was a necessary step, Carter believed that Americans should replicate the British constitution and reject republicanism. The British constitution was not at fault; instead it was that the actors had become corrupt, passing arbitrary policies designed to rob the colonists of their rights. Paine vehemently disagreed. He acknowledged that the British system had once been necessary because it had brought the English out of dark times. At the same time the British system was "imperfect, subject to convulsions, and incapable of producing what it seems to promise, is easily demonstrated." For Carter, rejecting the mixed English system was a "mere cookery among the Congress Republicans," born out of a tendency to falsify facts for corrupt purposes. For Paine, continued acceptance of the same system was madness. From their points on the spectrum, both men squinted at the other and saw inconsistencies and mental instability.

Despite the range of differences in Americans' feelings toward separation from Britain, by May 1776, Congress paved the way toward declaring independence, sending instructions to all of the "respective assemblies and conventions of the United Colonies" to form new governments to "best conduce to the happiness and safety of their constituents." Leaders in some colonies simply kept on under barely modified colonial charters, but others took the opportunity to build something new. Regardless of which avenue each colony chose, the health of the new body politic depended on the consent of the governed. In Pennsylvania, James Allen, who had been elected to that colony's assembly, worried about the danger that lurked in the new governments. In his diary he noted, "The Congress have resolved to recommend it to the different Colonies to establish new forms of Government." He also wrote of his fear of any government based on the will of the people: "A Convention chosen by the people, will consist of the most fiery Independents." He found these fiery independents obnoxious and noted that he had "openly declared my aversion to their principles & had one or two disputes at the coffee-house with them." In his diary's pages he vowed "to oppose them vehemently in Assembly, for if they prevail there; all may bid adieu to our old happy constitution & peace."[46] There was, of course, already no peace, but any move toward independence guaranteed further confusion and war.

While Paine asserted that only good would come from independence, men like Allen feared anarchy and disorder. Their fears grew when they examined the new governments that emerged and saw the imperfection of the men in power. In the end, Allen's fears that the newly elected were fiery independents were realized; on June 16, he despaired that "the Tide is too strong, we could not prevent a change of instructions to our Delegates."

The new government that emerged from the workings of these delegates, encoded in the Pennsylvania Constitution, was the most markedly different and democratic new form of government, written by "a plainspoken, largely unschooled group of men with work-toughened hands," according to historian Gary Nash.[47] Joseph Reed worried that the new Constitution would create illness in the body politic; he expressed concern that: "Government will sink into a spiritless languor, or expire in a sudden convulsion."[48] The Pennsylvania Constitution included a Council of Censors that would review the Constitution every seven years to suggest changes, but critics found this "as absurd and dangerous, as physic to a healthy body." One writer said that this provision was "composed in a hurry . . . by a fanatical school-master, while the wisest and best men in the state were in the field."[49] Fanatics were mad, unreasonable, and maniacal. In a disordered time, the body politic could become deranged by these madmen as they attempted to mold something new. This fear found voice in a petition published in the *Pennsylvania Gazette* on March 24, 1779. The authors of this petition gave vent to their worst fears. They believed that, under this system, there would be "a jubilee of tyranny to be celebrated at the end of every seven years.. . . When the foundations of government shall be torn up! When anarchy and licentiousness and force shall roam unawed and unrestrained!"[50]

For as long as they have been telling the story, historians have uncovered the tensions between the democratic and conservative elements in Revolutionary-era society.[51] Some Americans believed that as long as there was the possibility of creating something new, the people should want to expand the boundaries of political participation, create rights-based governments, and "remember the Ladies." Other Americans, often those with access to more-traditional forms of power, worried that their "Struggle has loosened the bands of Government everywhere," and, as we know, men like John Adams did not think that was a good thing. These tensions played out even in regions directly affected by military conflict. Americans were far from united in their philosophies of government or hopes for the future.[52]

In Massachusetts, these tensions were clear. In January 1776, John Adams had worked with the General Court to pass a Proclamation in preparation for a change in government. The Proclamation urged caution: "commending and enjoining it upon the good People of this Colony, that they lead sober, religious and peaceable Lives." It asked the people of Massachusetts to avoid many things, including "all riotous and tumultuous Proceedings." After all, the Proclamation concluded, this would be "for the good of the People, inculcating by their Public Ministry and private Example, the Necessity of Religion, Morality, and good order."[53] In May of 1776, James Sullivan, a hearty supporter of independence, wrote a letter to his friend Adams, also advocating for caution. He stated that he agreed with John Adams that Massachusetts should rely on the old form of government rather than creating something new from a whole cloth: "I have not the least Idea of dissolving the old and Making an entire new Form of Government," he wrote. "I think it would be attended with the greatest Anarchy as it would leave the people for a Time without any Government."[54]

Indeed, those in power had a strong preference for continuity rather than change. As historian John L. Brooke has shown, "In a very important sense, then, the opening phases of the Revolution [in Massachusetts] were continuous with recent provincial experience, rather than making a fundamental break with the past."[55] Many who kept or assumed positions of power believed that deference was due to them and, in fact, deference would be the only thing that kept anarchy at bay while men worked to fill "a governmental vacuum until traditional institutions could be restored."[56] These men urged restraint and caution. Yes, they wanted independence from Great Britain, but not at the expense of order, or at least as much order as possible in a countryside that experienced warfare.

Unrestrained government called to mind the fears of unrestrained people, and, to men like Adams and Sullivan, some of the residents of Massachusetts proved their point. The people in Berkshire County were filled with what more conservative men dismissed as a "rage for innovation." The Town of Pittsfield rejected the scheme to keep functioning under the colonial system of government. After all, through appointed governors "all manners of disorders have been introduced into our constitution, till it has become an instrument of oppression and deep corruption." In this petition, Pittsfield residents asserted that they were not unreasonable. Instead, they had listened with "decency and moderation" to the other side. In the end, they concluded that their request was "just and reasonable." They needed a new government, and they wrote: "we pray that it may be *de novo*."[57] In Taunton, Massachusetts, men armed with sticks kept the court there from sitting. These men wanted to be heard, but to the more-established leaders, like John Winthrop, they symbolized, simply "an unwillingness to submit to law, and pay their debts."[58] In part because of the differences, Massachusetts would not adopt a constitution until 1780 and although today it is the oldest constitution that continues to function, it remained a flashpoint of contention in the era of the American Revolution.

While other colonies faced a smoother transitions to new governments than Pennsylvania or Massachusetts, the unwillingness of colonists in 1776 to quietly accept governments on any level that seemed antithetical to liberty was widespread. Historians have written about the shift from the older more deferential political culture of the seventeenth and earlier eighteenth centuries to a more democratic political culture. In 1973, John Shy wrote, "It has always seemed slightly implausible that the American Republic was born out of congeries of squabbling, unstable colonies and that labor was induced by nothing more than a few routine grievances expressed in abstract, if elegant prose." To some observers, the squabbling of the colonists and the instability of the colonies were signs of derangement within the body politic.

That abstract and elegant prose Shy later referenced made an appearance in early July 1776 in the Declaration of Independence. The final version of that document managed to pull together many of the grievances that had been building both in the decade and the year that preceded its publication. When Congress approved the Declaration on July 2, it approved a document that, among other things, claimed a rational basis for separation and the creations of new governments, both already effected and ongoing. After all, these were self-evident truths that could be discovered through observation and while prudence had kept the colonists under a bad government for longer than it should have, that was part of human experience, that "all experience hath shown, that mankind are more disposed to suffer, while evils are sufferable, than to right themselves by abolishing the forms to which they are accustomed." Congress declared independence for the United States of America and declared that they would build government based on the rational principles of the social contract, that people would give up some liberties for the sake or order and good government, but those liberties could not be taken away without their consent. The signers adopted a theory that had been put in place only partially in existing governments. The challenge would be if they could win a war, adhere to those principles, and birth a rational state.

The questions of government during wartime were far from settled when Congress declared independence. As shown above, Massachusetts would not adopt a constitution for another four years and while Congress began working on the Articles of Confederation, differences in ideology, regional differences, and the various states' size and power would keep them from agreeing on a form of national government until the war was almost over. Americans had built governments around old colonial charters, republican principles, and notions of rights, but the governments were far from perfect and far from rational. Together with problems of economics, alliances, warfare or threatened warfare, irrational actors also would continue to plague the workings of these new governments often leading to more instability than stability. It was not clear that the republican experiment would last and history seemed to show that it would not.

NOTES

1. Pauline Maier addressed this fear in depth in her *From Resistance to Revolution: Colonial Radicals and the Development of American Opposition to Britain, 1765–1776* (New York: W. W. Norton & Company, 1972).

2. Thomas Gage to Josiah Martin, April 1775. https://docsouth.unc.edu/csr/index.php/document/csr09-0496. Accessed November 9, 2018.

3. Hulton, *Letters of a Loyalist Lady*, 72.

4. Peter Oliver, *Origin and Progress of the American Rebellion, 1781*. http://americainclass.org/sources/makingrevolution/rebellion/text2/oliverloyalistsviolence.pdf.

5. "Extract of a Letter from Roxbury, Dated April 23," *Pennsylvania Evening Post* (Philadelphia) May 9, 1775.

6. Andrew Eliot to his son, April 23, 1775. Miscellaneous Manuscripts, Massachusetts Historical Society.

7. Boston Town Meeting Minutes, April 22, 1775, Massachusetts Historical Society, MHS Collections Online, https://www.masshist.org/database/viewer.php?item_id=1903&img_step=1&mode=transcript.

8. Letter from Abigail Adams to John Adams, May 7, 1775 [electronic edition]. *Adams Family Papers: An Electronic Archive*. Massachusetts Historical Society. http://www.masshist.org/digitaladams/.

9. John Leach Diary, June 29, 1775, "Life during Siege of Boston Document Packet," Massachusetts Historical Society, https://www.masshist.org/2012/juniper/assets/ed-curricula/fernandez_document_packet.pdf.

10. Peter Edes Diary, https://www.masshist.org/database/1978.

11. Timothy Newell. Diary 1775–1776. Massachusetts Historical Society.

12. John Leach, "A Journal Kept by John Leach during His Confinement by the British, in Boston Gaol, in 1775," *New England Historical and Genealogical Register* 19 (1865): 260, https://books.google.com/books/about/New_England_Historical_and_Genealogical_html.

13. Peter Edes diary, June–October 1775. *Siege of Boston: Eyewitness Accounts from the Collection of the Massachusetts Historical Society*. https://www.masshist.org/online/siege/doc-viewer.php?item_id=1978&mode=nav.

14. Quoted in Peter Linebaugh and Marcus Rediker, "The Many-Headed Hydra: Sailors, Slaves, and the Atlantic Working Class in the Eighteenth Century," *Journal of Historical Sociology* 3 (1990): 234.

15. Quoted in John Adams, *Slavery, and Race: Ideas, Politics, and Diplomacy in an Age*, 5.

16. Henry Hulton, Boston, to Robert Nicholson, May 7, 1775. In Neil Longley York, *Henry Hulton and the American Revolution: An Outsider's Inside View* (Boston: The Colonial Society of Massachusetts, 2010), 320.

17. For discussions of eighteenth-century treatment of the mentally ill, see Robert Whitaker, *Mad in America: Bad Science, Bad Medicine, and the Enduring Mistreatment of the Mentally Ill* (Cambridge, MA: Perseus Publishing, 2002). Starvation and other harsh treatments are discussed on pp. 6–8.

18. Quoted in Provincial Congress, 181.

19. Hulton to Nicholson, May 7, 1775, York, ed., *Henry Hulton*, 320–321.

20. Archibald Neilson to Andrew Miller, January 28, 1775. https//docsouth.unc.edu.

21. Inhabitants of Anson County to Governor Josiah Martin, 1775. https://docsouth.unc.edu.

22. William Franklin, Speech to the New Jersey Assembly, January 13, 1775, in Sheila L. Skemp, *Benjamin and William Franklin: Father and Son, Patriot and Loyalist* (Boston: Bedford St. Martin's, 1994), 177.

23. William Franklin to Lord Dartmouth, 6 May 1775 in Skemp, *Benjamin and William Franklin*, 178–182.

24. *Conciliatory Address to the People of Great Britain and the Colonies, on the Present Important Crisis* (London: J. Wilkie, 1775). Reprinted in Harry T. Dickinson, ed., *British Pamphlets on the American Revolution, 1763–1785*, Vol. 3 (London: Pickering & Chatto, 2007), 251–310.

25. Samuel Langdon, *Government Corrupted by Vice, and Recovered by Righteousness. A Sermon Preached before the Honorable Congress of the Colony of the Massachusetts-Bay in New England, Assembled at Watertown, On Wednesday the 31st Day of May, 1775. Being the Anniversary Fixed by Charter for the Election of Counsellors.* (Watertown: Benjamin Edes, 1775), 25–26, Evans Early American Imprint Collection.

26. William Hooper to Samuel Johnston, May 23, 1775 in Paul H. Smith, ed., Letters of Delegates to Congress, 1774–1789 (Washington, DC: Library of Congress, 1976), 398.

27. Benjamin Franklin to Jonathan Shipley, May 15, 1775, in William B. Willcox, ed., *The Papers of Benjamin Franklin*, Vol. 22 (New Haven: Yale University Press, 1982), 42.

28. James Duane, "Notes on the State of the Colonies," in Edward C. Burnett, *Letters of Members of the Continental Congress*, Vol. 1 (Washington: Carnegie Institution of Washington, 1921), 99, https://books.google.com/books?id=4AmKAA AAMAAJ.

29. John Dickinson, in Smith, ed., *Letters of Delegates to Congress*, 376.

30. "From John Adams to Moses Gill, 10 June 1775," *Founders Online*, National Archives, https://founders.archives.gov/documents/Adams/06-03-02-0014.

31. Thomas Willing to John Dickinson in Smith, ed., *Letters of Delegates to Congress*, 431.

32. "Nothing Is Heard Now but the Trumpet and Drum," in *The Spirit of Seventy-Six*, 94–96.

33. Gage to Lord Barrington, June 23, 1775. *The Spirit of Seventy-Six*, 134.

34. John Adams to Joseph Warren, July 6, 1775 in Robert J. Taylor, ed., *The Adams Papers, Papers of John Adams*, Vol. 3 (Cambridge: Harvard University Press, 1979), 60–63.

35. John Adams to William Tudor, July 6, 1775, in Taylor, ed., *The Adams Papers*, 59–60.

36. John Dalrymple, *The Rights of Great Britain Asserted Against the Claims of America: Being an Answer to the Declaration of the General Congress* (Philadelphia: R. Bell, 1776), 86, Evans Early American Imprint Collection.

37. Joseph Hewes to Samuel Johnston, July 8, 1775, *Documenting the American South*, https://docsouth.unc.edu/csr/index.html/document/csr10-0034.

38. "Dialogue on Civil Liberty, Delivered at a Public Exhibition in Nassau-Hall. Jan. 1776," *The Pennsylvania Magazine* 2 (April 1776): 167.

39. Maier, *From Resistance to Revolution*.
40. Constitution of New Hampshire, 1776, http://avalon.law.yale.edu/18th_century/nh09.asp.
41. Quoted in W. F. Dodd, "The First State Constitutional Conventions, 1776–1783" *American Political Science Review* 2 (1908): 547, https://jstor.org/stable/1944479.
42. Junius, "The Congress at Exeter," *New Hampshire Gazette,* January 9, 1776. Reprinted in Nathaniel Bouton, ed., *Documents and Records Relating to the State of New-Hampshire during the Period of the American Revolution, from 1776 to 1783,* Vol. VIII (Concord: Edward A. Jenks, 1874), 25, http://catalog.hathitrust.org/Record/101782272.
43. John Sparhawk, Danbury, to Joseph Whipple, Portsmouth, June 11, 1776. Charles Lowell Papers, 1657–1853. Massachusetts Historical Society.
44. See for instance, Eric Foner, *Tom Paine and Revolutionary America* (New York: Oxford University Press, 1976); J. C. D. Clark, *Thomas Paine: Britain, America, and France in the Age of Enlightenment and Revolution* (New York: Oxford University Press, 2020); Craig Nelson, *Thomas Paine: Enlightenment, Revolution, and the Birth of Modern Nations* (New York: Penguin Books, 2006).
45. Jack P. Greene, ed., *The Diary of Colonel Landon Carter of Sabine Hall, 1752–1778,* Vol. II (Charlottesville: University Press of Virginia, 1965), 1042, 1046.
46. May 15, 1776, in "Diary of James Allen, 187.
47. Gary B. Nash, "Philadelphia's Radical Caucus That Propelled Pennsylvania to Independence and Democracy," in Young, Gary. Nash, and Raphael, eds, *Revolutionary Founders*, 67.
48. William B. Reed, ed., *Life and Correspondence of Joseph Reed*, Vol. 1 (Philadelphia: Lindsay and Blakiston, 1847), 302, https://catalog.hathitrust.org/Record/000364985.
49. *A Candid Examination of the Address of the Minority of the Council of Censors to the People of Pennsylvania* (Philadelphia: 1784), 23.
50. *A Candid Examination*, 22.
51. This literature goes beyond what a single footnote can cover, but includes Bernard Bailyn, *The Ideological Origins of the American Revolution* (Cambridge: Harvard University Press, 1967); Pauline Maier, *From Resistance to Revolution: Colonial Radicals and the Development of American Opposition to Britain, 1765–1776* (New York: W.W. Norton & Company, 1972); Rhys Isaac, *The Transformation of Virginia, 1740–1790* (New York: W.W. Norton & Company, 1982); Gordon S. Wood, *The Radicalism of the American Revolution* (New York: Random House, 1991).
52. Letter from Abigail Adams to John Adams, 31 March–5 April 1776, and letter from John Adams to Abigail Adams, April 14, 1776, *Adams Family Papers: An Electronic Archive.* Massachusetts Historical Society, http://www.masshist.org/digitaladams/.
53. Written in John Adams's hand, "A Proclamation by the General Court," in Taylor, ed., *Adams Papers*, 83–388.

54. James Sullivan to John Adams, May 9, 1776, *Founders Online,* https://founders.archives.gov/documents/Adams/06-04-02-0075.

55. John L. Brooke, *The Heart of the Commonwealth: Society and Political Culture in Worcester County, Massachusetts, 1713–1861* (New York: Cambridge University Press, 1989), 157.

56. Brooke, *Heart of the Commonwealth,* 157.

57. "The Petition, Remonstrance, and Address of the Town of Pittsfield to the Honorable Board of Councilors and House of Representatives of the Province of Massachusetts Bay, in General Assembly, now sitting at Watertown," reprinted in J. E. A. Smith, *The History of Pittsfield, (Berkshire County,) Massachusetts, from the Year 1734 to the Year 1800* (Boston: Lee and Shepard, 1869), 343–345, http://books.google.com/books/about/The_History_of_Pittsfield_Berkshire_Coun.html.

58. John Winthrop to John Adams, June 1, 1776, in Taylor, ed., *The Adams Papers,* Vol. 4, 222–225.

Chapter 6

An Irrational State, 1783–1787

By 1783, the Revolution was all but over and many hoped with Phillis Wheatley that Americans could, "Now sheathe the Sword that bade the Brave attone/With guiltless Blood for Madness not their own."[1] The instability of the post-war world, however, unnerved the citizens of the new nation and brought about forms of madness that they could not blame on anyone other than themselves. After all, the war had resolved the question of independence but little else. Tensions and divisions caused by the disruption of war did not disappear but sometimes grew and multiplied. The new Americans seemed prone to the fevers of enthusiasm, the frenzy of leveling, and madness of party. They worried that they had created an irrational state, one which might not survive and prosper. Americans celebrated the freedom from former strictures imposed by the British Empire but feared the absence of the support that empire had provided. What had they created during the frenzy and madness of war? Could the ideology that had served them on paper also serve them in real life? These and other questions confronted the country as it stumbled into peacetime with grand hopes and dreams but a scaffolding that many believed had been too hastily raised and therefore inadequate for the challenges ahead.

From different vantage points, most Americans worried about the state of the nation and their individual states. Many had hoped on some level that the war for independence would create a better world. The war over, Americans from different backgrounds wondered what they had wrought. Both the confusion and bloodshed of war and the economic depression that followed created conditions that might doom the republic. Mercy Otis Warren complained to Abigail Adams that despite the "Governments of our own Forming" and "Magistrates of our own Electing," the American people did not seem to have enough "Energy and Decission on their part" to become "wholly independent."[2] The British philosopher Richard Price wrote that now that peace had come, Americans who had been relatively united in their war against Great Britain were now "in danger of fighting with one another" and if that happened the new country would be "turned into a scene of blood; and instead of being the hope and refuge of the world, may become a terror to it."[3] There was the possibility that the United States as a body politic was in danger of going furiously mad.

In the years leading up to the war, colonists had clamored that only representative governments could pass laws acting on the people. Now they had those representative governments but the men elected failed to check their baser impulses and failed to build a self-reliant nation. If the individual actors lacked vital energy, as Warren argued, representation would not be enough; the body politic would sicken and its mind begin to show signs of disorder. In fact, Dr. Benjamin Rush believed just that. In his estimation, Americans were "wholly unprepared for their new situation."[4] The chaos and confusion that followed the war, when combined with continued democratic impulses among ordinary people, precipitated the conditions in which insanity could take hold and thrive. Doctors theorized that excessive passions, opposition or competition, and joy, among other things, led to mental disorders in some individuals. With these conditions in place, some Americans became lunatics. Without individuals sound in mind, the thirteen clocks that struck together to successfully conclude the war would be unable to come up with solutions for problems that continued to plague the new nation.

The evidence was everywhere that while states had formed new governments and covenanted together in a firm league of friendship under the Articles of Confederation, disorder abounded. History provided no comfort, for history told stories of the failures of once-great republics. Writing to her husband in Paris, Abigail Adams worried "that like the Greek Republicks we should by civil discension weaken our power, and crush our rising greatness." In that case, all of the bloodshed and strife during the years of war would have been in vain. Adams saw two paths available to the new United States, one of "honour, and Fame," the other of "disgrace, and infamy."[5] She was not alone in this assessment for the country lay in a delicate balance. A single misstep could tilt the country toward ruin rather than prosperity.

It did not help that the Confederation Congress, one of the mechanisms of government that had been crafted in war, functioned poorly in the immediate aftermath of the war. Men and women worried that the energy exerted by members of Congress while the revolution raged had dissipated. They worried that the covenant into the states had voluntarily entered during the war, "binding themselves to assist each other," had begun to dissolve. Maryland delegate James McHenry complained to Alexander Hamilton that Congress was "a council composed of discordant elements." A generation educated to believe that intrigue, influence, and a lust for power destroyed the fabric of government saw corruption everywhere in the political world around them. "The Prostitutes to Influence are capable frequently of making the wrong seem to be Right," Samuel Osgood wrote to John Adams. They held onto the slender hope that "a Jealous, well informed People" would keep watch, and that "Truth will prevail."[6] For there to be hope, the people could not relax but had to stay on guard to protect what had been so hard won.

The bonds that had tied Americans together during the war did loosen and sometimes even dissolved. One example of this can be seen in the inability for Congress to quickly and efficiently ratify the Paris Peace Treaty. Ratifying the treaty was an important step for the new country to take toward standing on the world stage, to becoming a nation with which other nations would enter into economic or diplomatic relationships.[7] Would this step falter because of the lack of energy? The signs pointed in that direction, worrying observant Americans. Congress could not ratify the treaty immediately because they did not have a quorum. They needed delegates from nine states to proceed but were slow to reach that number. The delegates who did show up filled their correspondence with their frustration at the inability of Congress to get the work of a nation done. Only on April 15, 1783, just a few days short of the eight-year anniversary of the Battles of Lexington and Concord, did Congress finally ratify the preliminary articles of the treaty.

Perhaps the problem was that the men in power during the war had been mistaken in wanting a republic. Lawyer Timothy Ford linked the adjective "republican" with the noun "caprice," fretting that a system based on government by the people led only to "very confused" politics and "opinions & interests various & adverse," creating unstable legislatures. The door to political participation opened wider than ever, allowing new men to take part in politics. Ford worried that the door had opened too wide and had erased too many of the distinctions that had previously qualified men as political actors. In addition, Ford believed that the war had led to increased numbers of people who experienced mental instability for "war corrupts the human mind & tends to erase the salutary ideas of honesty & good faith." In his opinion, a virtuous state had not emerged from the war, at least not yet. War had thrown Americans back into a state of nature that lacked a coherent government, one where men had bloodied their hands in their brothers' blood and where, with the lack of a legitimate government, "civil contracts were broken up & property set afloat upon the sea of a fluctuating paper."[8] The job now was to find a medicine that would cure the corruption of mind and to do what was needed to right the ship of state. Even before the war had ended, some Americans had called for a more centralized form of government. Now those calls increased. From Massachusetts, Benjamin Hichborn celebrated the ninth anniversary of the Declaration of Independence in an oration where he stated that "without an adequate power" to provide the new country "a proper direction," the

United States could "only operate like a mass of unanimated matter."⁹ The body politic would lose its vigor and die.

Thus it was that Americans approached official independence with a mixture of joy and caution. They had won independence but they might not manage to keep it. When George Washington made his preliminary announcement that he would return to private life once the peace treaty was ratified, he wrote that the individual states within the new country could "establish or ruin their national Character forever." He feared the legacy of the American Revolution would be a curse unless the states agreed "to delegate a larger proportion of power to Congress." If they did not take this step, he believed, "every thing must very rapidly tend to anarchy and confusion."¹⁰ The fear of failure was not mere speculation. With good reason, Americans saw threat everywhere they looked: in the economy, in the political world, and in the upheavals in Europe. Every change, every hiccup, every innovation led to fears that the new United States would not survive long, that irrationality or insanity would overcome the rationality needed for the new social compacts to work. For some, it was an excess of liberty unleashed by the democratic elements of the Revolution that would bring about ruin. For others, it was the aristocratical tendencies already present and rising. Men like William Samuel Johnson, serving in the Confederation Congress in 1785 believed Americans had a "Strong propensity" to "run into . . . lunacy & dissipations of every kind."¹¹ Checking the madness of the people—either democratical or aristocratical—seemed difficult if not impossible as the new governments moved from peace to war.

Was the nation Americans had created the one that they had wanted to create? Soldiers were among the first to raise this question. They had faced hardship and the possibility of death but hoped that their service provided a way to position themselves better both socially and economically. Instead, many of them worried about how to put clothes on their backs or to find jobs that could earn them a decent living. When veteran Joseph Plumb Martin published his memoir of his military service decades later, he did so in part to remind his fellow Americans that the men who had helped to win independence were often left with nothing. Although no longer on the field of battle, they faced the same hardships they had during wartime including insufficient food, shelter, and clothing. Soldiers often sold their final settlement certificates as a survival tactic. With nothing more than the clothes they wore and a small sum of money, they then had to find their way in peacetime society. As Martin later wrote, "When the country had drained the last drop of service it could screw out of the poor soldiers, they were turned adrift like old worn out horses, and nothing said about land to pasture them on."¹²

As their former commander in chief, George Washington believed that soldiers' service should have meant both praise and reward. At the same time, Washington was well aware that many of the men who served under him would be hard-pressed to make ends meet in the aftermath of the war. Washington spoke of the soldiers' "well earned *laurels*," but he also cautioned and then threatened the men serving under him. He cajoled them to leave the service with "no disorder, or licentiousness" and told them that patience would be needed as Congress acted.[13] He continued that looting or other "Military neglects, or excesses" would be punished. Like he had many times before he held out a carrot of praise and a stick of threat. At least some of his hearers would have been aware that Washington had executed two mutineers without even a court martial in 1781. It is easy to imagine that Washington believed he spoke for the new nation in a rational and reasoned manner. It is also easy to imagine that the men who heard him would be mixed in their response to his words and might have rankled at the idea that it was rational for men who had served to continue suffering into peacetime.

Officers generally had more financial wherewithal than the men they had commanded, but they too were worn out from years of battle in grim circumstances. They thought that the citizens of the new United States, including the members of Congress, should be grateful for their service and should therefore reward them. In December 1782, officers sent a memorial to Congress complaining of the "great distress" of their financial hardship. They had suffered more than "any other citizens of America" for they had endured the folly and madness of war while putting their lives on the line for independence. However, they now found themselves at a point where they had "borne all that men can bear." They begged for money and rations. Like Martin, they noted that they should be honored for their service but instead the officers who had already retired found themselves "the objects of obloquy."[14] They informed Congress that anger was growing in the army because independence should not mean that those who had served in the military ended up in ruined circumstances. This resonated with some members of Congress who raised the alarm within that body and with powerful friends. It also resonated with other leading men. Alexander Hamilton urged General Washington to act quickly "to keep a *complaining* and *suffering* army within the bounds of moderation."[15] Washington initially ignored this advice, only to find more anger among the officers when Congress rejected a measure to commute officers' pension for six years' full pay.

Fed up, Major John Armstrong wrote an anonymous address to other officers. He wanted to know, he wrote, if the emerging government embodied the principles for which they had fought. Was the new country willing to help them with their transition to private life, or was it "rather a country that tramples upon your rights, disdains your cries and insults your distresses?" He urged the officers to "assume a bolder tone." Using the language of physical illness, he remarked "that the wound often irritated, and never healed, may at length become incurable."[16] In Armstrong's view, they should not simply try to survive this irritated and unhealed wound but instead should use strong, preventative medicine. This meant that officers needed to be willing to act again with force if necessary. On March 15, 1783, officers under Washington's command met to discuss this address in what became known as the Newburgh Conspiracy.

With this address circulating and his officers meeting, Washington jumped back into the fray, condemning the anonymous address for working to disorder minds. The writer "intended to take advantage of the passions ... without giving time for cool deliberative thinking." In other words, this shaky new government that was supposed to be ruled by rationality threatened to come undone because of the irrationality of one "insidious foe" or "designing emissary." As Nicole Eustace has shown, many in Washington's generation believed emotions or passions were "an essential animating force" but only if guided by reason and held in check.[17] Although ideas about the benefits of passions circulated widely, many Americans still held onto classical beliefs that anger led to madness. In Washington's view, the passion of the officers was misguided and unchecked. If other officers listened to this writer, the only consequence would be ruin for the new republic and an opening of "the flood-gates of civil discord" to "deluge our rising empire in blood."[18] The body politic would become a furious lunatic. Washington's impassioned plea and the fear he raised in his fellow citizens worked to a degree: Congress responded with a compromise agreement that funded some back pay and granted soldiers five years of full pay.

Although Washington managed to squelch Armstrong's call for disobedience, other soldiers grew uneasy. When Congress began to furlough soldiers with less than complete pay, militiamen in Lancaster, Pennsylvania marched to Philadelphia where they were joined by hundreds of others demanding payment for their services. There were rumors that the furloughed soldiers were going to rob the Bank or the Treasury in order to obtain the funds promised to them. Members of Congress called on John Dickinson, then President of Pennsylvania, and the rest of the Pennsylvania government to call out militia to put the rebellion down. Always in favor of the olive branch, Dickinson argued that the soldiers were not acting in a disorderly fashion and that negotiation was the better course. While Dickinson kept a cool head and the soldiers engaged in a well-regulated protest, some members of the Confederation Congress became so sure that the protest posed a threat to good government that they convinced other members of that body to leave Philadelphia and reconvene in Princeton. In the end, the protest dissolved under a combination of negotiation and threat of military force but it demonstrated one potential for distress and disease in the body politic.

The problem with soldiers' pay and the potential for mutiny portended long-standing economic struggles. The arguments that had helped sell the American Revolution about the resources in and economic strength of North America were better propaganda than truth. As Kariann Akemi Yokota has shown, the new United States was rich in raw materials but newly crafted American citizens still wanted and relied on British manufactures.[19] When the ports reopened to foreign trade, the nascent North American manufacturing economy collapsed on its head as Americans rushed to procure the European goods and services they had been largely denied during the war. With little basis for a strong domestic economy, Americans relied on risky credit or continued to rely on older forms of trade and barter. If the medical doctors were to be believed, this shaky economy was a fruitful source of mental illness. Doctors listed the highs and lows of commerce as one of the primary causes of insanity. English physician Thomas Arnold had written that commerce caused insanity by "giving birth to the desires, fears, anxieties, disappointments, and other affections which accompany the pursuit, or possession, of riches."[20] The fears, anxieties, and disappointments in the American economic world created an unstable world with the potential to drive Americans insane.

By the mid-1780s, madness swept throughout the new United States, at least according to some observers. Struggling under tax debts, rural Americans called on the tactics of pre-revolutionary protest by raising liberty poles, preventing courts from sitting to foreclose on their property, holding town meetings, and petitioning their governments. In Maryland, South Carolina, Virginia, New Jersey and other states, protesters--many of them Revolutionary War veterans--took matters into their own hands. Like the Schenck brothers in New Jersey, these protesters felt that they were driven to action by the "madness of poverty."[21] To men and women unable to make ends meet through hard work and honest means, the state created by the Revolution seemed far from rational and the promises of liberty and good government unobtainable. First war and then poverty had disrupted their lives and shackled them against their wills in untenable economic circumstances.

As poor and debt-riddled protesters tried to take matters into their own hands and register their discontent with the new social and economic order, men with political or legal power feared that the Revolution had opened the doors to a world in which law and order would not be able to function. In Camden, South Carolina, for example, Judge John Grimke found himself a virtual prisoner in the courthouse. He had arrived in Camden on April 25, 1785 to hear debt cases. Although he had heard rumors that a crowd would try to stop the court from sitting, he dismissed those rumors. Even if a crowd gathered, he believed that the gentlemen in the community would intervene on his behalf to uphold the law and stop any illegal actions. When Grimke started the court proceedings on April 27, a man identified as Hill called out names, interrupting the court proceedings. At first, Grimke could not figure out what was going on, but noticed that more and more men gathered to prevent the sheriff from stopping Hill's recitation. Still, he felt relatively secure because he was an important man, high up on the hierarchical ladder, a gentleman who was used to having control over those of the lower sort. Because of this, Grimke's first tactic was to look at the man interrupting him in the eye and to tell him he was insulting the court. In the days before the American Revolution this may have worked to reestablish deference and order; it no longer did. Grimke wrote, "I questioned him concerning his behaviour and the Insult he was offering to the Court; hoping that it would daunt himself, prevent others from supporting him." Instead Hill replied with a taunt, "It was not many words that could fill a bushel," he said, thus rejecting Grimke's attempt to establish his own control and Hill's obedience. Grimke then left the bench and tried to persuade others to join him in seizing Hill. Hill and the others fled but no one came to Grimke's aid. With the so-called malcontents gone, Grimke tried to return to business but found there were not enough jury men available because of the confusion that reigned. In the end, he adjourned the court until November. The adjournment achieved what Hill and others in the crowd desired. Because they had made it impossible for the court to proceed, they also had made it impossible to punish anyone for nonpayment of debt.

What most disconcerted Grimke, as we can see in his report to the governor, was that no one helped him, or, as he wrote, that he "received no offer of support from the Gentlemen of the District." According to the unwritten rules of society, gentlemen were supposed to help each other keep the lesser sort in their place. When he talked to one of the men he trusted, Grimke was informed that while gentlemen might condemn "the mode which Hill and his Party had adopted," they agreed with the result of Hill's actions: the closing of the court. What Grimke had not understood is that while the better sort distanced themselves from the tactics of the lower sort, they simultaneously allowed the lower sort to act to do the work and accept the blame in achieving the end result they desired.

According to the rules of behavior, gentlemen could not stop the court from sitting therefore they allowed poorer men to do so instead. Planters had status, but their wealth was chimerical. They had land but not cash, and their good names allowed them access to lines of credit. Their future, planters believed, lay in a continued intensive monoculture economy that would allow them to sell their crops at a profit in order to continue to invest in property, increasing their status and wealth. In order to achieve this, planters panted after slave labor. Timothy Ford, an observer of South Carolina society noted in his diary that planters "viewed their forlorn situation as the prelude of their speedy ruin unless they immediately availed themselves . . . on some mode of procuring negroes."[22] The only way for these same men to procure enslaved people was to rely on credit beyond their means to pay off their debts. If their debts were called in, planters faced the prospect of ruin. Just like Hill and the other mobbing men in Grimke's courtroom, planters did not want the court to punish them for their financial hardship because that could mean the end of their good name, so vital to keeping the illusion of wealth and status in place. Through their inaction in the courthouse, an inaction that had baffled Grimke, they argued that their pursuit of happiness and the creation of a rational state and economy stood on human property and the exploitation of unfree labor and thus also on the stoppage of the court which allowed them to continue to acquire enslaved people.[23]

While Hill and his followers' main purpose was to continue to hold onto their means of production in order to eke out a living from the soil, the planters' main purpose was to continue to hold onto the framework of a hierarchical society that kept them at the top, a framework that rested on the foundation of slavery. Their American Revolution, the history of which they revised to suit their purposes, was a revolution that protected all forms of property from government interference. In Lunenburg County, Virginia, petitioners made this connection plain. Because of the war, the petition stated, Virginians were "happily possess'd of all the rational rights of freedom" which included the sacred rights of property."

To our ears, nothing sounds more irrational than American men and women who had earlier crafted a rhetoric of resistance based on the rejection of being made slaves by British policy, turning immediately to an equally powerful rhetoric that linked their own liberty to the brutal exploitation of slave labor. Proslavery Americans, however, argued that there was nothing more rational and scientific than this stance. They turned to existing tropes of biological difference and developed them further, strengthening the foundation of an American form of racism that embedded slavery into the new nation for many generations to come. Proslavery whites also played on Americans' anxiety in an unstable time, arguing that any threat to slavery unleashed further possibility of disorder. As the Lunenberg County petitioners wrote, any movement toward emancipation was misguided madness prompted by "the chimerical Flights of a fanatic Spirit."[24] After all, they argued, freed people were dangerous, criminal, and disorderly and therefore posed even further danger to the new nation. Slavery kept this criminal element in check according to those invested in buying enslaved people and exploiting their labor. Grimke's informants could not have articulated the layers of experience and desire that lay behind their lack of action and Grimke did not understand what shaped his frustrating experience. The lower sort wanted a chance at economic liberty, the upper sort wanted to keep in place an unequal society with slavery at its foundation, and both these groups saw the courts as an enemy to liberty.

With examples like this before them, more conservative Americans like Ford worried that the war and the ensuing depression had unleashed anarchy. In New Jersey, Joseph Lewis wrote in his diary, "A spirit of rebellion or uneasiness subsists in the greatest part of the community," but hoped the "the most thinking part of the society" would realize they could not operate outside the law.[25] In his correspondence with his fellow Massachusetts citizen Theodore Sedgwick, Rufus King wrote that perhaps the leaders had placed too much faith in the people. If it turned out that people were not virtuous, "and not governed by any internal Restraints of Conscience," that is, if they continued to exist in a state of nature, then there was "far too much reason to fear, that the Framers of our constitutions, & laws have proceeded on principles that do not exist."[26] Or, as Sedgwick then wrote to his wife Pamela that without a reform in government, nothing more than "accident will determine the state of our future existence."[27]

The thought that the future would be determined by accident rather than choice terrified Sedgwick and others. After all, one of the attractions for independence had been the possibility that they could "begin the world over again," as Paine had argued in 1776. In *Common Sense*, Paine conjectured that creating a government based on "the legal voice of the people in Congress" meant Americans had the opportunity "to form the noblest, purest constitution on the face of the earth." Instead, by 1786, Sedgwick and others found the new governments far from noble and, in particular, were terrified that these governments coped poorly with the financial difficulties that followed the war. Sedgwick wrote that their state of Massachusetts felt "pressed with an almost intolerable burden of taxes."[28] Other states felt the hardship along with Massachusetts. From South Carolina, David Ramsay wrote to a friend that "the madness of speculation & the weakness of government had made his state "a theatre of discontent & confusion."[29] Even if individuals wanted to pay their new taxes, there was little currency with which to do so. With no solution, Sedgwick worried, "how easily are . . . [the] passions agitated even to a degree of frenzy." Made sick by the disease of economic worry and the subsequent rise of emotion, the passions became a disease agent infecting the body politic. The new nation was in desperate need of a physician to bring it back to health.

The medicine most needed for the United States to survive was for the new nation to pay its debts. In a 1786 Fourth of July oration, lawyer Jonathan Austin spun out the worst-case scenario. If the government did not pay back the money it had borrowed during the war, no credit would be extended in the future. This would make it impossible for the economy to ever prosper. The extension of credit went hand-in-hand with the circulation of specie. Paper money could not substitute for specie; as experience had shown, paper money deepened the financial crisis. Austin concluded that if the United States continued along this path, it would "occasion, in many instances, excessive usury, and finally plunge such a government into the greatest distress."[30] Once plunged into distress, the danger was that rational government would dissolve. What would be left in the aftermath of this dissolution was anyone's guess, but Americans hypothesized everything from the madness and confusion of anarchy to the establishment of a fully tyrannical state.

The worst of the disease in the body politic came in the late summer of 1786 in Massachusetts in an uprising that became known as Shays's Rebellion. Massachusetts merchants, initially optimistic about their chances of competing in the world of transatlantic trade had overextended themselves. When British merchants called in their debts from their American counterparts, American merchants tried to collect debts from their consumers. However, there was not enough circulating specie to make this possible. As historian David P. Szatmary has shown, "merchants increasingly chose legal action" and turned to the courts to recover money owed to them. Almost a third of the men in Hampshire County in western Massachusetts were involved in debt cases in the years from 1784 to 1786.[31] To make matters worse, in 1785 the Massachusetts legislature levied an additional property tax to raise funds to help pay off the commonwealth's share of war debt. For western Massachusetts farmers, these actions signaled total financial ruin. They could no longer rely on barter or delayed payment as they traditionally had because the courts and their government demanded payment in hard currency.

Daniel Shays was one of the leaders of the rebellion, a Revolutionary War veteran who did not believe the world that emerged after the war was the world for which he and others had fought. Shays's Rebellion began like other rebellions had. Individuals feeling overburdened with taxes they could not pay and in danger of losing their land and therefore their livelihood, began to hold conventions and then to stop the courts from hearing foreclosure cases. For Shays and others, debt relief rather than debt foreclosure was the obvious cure for their disease that was ravaging the body politic. Old Plough Jogger wrote that he had been ruined by the taxes forced upon him. "I have been obliged to pay and nobody will pay me," he wrote. As far as he could tell, the poor suffered while the rich, or the "great men," got "all we have." Old Plough Jogger figured that "it is time for us to rise and to put a stop to it." Revolutionary language had promised no free man would be made a slave through the economic policies of a government based on the consent of the governed yet here were hardworking Massachusetts farmers being crushed under the tyrannical heel of the men in power.

Old Plough Jogger was not alone. Even some better off citizens like Dr. William Whiting, who was both a physician and the Chief Justice of Berkshire County Court of Common Pleas, saw injustice when he looked at the government's policies. He believed the anger of the people against the government of Massachusetts was justified. Unlike many of the better sort, Whiting did not see any unruly mob when he looked at the protesters. Instead, he saw hardworking farmers and mechanics who, for no fault of their own, could not pay their debts. He characterized them as "the poor and most Laborious part of the people" who started life with little or nothing but now faced harassment and injustice. He reasoned that "it is much Better that the Courts of Law Should be Suspended until" the system should be examined and "Remedied."[32] Instead of a rush to judgment or punitive measures, Whiting advocated for a reasoned and deliberative approach, one that would bring the systems back to health rather than causing further harm.

The government refused to take Whiting's advice and continued the path of court seizures of property for nonpayment of debt. For some of the Massachusetts citizens faced with financial ruin, the only path was to seize control of local governments as a way to register protest as they had during the era of the Coercive Acts. In some counties, men called county conventions and spoke out against the Massachusetts government. Like the colonists in the 1760s and 1770s, they believed their actions lawful, conforming to the long-standing tradition of regulation. They hoped they could bring the government back to good health and away from disorder and the disease caused by unpayable taxes. In the conventions they held, these men denounced mob actions but also addressed their grievances forthrightly, condemning the lack of circulating money, "abuses in the practice of the law," overly high salaries for elected officials, and other problems. They petitioned their government for redress but when there was little or no movement to meaningfully address their complaints, some of these citizens willingly took the next step toward more militant action.

In August of 1786, approximately 1500 men, some of them armed, assembled to prevent the Court of Common Pleas from sitting in Northampton, Massachusetts. In September, protesters prevented five more courts from sitting. Governor James Bowdoin was outraged. To Bowdoin these actions were a "high-handed offence" that "must tend to subvert all law and government, to dissolve our excellent constitution, and introduce universal riot, anarchy and confusion, which would probably terminate in absolute despotism, and consequently destroy the fairest prospects of political happiness that any people was ever favored with."[33] He feared that the actions taken to shut down the courts would escalate and that these actions had the potential to bring down the government of the commonwealth and perhaps the government of the United States. James Bowdoin and the legislature took measures to stop this from happening but, just like Thomas Gage's actions in 1775, their actions made matters worse rather than better. After warrants were issued for the arrest of some of the leading protesters and a posse not only chased down but wounded Job Shattuck, some of the protest leaders began to call for the overthrow of the "tyrannical government of Massachusetts."[34]

In the face of this crisis, the physician tending the body politic needed to be able to find a cure that would not destroy the body in the meantime. William Whiting continued to believe he had the solution. As a doctor and a judge he might be able to "Soothe and Quiet" the protesters before their actions got out of hand as he would soothe and quiet a fever patient to try to work a cure. He wrote a long piece entitled, "Some Remarks on the Conduct of the Inhabitants of the Commonwealth of Massachusetts in Interrupting the Sitting of the Judicial Courts in Several Counties in the State." In this address, Whiting used his doctorly knowledge to analyze the situation around him. He first addressed the lawmakers, writing that their governments were "Very Subject to feverish fits, to Caprice Petulance and Wrangling with each other." Government in this case acted as a disease conduit rather than soothing and curing, setting politicians against one another in damaging ways. Whiting warned the "Political Physicians" that heroic medicine, and particularly bloodletting, would worsen the disease and therefore they should instead rely on "Light Medicines and moderate Correction." However, as a man of the better sort, while Whiting could sympathize with the frustration of the debtors, he also feared a system in which the people subverted the rule of law. He understood the impulse toward holding conventions and believed the people had the constitutional right to take that step, but thought that it was a step taken in error. In addressing the people, he asked them, "Immediately to Desist, and pursue only those Legal and peaceable measures for obtaining the Redress of your Grievances." Ever the physician, he likened the thirteen demands of the Worcester County Convention to thirteen different pills. If they were "Crammed into our General [Court] at once" they would make the "political Distemper" worse because each one of the pills was created to target a different element of the illness and that each needed to be given time to act on that element. The pills would work better in "Smaller Doses and at proper intervals," so that the body politic could digest them and they could work a cure.[35]

While Dr. Whiting believed the insurrectionists had just cause for complaint, other Americans disagreed. Theodore Sedgwick felt personally attacked by Whiting's analysis that the rich and powerful had used their "Power by Compulsion to enrich themselves by the same means that impoverishes and depresses some other Orders of people" and were therefore largely to blame for the troubles. Sedgwick believed Whiting's stance helped further the madness in the body politic. He wrote a long letter to Whiting censuring him for neglecting his duty "to the happiness and prosperity of his country." In Sedgwick's opinion, Whiting "condescend[ed] meanly to sacrifice" the country's happiness "to a momentary popularity arising from the frenzy of the times." Whiting was in error if he believed his essay would "sooth [sic] and quiet the turbulence of" the people's "already heated passions."[36] To Sedgwick, Whiting was neither an upstanding politician nor a competent doctor. Instead of curing the patient, Sedgwick believed he sickened it further.

Elite men took to print to argue over why some Massachusetts citizens were in revolt while the convention-goers tried to convince anyone who would listen that they were good, hardworking people. They had a hard task before them as evidenced by the large number of personal and private writings from 1786 to 1787 that condemned the protesters for their immorality and lack of reason. Noah Webster, writing as Tom Thoughtful, started one piece by reminding his readers, "That the political body, like the animal, is liable to violent diseases." However, the patient, in this case the body politic, was to blame for its illness because "most of the disorder, incident to the human frame, are the consequence of an intemperate indulgence of its appetites."[37] Webster's piece reflected the prevailing rhetoric that the western farmers did not suffer because of an unjust system or because designing men corrupted by power lined their own pockets at the expense of the poor. According to Webster, these farmers suffered because of their overconsumption of goods which ran them into debt and because of their laziness which prevented them from making enough to pay their debts like any good citizen should. Sampson Rea agreed that while "their taxes comes hard upon them," if they only "should adopt a way of living that would tend more upon economy," they would find a way to pay those debts.[38]

Webster, Rea, and others placed the blame for the financial troubles not on new and relatively untried governments bound to make mistakes, but on the habits of the people within the commonwealth. In October 1786, the town of Haverhill, Massachusetts circulated a letter in the wake of a town meeting. The writers understood that the times were troubled and felt the grievances "in common with our fellow citizens," but they also believed that there were constitutional remedies available. Because there were remedies available, the troubles were made worse by the bad behavior of some citizens. They traced the grievances to "luxurious, dissipated living," to "idleness, . . . [and] want of temperance, honesty, industry, frugality and economy." Anyone who believed otherwise was delusional, a madman who had been led in an improper direction by "the arts and intrigues of wicked and designing men." If they turned to "a cool and dispassionate consideration of the evil consequences of such measures," government could continue to work for a solution.[39] Or, as an anonymous writer argued in a letter to the *Hampshire Gazette*, the rebellion was like a disease "in the head." The only solution was to remove the disease, otherwise the rebellion "may bring on political dissolution."[40]

From his home in Virginia, George Washington read about these tumults with alarm. He wrote to General Benjamin Lincoln in Massachusetts, "Are your people getting mad? Are we to have the goodly fabrick that eight years were spent in rearing pulled over our heads?"[41] The specter of disorder and irrationality in the nation Washington had helped create terrified him. Lincoln replied that "the State is convulsed, and the bands of government, in some parts of it, are cast off." He then directly responded to Washington's question, "Are your people getting mad?" Lincoln answered, "Many of them appear to be absolutely so, if an attempt to annihilate our present constitution and dissolve the present government can be considered as evidence of insanity."[42] Only madness could explain the protesters' response to a government truly based on the consent of the governed. For Washington, Lincoln, and others, the growing rebellion could portend a downfall of the republic, a destruction of their experiment, and a destruction of a social order which made sense to them. The author of a song published in the *Worcester Magazine* in 1787 mocked the Massachusetts rebels. For the author it was ridiculous that: "The mobmen shall rule, and the great men obey." It would lead to "The world upon wheels shall be all set agog/ And blockheads and knaves hail the reign of king log."[43]

The world was set agog, but perhaps a course of governmental interventions could help set it right again. Like the British diplomats who came to negotiate peace in 1778, the Massachusetts General Court tried a combination of gentle and heroic medicine to cure the body politic. They suspended the writ of habeas corpus but also offered amnesty to those who would distance themselves from the rebellion and pledge fealty to the commonwealth. Although some regulators came in from the (literal) cold, for those who supported the government even the gentle measures seemed to make things worse. On November 25, 1786 Governor Bowdoin issued a proclamation to that effect. The gentle measures "(instead of giving quiet to the mal-contents) have been added to their catalogue of grievances, and furnished them with new pretentions of complaint."[44] Because of this, Bowdoin concluded, the gentle medicine would not work. Bowdoin and others thought it was clear that the leaders of the insurrection were bent on destroying government altogether and had laid out a clear path to anarchy. The only solution was bleeding in the form of military action.

Black freemason Prince Hall offered his and his brothers' services to take part in any military campaign directed toward the rebels. In a letter to Governor Bowdoin, Hall wrote that he and his masonic brothers were "willing to help support, as far as our weak and feeble abilities may be necessary in this time of trouble and confusion."[45] Bowdoin ignored this offer of service without giving a reason. Historian Sidney Kaplan tackled the question of why the offer was ignored, but could only speculate that armed black men mustering together was a frightening idea not just in the slave-intensive states in the south but in Massachusetts as well. At the same time that Massachusetts dealt with their small-scale civil war between white residents, the British colony of Dominica faced slave rebellion, a fact that was widely reported in New England's newspapers. Consciously or unconsciously the fear of armed black men and the imagined consequences thereof may have played a part in Bowdoin's equation.

In the midst of mustering troops and small-scale guerrilla warfare, conspiracy theories of various kinds abounded about the motives of Daniel Shays and the other insurgents. The most generous of the conspiracy theorists were those who tapped into the eighteenth-century ideology about the corruptibility of the impoverished. While these poor men and women were obviously deluded, they were not to blame for they could not think for themselves and therefore had been led down a path to madness by the words and actions of powerful "corrupt and designing men."[46] Poor people were corruptible, according to this theory, because their poverty made them open to bribery or other incentives. As John Adams had written in 1776, the poor were "too dependent upon other men to have a will of their own."[47] The poor had been led astray by a group of corrupt men who "having no Character, or Property to lose, mean to bring on Riot, Confusion, Injustice, and Civil War."[48] These designing men were levelers bent on abolishing distinctions, including distinctions created by property ownership.

Another strain of conspiracy theory argued that the British were behind the rebellion, that they rankled the passions of some to destroy the possibility of success for the new nation. While British ministers certainly paid close attention to the rebellion and considered military aid, this conspiracy ignored the fact that the insurgents needed no provocation from outside. Their beef with the government was born out of pre-revolutionary protest and then reborn at the end of a war that had promised much but had failed in fulfilling those promises. The conspiracy theorists concluded, however, that British agents offered financial reward to those who "have rather get their living in any other way, than be obliged to obtain it by industry." To the writer Publicus, the men who participated had either been loyalists during the war or were poor men who wanted to avoid the payment of debt.[49] An acrostic that spelled out "INSURGENTS" characterized the participants in a number of ways. The I in insurgent was for "Insolvent debtors, aiming ne'er to pay." And the T was for "The vicious ign'rant herd." The acrostic's composer did acknowledge that some of the protesters might be honest, but most were "deluded fools."[50] Those deluded fools had upset the commonwealth. Only time would tell "where popular Tempest will carry us." While "the Disease [might] produce its own Cure" it could also "end in the total Overthrow of Liberties of the People."[51]

Like with other diseases, including the diseases of the head, the delusion and acts "of madness and extreme folly" exhibited by those closing the courts were catching. The insurgents used the economic depression to lend an air of legitimacy to their protests, but according to their opponents, they exaggerated the badness of the government with false reports. A letter appeared in the *Worcester Magazine,* in which the author claimed he had been one of the protesters but had come to his senses. He had been deluded but had since regained reason and accepted that the present government and lawful authority were the answers he had sought. He saw that while he and others were aggrieved "in some instances," that the folly and madness of those who shut down the courts exacerbated the problems and allowed them to spread.[52] Unless friends to government could put a stop to this uprising, the republican experiment would fail. They needed to administer a course of medicine to the body politic that would cure the disease.

Bowdoin called on sanctioned militia leaders to form divisions to move against the rebellion.[53] At the end of the year, Samuel Savage wrote in his diary, "our greatest Calamity has been among ourselves—an unnatural Insurrection hath been raised in the County of Berkshire, Hampshire, Worcester, Middlesex and Bristol by a no. of cruel and unreasonable men headed by a Sheriff." His language is telling. The insurrection was "unnatural." It was a monstrous stillbirth that would be recorded but then, he hoped, buried. The leaders were unreasonable men who needed to be killed or confined. In January 1787, Governor Bowdoin put General Benjamin Lincoln in charge of the Massachusetts militia. Faced with the might of an organized military response, in the bitter cold of winter and without proper resources, many of the insurgents accepted amnesty. Some continued to fight and were killed or captured. Thousands of the insurgents, including Shays, managed to escape into Vermont, New Hampshire, or New York where they remained uncaptured and, in some cases, continued guerrilla attacks on prominent leaders in western Massachusetts.

The men who were captured and put on trial for taking part in the insurrection were charged with treason, as traitors to both the government and the people. According to their charges, they had renounced their allegiance to the commonwealth and to the United States and levied a war "with design to subvert the Government." Those charging them with crimes believed their goal had been to "reduce the Inhabitants to lawless power, Anarchy & confusion." As the insurrection was put down and men were arrested for their part in it, some outsiders to the insurrection pled for leniency. In early February 1787, the town of Princeton sent a petition to the Massachusetts Senate and House. While the petition denounced the actions of those who had taken part in the insurrection, it acknowledged that real hardship had motivated the men who had joined. These men had been made temporarily mad while "under the Influence of an impetuous Tempest heated Imagination," but now that they were restored to rationality, the petitioners hoped that the court "would extend the Benefits of Indemnity to those unhappy misguided Offenders."[54] In fact, most of the men who came to trial in early April of 1787 were acquitted. As Justice Increase Sumner wrote to his wife, most pleaded guilty to "Crimes *below treason*," and were then "pardon'd on Condition of their Exertions to promote order & good Gov[ernmen]t."[55] Thirteen total men were charged and sentenced to death. Only two men, John Bly and Charles Rose were hanged; the others were eventually pardoned.

What is sometimes lost to us in the classroom telling of Shays's Rebellion are the voices of those who were not profligate and deluded men but had real grievances they thought they could redress in the same ways they had in the 1760s and early 1770s. Their opponents dismissed their complaints, attacking the characters of the regulators or arguing that they now had a government that recognized their sovereignty. According to this version, the men in power were "Their own rulers, whom they themselves raised to power," or, in other words, the Revolution had built a social compact truly based on the consent of the governed.[56] The men who called themselves regulators saw it differently. In their version, the members of the General Court did not represent or listen to them but were bent on filling jails with debtors. In December 1786, some of those who had taken up arms wrote that the tactic of jailing debtors made it impossible for men to participate in their communities or the economy. As men in power condemned the early conventions, George Brock, an Attleborough farmer took to his pen, defending the conventioneers as patriotic war veterans, prosecuted simply "for daring to inquire into the present gross mismanagement in our rules." The regulators were hardworking people who had "their hard earned property taken from them by excessive rates," and like the Irish who were oppressed by their English landlords, were expected to "live wholly on skimmed Milk & Potatoes."[57]

The government had suspended the writ of habeas corpus, one sign of a growing tyranny. With this step, those in positions of power found they held that power with few limits and therefore they could use it to prosecute their enemies "from a principle of revenge, hatred and envy."[58] The regulators were not loyalists, working to bring Britain back to North America, they were standing up, again, against an oppressive government and doing what they could to support and secure a republic. When they petitioned the Governor, they insisted they were "not of the wicked, dissolute and abandoned," but were working to provide for their wives and children. In an unsigned letter in the Robert Treat Paine papers at the Massachusetts Historical Society, a writer compared the wealthy to millers, except instead of grinding grain, they "have been grinding the faces & estates of ye poor people."[59] John Healy's April 1787 testimony in front of Judge Sumner recounted a conversation from the previous October with Jacob Chamberlain about closing the courts. According to Healy, Chamberlain had said the regulators, "were not too rash in taking up Arms." After all, "the poor were dying & they had as good die one way or another." They were dying because, "Great ones" were "eating up little ones . . . [and] if they didn't carry their points the poorer sort of people would be undone." Others spoke of their Captain, Henry Gale, who convinced men to join the regulation because "the Salvation of the State depended upon a rising of the people to stop the Courts and make an Alteration in the times."[60] Gale and others exhorted those who joined that they would be crafting a more just future, one that would not trample the rights and financial solubility of ordinary people.

What Gale and others imagined remains part of the legacy of the American Revolution, a vision of a more just future where the poor as well as the rich have rights and governmental support. But at the time powerful men shaped the narrative to reject those who envisioned the future in this way as deluded at the very least and madmen at the extreme. Park Holland gave one of the more gentle interpretations of these events in his 1832 hand-written memoir. He had served with Daniel Shays during the Revolution and knew him to be a good and brave soldier. In 1786 and 1787, however, Holland believed Shays's followers were misled. As a Grand Jury-man during the trials, Holland had to focus on their misdeeds although he could also summon sympathy. Whatever his feelings at the time, almost half a century later it was that sympathy he remembered. He could relate to the men in front of him charged with the blackest crimes but would rather "remember the *good service* they rendered their country than dwell upon what historians have set down as a *black spot* upon this country's pages." He reminded his reader or readers that "our government was a *new untried ship*, with many joints that needed oiling to say the least—no chart of *experience* to guide us nor map of the past by which to lay our course."[61] Decades later, Holland acknowledged that the path Shays and his followers marched along was one of the many possible paths available to a new nation with new and unstable governments in place.

While Holland could summon sympathy in 1832, in 1787 many Americans could not. The future Henry Gale and others imagined frightened the great ones. The trial testimony provided evidence to those who had argued for a stronger national government from the beginning of the war for independence that those who rose against the republican governments were men who wanted to bring the commonwealth and country into a state of anarchy and erase the distinctions in society. These Americans wanted to crush this alternative vision and replace it with a different one, one that still contained deference, due submission, and order. For these Americans, the crushing of the rebellion and the establishment of a more centralized and powerful government were the medicines for which the ailing body politic called.

NOTES

1. Phillis Wheatley, "Liberty and Peace, a Poem" (Boston: Warden and Russell, 1784), Evans Early American Imprint Collection.
2. Mercy Otis Warren, Milton Hill, to Abigail Adams, April 30, 1785. In Richard Alan Ryerson et al., *Adams Family Correspondence*, Vol. 6 (Cambridge: The Belknap Press of Harvard University Press, 1993), 114.
3. Richard Price, *Observations on the Importance of the American Revolution, and the Means of Making it a Benefit to the World* (Boston: Powars and Willis, 1784), Evans Early American Imprints.
4. Benjamin Rush, *Medical Inquiries and Observations* (Philadelphia: Prichard & Hall, 1789), 196, Evans Early American Imprint Collection.
5. Letter from Abigail Adams to John Adams, June 20, 1783 [electronic edition]. *Adams Family Papers: An Electronic Archive*. Massachusetts Historical Society. http://www.masshist.org/digitaladams/
6. Samuel Osgood to John Adams, December 7, 1783 in Gregg L. Lint et al., eds, *The Adams Papers, Papers of John Adams*, Vol. 15 (Cambridge: Harvard University Press, 2010), 398–414.
7. Eliga Gould writes about treaty worthiness in *Among the Powers of the Earth: The American Revolution and the Making of a New World Empire* (Cambridge: Harvard University Press, 2014).
8. Timothy Ford, "Diary of Timothy Ford, 1785–1786," *South Carolina Historical and Genealogical Magazine* 13, no. 3 (July 1912): 196, 202, https://www.jstor.org/stable/pdf/27575338.pdf.
9. Benjamin Hichborn, *An Oration, Delivered July 5th, 1784 at the Request of the Inhabitants of the Town of Boston; in Celebration of the Anniversary of American Independence* (Boston: John Gill, 1784), Evans Early American Imprint Collection.
10. George Washington, *A Circular Letter, from His Excellency George Washington, Commander in Chief of the Armies of the United States of America; Addressed to the Governors of the Several States, on His Resigning the Command of the Army, and Retiring from Public Business* (Philadelphia: Robert Smith, Jr., 1783), Evans Early American Imprint Collection.
11. William Samuel Johnson to Benjamin Gale, February 2, 1785, in Smith, ed., *Letters of Delegates of Congress*.
12. Martin, *A Narrative of a Revolutionary Soldier*, 243.
13. "Proclamation for the Cessation of Hostilities, April 18, 1783," *Founders Online, National Archives*, last modified June 13, 2018, http://founders.archives.gov/documents/Washington/99-01-02-11104.
14. "The Address and Petition of the Officers of the Army of the United States," April 1783, *A Century of Lawmaking for a New Nation: U.S. Congressional Documents and Debates, 1774-1875*, memory.loc.gov/ammem/amlaw/lawhome.html.
15. Quoted in *The Spirit of Seventy-Six*, 1283.
16. *The American Museum, or, Repository of Ancient and Modern Fugitive Pieces, &c. Prose and Poetical, for January, 1787*, Vol. 1 (Philadelphia: Carey, Stewart, and Co., 1790), 304.

17. Nicole Eustace, "Emotion and Political Change," in *Doing Emotions History* (Champaign: University of Illinois Press, 2014), 165.

18. George Washington, "Newburgh Address," https://www.mountvernon.org/education/primary-sources-2/article/newburgh-address-george-washington-to-officers-of-the-army-march-15-1783/.

19. Kariann Akemi Yokota, *Unbecoming British: How Revolutionary American Became a Postcolonial Nation* (New York: Oxford University Press, 2011).

20. Thomas Arnold, *Observations on the Nature, Kinds, Causes, and Prevention of Insanity, Lunacy, or Madness*, Vol. I (Leicester: G. Ireland, 1782), 21, https://archive.org/details/b21440712_001.

21. Quoted in David P. Szatmary, *Shays' Rebellion: The Making of an Agrarian Insurrection* (Amherst: University of Massachusetts Press, 1980), 125.

22. "Diary of Timothy Ford," 194.

23. The classic work on this is Edmund S. Morgan, *American Slavery, American Freedom* (New York: W.W. Norton & Company, 1975).

24. "The Remonstrance and Petition of the free Inhabitants of the County of Lunenberg," in Fredrika Teute Schmidt and Barbara Ripel Wilhelm, "Early Proslavery Petitions in Virginia," *William and Mary Quarterly* 30 (1973): 141–143, https://www.jstor.org/stable/1923706.

25. "The Diary of Joseph Lewis," *Proceedings of the New Jersey Historical Society* 60 (January 1942): 61.

26. Rufus King, New York, to Theodore Sedgwick, October 22, 1786. Sedgwick Family Papers. Massachusetts Historical Society.

27. Theodore Sedgwick to Pamela Sedgwick, June 24, 1786, Sedgwick Family Papers, Massachusetts Historical Society.

28. Theodore Sedgwick, New York, to Pamela Sedgwick, June 24, 1786. Sedgwick Family Papers. Massachusetts Historical Society.

29. Quoted in Huw David, *Trade, Politics, and Revolution: South Carolina and Britain's Atlantic Commerce, 1730–1790* (Columbia: University of South Carolina Press, 2018), 155.

30. Jonathan L. Austin, *An Oration, Delivered July 4, 1786, at the Request of the Inhabitants of the Town of Boston, in Celebration of the Anniversary of American Independence* (Boston: Peter Edes, 1786), 14, Evans Early American Imprint Collection.

31. Szatmary, *Shays' Rebellion*, 29.

32. Quoted in Stephen T. Riley, "Dr. William Whiting and Shays' Rebellion," *Proceedings of the American Antiquarian Society* 66 (1956): 135, https://www.americanantiquarian.org/proceedings/44539282.pdf.

33. James Bowdoin, "A Proclamation," reprinted in *The New-Haven Gazette, and the Connecticut Magazine* September 14, 1786, 1, 31. *American Periodicals*, p. 242.

34. Quoted in Szatmary, *Shays' Rebellion*, 97.

35. Riley, "Dr. William Whiting," 159.

36. Riley, "Dr. William Whiting," 137.

37. Tom Thoughtful [Noah Webster], "The Devil is in You," *Worcester Magazine* 2 (November 1786): 382.

38. Sampson Rea, Philadelphia, to Samuel Phillips Savage, November 21, 1786. Lemuel Shaw Papers. Massachusetts Historical Society.

39. Quoted in George Wingate Chase, *The History of Haverhill, Massachusetts* (Haverhill: New England History Press and the Haverhill Historical Society, 1983, originally printed in 1861), 437.

40. Letter to the Editor, *Hampshire Gazette*, February 14, 1787. http://shaysrebellion.stcc.edu/shaysapp/artifact.do?shortName=gazette_dg27dec86.

41. George Washington to Benjamin Lincoln, November 7, 1786 in W. W. Abbot, ed., *The Papers of George Washington*, Confederation Series, Vol. 4 (Charlottesville: University Press of Virginia, 1995), 339.

42. Benjamin Lincoln to George Washington, in Abbot, ed., *The Papers of George Washington*, 418.

43. "A Song for the Massachusetts Insurgents," reprinted in *The American Museum, or, Repository of Ancient and Modern Fugitive Pieces, &c., Prose and Poetical, for January, 1787*, Vol. 1 (Philadelphia: Carey, Steward, and Co., 1790), 485.

44. James Bowdoin, *A Proclamation* (Boston, 1786), https://shaysrebellion.stcc.edu/shaysapp.

45. Quoted in Corey D. B. Walker, *A Noble Fight: African American Freemasonry and the Struggle for Democracy in America* (Champaign: University of Illinois Press, 2008), 78.

46. "Circular Letter," *Boston Gazette*, September 18, 1783.

47. John Adams to James Sullivan, May 26, 1776 in Charles Francis Adams, ed., *The Works of John Adams, Second President of the United States* (Boston: Little, Brown, and Company, 1854).

48. "To the Free, Virtuous, and Independent Electors of Massachusetts (Boston, 1787).

49. Publicus, "From the *Independent Chronicle*," reprinted in the *Hampshire Gazette* 20 September 1786.

50. "A Crostick" *Hampshire Gazette*, June 6, 1787, http://shaysrebellion.stcc.edu/shaysapp/artifact.do?shortName=gazette_crostick6jun87.

51. "The Free, Virtuous, and Independent Electors of Massachusetts."

52. Letter to the Editor, *Worcester Magazine*, January 1787, Massachusetts Historical Society.

53. James Bowdoin, "Commonwealth of Massachusetts," November 25, 1786. Israel Keith Collection, Massachusetts Historical Society.

54. Petition from the town of Princeton, February 1, 1787. Shays Rebellion Collection. Clements Library.

55. Increase Sumner to Elizabeth Sumner, April 8, 1787. Amory Family Papers. Massachusetts Historical Society.

56. "From the Independent Chronicle."

57. George Brock, "To the Yeomanry of Massachusetts." Copy in the Robert Treat Paine papers, Massachusetts Historical Society.

58. "An Address to the People of the Several Towns in the County of Hampshire, from the Body Now at Arms," December 7, 1786.

59. Robert Treat Paine Papers, Massachusetts Historical Society.

60. Testimony of Eli Allen, Amory Family Papers, Massachusetts Historical Society.

61. Park Holland, handwritten memoir, 1832, Holland Family Papers. Massachusetts Historical Society. Emphases in the original.

Chapter 7

"The Temple of Tyranny Has Two Doors," 1787–1791

In 1783, with the Paris Peace Treaty ratified, Thomas Paine had exalted that "The times that tried men's souls are over and the greatest and completest revolution the world ever knew, gloriously and happily accomplished."[1] By 1787, however, many Americans believed that the times still tried men's souls and that the revolution was far from complete. In that year, Benjamin Rush published an address to the American people that was widely reprinted, cautioning his fellow citizens that while they had won the war for independence, the revolution was ongoing. He reassured his readers that the bumps that Americans had experienced in the four years since the definitive peace treaty had been signed, while serious, were to be expected. After all, during the war Americans had been so focused on defeating the British and winning their independence that laying the foundation for a good government had been secondary. Rush reminded his readers that at the time, "the British army was in the heart of our country, spreading desolation wherever it went." While the states and the nation had crafted new governments to see them through the war, these governments' first priority had been shutting the door on the British system. Reacting to the circumstances, "we forgot that the temple of tyranny has two doors." According to Rush, they had bolted the door against monarchy but neglected "to guard against the effects of our own ignorance and licentiousness."[2] For men like Rush, the four years that followed the war had brought incidents of ignorance and licentiousness to the fore in states like Massachusetts. He believed it was past time to bolt that door as well. In a time of relative peace, the people had the opportunity to sit down and coolly deliberate, to come up with a better solution to governance.

Rush repeated a conservative orthodoxy when he presented his analysis of the world around him. Like others, he found the post-war world unsettling and saw the experiment that was the United States in danger of failing. In 1787,

Noah Webster delivered a lecture series on American attitudes and manners that reinforces for us that the attitude Rush had articulated was prevalent in some circles. In words almost identical to Rush's, Webster told his audience that it was a "fundamental mistake" of the Americans that they "considered the revolution as completed when it was but just begun." They had only "raised the pillars of the building," and then "ceased to exert themselves and seemed to forget that the whole superstructure was then to be erected."[3] The words of Rush, Webster, and others like them reflected one American worldview that emphasized the dangers of democracy and the threats of anarchy, a world view where the people needed to be kept in check and proper leaders put in place. Webster and Rush were two of the many American men and women who distrusted the ways that the American Revolution, despite its conservative elements, had unsettled the natural order of things.

The Revolution had not turned the world upside down but it had tilted it sideways. For conservative Americans, the sideways tilt was apparent in the off-kilter economy and the accompanying protests and insurrections, in the presence of new and unpolished men assuming the trappings of political power, and in "female politicians" among other phenomena. As historian Charlene Boyer Lewis has written, "Americans had to rethink the relationship of the self not only to a new nation, but also to a new society and changing family."[4] The allegedly leveling Shaysites were the clearest symbol of this world tilt but other symbols were everywhere as conservatives found that they had created not only an independent nation but also a nation where older rules of behavior were rewritten or disappeared. For the nation to be mended, they believed, the economy needed to be fixed, the poorer sort needed to defer to the better sort, fathers needed to rule within the household, and women needed to remain within what Mercy Otis Warren called, "The Narrow Bounds prescrib'd to Female Life/ The Gentle Mistress and the Prudent Wife."[5] Instead, the economy remained broken and patriarchal authority was challenged although not discarded.

Conservative Americans could make peace with the tilted world if they altered their readings of the changes around them in a way that allowed them to see a more sane and rational reality behind deceptive appearances. One example comes to us from Elkanah Watson who, in 1786, was disconcerted by his initial reading of events at a local polling place only to learn that order and deference had not been overthrown as he had suspected. An outsider, and not eligible to vote in the local election, Watson was interested in the political culture of the town he visited. As he made his way through the polling place, Watson was astonished when "the most obese woman I ever had seen . . . appeared to be an active leader at the polls."[6] To him, both her size and her role as an active player in the male sphere of politics was a grotesque mockery of the political system. It was at least a laughable if not a horrifying symbol of the new political world the American Revolution had created. Coming upon one of his acquaintances, Watson expressed his dismay at what he had seen. His acquaintance did not respond to Watson's astonishment but invited Watson to visit him at his home. The next day Watson showed up at his acquaintance's house where he found that the obese woman was a respected member of the family. What Watson learned, however, was that this woman did not represent a breakdown of society. She participated at the polls with the full knowledge and confidence of one of the leading families only because "she had more political influence, and exerted it with greater effect, than any man in her county."[7] She was the exception rather than the rule and therefore did not represent disorder, anarchy, madness, or the overturning of society but was simply a remarkable woman who was allowed access to a process that other women were denied. In his journal, Watson reread and rewrote the situation, coming to see the woman's participation as part of an ordered, rational, and sane world. Her wealth and connections opened a door that was closed to others.

While Watson could make his peace with one female politician who occupied an elevated position in society, other men found it impossible. In Maryland, Philantropos wrote a long letter damning women in politics. He claimed that women should not be political actors because even virtuous men could not resist the power of women's sexuality. The temptations offered by women orators "might reasonably yield to what it would be hardly possible for *man* to refuse."[8] The assumption was any woman stepping into the political sphere could not possibly covenant together for the common good; instead she would be angling to overthrow societal norms and disrupt the political community. Succumbing to the wiles of these female politicians, men's sexual desire would override their reason, transforming them from rational to irrational actors. Philantropos did not, of course, question men's fitness for political life or ask if perhaps men were unfit to rule if they could be so easily maddened by the temptation of female orators.

For those Americans who had agitated for a stronger national government even before the war was over, all of the changes they witnessed and all of the things that seemed out of order added fuel to their paranoia that the republic would not last long. The "morn" of independence had "dawned more favourable," according to George Washington, but "no day was ever more clouded than the present!" If "some alteration" was not made, and quickly, "the superstructure . . . must fall."[9] From London, Abigail Adams wrote to her sister Elizabeth Shaw that she was anxious to be back in the United States for her separation from her native land meant that she always imagined the worst. Adams could not interpret the shifts and changes in the United States for herself or find comfort in the ordinariness of everyday life. Instead she only had the words in the letters her friends and family members wrote to her. The inevitable delays of correspondence and the incompleteness of the accounts fed her fears. "I have seen my Countrymen armed one against the other," she wrote, "and the divided house falling to the ground."[10] From an ocean away, she fretted that the experiment her husband helped to launch from the political sphere and that she supported with her work at home would fail. She and other Americans shared a common core of fears about the longevity and ultimate survival of their new country.

One of these fears was that "party rage," or the division of political actors into opposing camps, would destroy the republic. Rage can mean a number of things, including anger. As Nicole Eustace shows, rage also had class connotations. In the first part of the eighteenth century, the word rage "clearly signaled capitulation to passion" and was "seldom if ever used to describe the anger of an elite man or woman."[11] Rage could be tempered with reason, but the lower sort were considered less reasonable than the elite. *Party rage* indicated anger without restraint and fueled by unnecessary and dangerous political divisions. When one leveled the charge of party rage against political opponents, it indicated that they were too guided by party leaders who deluded them and led them into the mazes of error. For conservative writers, it became an easy way to paint their opponents as, at the very least, too overcome by emotion to make good decisions, and at the most extreme, madmen who threatened to unhinge society and government further. To participate in the work of government and to benefit from unalienable rights, political actors needed to be rational.

The fear of party rage had a long genealogy in the British Atlantic world. Advocates for a stronger national government often went back to pre-revolution writings of American patriots to put the weight of history behind their arguments. The *American Museum* reprinted a piece by William Livingston who had served as the governor of New Jersey during the American Revolutionary War. Well before the war, Livingston had published an essay on party divisions. According to Livingston, parties led men to "abandon their reason," and be "led captive by their passions." Parties could lead a citizen to be overly attached to a fanatical leader and then become a madman, "confirm[ed] in his delirium."[12] That the editor of the *American Museum* felt this was a fit piece to print almost forty years after it first appeared shows the prevalence of this opinion and the desire to reach back to patriotic forbears for evidence that confirmed the prejudice against parties. Americans tended to believe that, as members of parties, men ceased to act on a rational assessment of the world around them. Instead they were guided or misguided by the passions of the leaders, allowing their minds to become corrupted. That delirium or madness instead of reason would guide these party men worried them.

Party rage went hand in hand with democracy. While many Americans in this era embraced forms of democracy, conservatives believed that if democracy prevailed licentiousness would take over and the system they had fought to establish would fail. Rufus King wrote to his friend Thomas Sedgwick that he was pleased Sedgwick had been elected to the Massachusetts legislature. In the midst of Shays's Rebellion, King hoped that Sedgwick would "be able to check the madness of Democracy."[13] Sedgwick replied that all rational men would agree "that the end of Government security cannot be attained by the exercise of principles founded on democratic equality."[14] According to King and Sedgwick, during Shays's Rebellion the people had been driven mad by democracy, which led to a rage for leveling and the destruction of the distinctions of property and standing within their state. This madness had infected all ranks of government. When Sedgwick looked around at the other members of the legislature, he saw some other good and virtuous men—as he believed himself to be—but he also saw men filled with "stupidity, vice, [or] meanness." In North Carolina, men like James Hogg and James Iredell felt as if some of their political opponents were nothing more than a "set of unprincipled men" who would be pushed along by the winds of party faction. Throughout the United States, some Americans worried that stupid, mean, and unprincipled men in power would cultivate sycophants rather than working to preserve the republic

For conservative Americans with the requisite trappings of distinction like property and distinguished marriages, the democratic elements that had attended or followed the American Revolution were disease elements overturning the established order in ways that threatened the future. The decentralized nature of government under the Articles of Confederation meant that there was no larger machinery to check the madness of democracy in any of its forms. A more centralized form of government might help contain the mental illness of the body politic. Thus, an initial step in this direction came with the 1786 call for a convention in Annapolis by James Madison. Madison framed his call for a convention cautiously for he knew some Americans would see faction and cabal in a meeting of elite men outside the institution of Congress. He stated, simply, that political leaders needed to come together to stabilize the economy, a feat yet to be accomplished by the sitting Congress.

The twelve men representing five states who attended the Annapolis Convention did little more than identify some defects in the system of commercial regulations and other barriers they believed kept them from national greatness. The report from the convention acknowledged that they might have "exceed[ed] the strict bounds of their appointment," but they did so only because they were "dictated by an anxiety for the welfare, of the United States." They called for a second convention to be held in Philadelphia the next year to address the numerous and "important defects in the system of Federal Government."[15] Although these men were frightened by the world they observed, they understood with so small a number and so few states represented that they could do little more than to call another meeting in hopes that enough delegates would attend to make a difference. Their call was deferential to the people and to the states, couched simply in the language of the need for a reform in the Articles of Confederation.

What came next is well known. The states sent representatives to Philadelphia for the convention that began in May 1787, although the meeting did not reach a quorum of seven states for more than a week after the original convening date. The men who attended agreed that their meeting would be held in secret and they nailed shut the windows of the hall to keep the prying eyes of the public away. In the end, they threw out the Articles of Confederation and set to work on a new constitution, quibbling and then compromising over everything from the power in the states, to representation, to slavery before presenting a final version for a ratification process. They wrote this ratification process into Article VII of the very document they had created: the new framework would be established when nine states had voted to accept it. The men who attended the Philadelphia convention were committed to compromise, to hammering out the best system for which imperfect men could hope. James Madison had come prepared with a plan but allowed that even the plan he had labored over could be modified and changed in the process of the convention.

When the men who had gathered in Philadelphia opened the windows and doors and revealed a new constitution rather than a revised Articles of Confederation to the American people, a heated national debate ensued in which Americans on both sides attempted to dismiss their political opponents for being wrongheaded, crazy, or undone by party rage. This tactic has a long and ongoing history, of course, but in an era when so many agreed that rationality was one of the cornerstones of government, it was a powerful weapon. A lunatic could stand the social order on its head, breaking the link between the individual person and the whole people. In Mercy Otis Warren's brief description of this moment in her long *History of the Rise, Progress, and Termination of the American Revolution* the convention at Philadelphia had raised suspicions from the start. For some people, the policing of information that included instructions to keep the debate from "the scrutinizing eye of a free people," must be "the result of the passions of a few." After all, "truth, whether moral, philosophical, or political, shrinks not from the eye of investigation."[16] Warren, like so many other Americans of that era, saw conspiracy in many of the corners into which she peered. The more hidden those corners, the more likely it was that the unvirtuous were acting in a way to seize power and to subvert the liberties of the people. Their fears, Warren wrote, were that the republican system they had fought for "might be annihilated by views of private ambition."[17] For Warren, that the indomitable Benjamin Franklin had doubts about the system onto which he signed was proof positive that the system was in error. She (inaccurately) wrote him with tears in his eyes, apologizing for signing on to the Constitution even as he did so. Franklin certainly expressed doubts, admitting that he did "not entirely approve of this Constitution at present," but he also said that it astonished him "to find this system approaching so near to perfection as it does." Warren focused only on the doubts of the old scientist, philosopher, and politician. His beginning with an expression of doubt resonated with her own fears and with her mission to keep the new frame of government from being ratified.

The most generous of the Constitution's opponents argued that the framers were poor physicians to the body politic who sought to cure the illness by killing the patient.[18] A writer going by the pseudonym Republican Federalist believed that if the proposed constitution was medicine, "the remedy proposed will . . . prove at least equally distressing with the disease itself."[19] The least generous opponents assigned motives of greed and ambition to them, arguing that those who supported the new framework of government did not seek a cure to the problems the nation faced but sought personal gain. Opponents did not reject the idea that serious problems existed under the Articles of Confederation, but they believed that the proposed constitution was attended by dangers they had distanced themselves from with the successful completion of the American Revolution. When they read the text of the new document carefully, they saw a consolidated government that opened the doors to an aristocratic system that would not keep them free but would enslave them.

To the opponents of this new government, the framers were conspirators set on shackling the rational and free men and women of the United States like the mad doctors who shackled or confined sane men and women. In a series of letters penned by Centinel, those who supported the new government "assume the pleasing appearance of truth" and then "bewilder the people in all the mazes of error."[20] The circular arguments of the proponents of the Constitution were enough to drive any rational American mad. In the end, those who were driven into the mazes of error by the Constitution's supporters would become convinced that the problems apparent in the new government were so severe that the only solution was to throw the system out in its entirety. Alternatively, like enthusiastic and deluded madmen, the framers led the people down a dangerous road to party rage and used the people's bewilderment to their own advantage. By raising fears of anarchy and confusion, the supporters led "the affrighted mind . . . to clasp the new constitution as the instrument of deliverance, as the only avenue to safety and happiness."[21] The proposed constitution was not the work of rational actors but of a group of men who were determined to make their followers irrational.

The men who believed this new government was a needed remedy to the weaknesses in the new United States tried to answer the fears about consolidation of power and the potential for a tyrannical government by pointing to the amendment process written into Article V; even if there were problems, they had also provided a way to fix those problems. This was not enough for Patrick Henry. Calling on his fellow Virginians to vote against ratification, Henry told his listeners, "I should be led to take that man for a lunatic, who should tell me to run into the adoption of a government avowedly defective, in hopes of having it amended afterwards." For Henry, the Constitution was a deformed beast that "squints toward monarchy," one that relied too heavily on the virtue of men to work.[22] Henry could imagine a near future where ambitious men made themselves more powerful through the proposed system of government, harming the liberty of the people as he went. In New York, Governor George Clinton echoed these sentiments. There were weaknesses in the Confederation, and yet his opponents used "the experience of its weakness" to "drive the people into an adoption of a constitution dangerous to our liberties." Again and again, the opponents of the constitution tried to get their listeners to hear what they believed were their rational arguments for fixing the current system rather than erasing it entirely. They tried to paint their opponents as irrational actors bent on either accumulating power and glory to themselves or as too blinded by their ideas to understand the problems that would arise in the future under the system proposed.

On the opposite side, the proponents of the Constitution also painted their political opponents as driven mad by faction and their own supporters as rational beings who stood above faction. One clear example of this reasoning from a proponent of the Constitution was Francis Hopkinson. In a long allegory he titled, *The New Roof*, he painted Americans who opposed the Constitution—the new roof for the republic—as badly misguided. In his allegory he took aim at a female critic of the Constitution, perhaps Mercy Otis Warren.[23] Whether or not Hopkinson specifically targeted Warren, that he put the character of a female critic prominently in his allegory shows us that he believed women could be disruptive forces in the political realm, capable of unleashing lunatic forces.

In *The New Roof*, the United States was a house with a roof, but a faulty one. Architects proposed building a new, stronger roof but members of the household did not agree on the necessity of such a project. One of the residents of the house was Margery. "Margery was, for many reasons, an irreconcilable enemy to the new roof and to the architects who had planned it." Margery herself was not a lunatic, but rather displayed irrational female characteristics. Any late eighteenth-century reader would recognize the behaviors of a woman not adhering to proper social norms: Margery had "unavoidably acquired an influence in the family," but instead of channeling that influence in proper womanly ways, she subverted the norms of the proper woman and "had long kept the house in confusion and sown discord and discontent amongst the servants."

Margery was not above employing a lunatic, a man obviously incapable of rationally accepting the need for a new roof. Margery sent this lunatic to further sow discord into an arena where she, as a woman, did not have ready access. As an audience member to the debates over the new roof, Margery saw a "harmless lunatic" among the observers. She thought "he might be a serviceable engine in promoting opposition to the new roof. . . . [S]he exasperated this poor fellow against the architects and fill'd him with the most terrible apprehensions . . . making him believe that the architects had provided a dark hole in the garret where he was to be chained for life." Once he was filled with rage and terror "she set him loose among the crowd, where he roar'd and bawl'd to the annoyance of all bystanders."[24] The lunatic stood in for Margery on the floor of the state house because Margery herself could not stand their roaring and bawling against the roof. In this way, Hopkinson deftly tied the irrational female mind, a mind that could not see the necessity for a new framework of government, a mind that opposed the proposed government on unreasonable terms, to lunacy. These opponents, absent rational arguments or a solid alternative, relied on sound and fury, or roaring and bawling, to distract those around them from the unavoidable destruction of their new republic under the Articles of Confederation.

Hopkinson's long allegory substituted fictional characters and objects for real actors and a proposed framework of government. Other proponents of the new constitution focused on real people and institutions. For Henry Knox the problem was the state governments. Writing to Rufus King he called these governments "vile" and "sources of pollution, which will contaminate the American name perhaps for ages."[25] On the small scale of the states, it was too easy for a deluded mob to wreak havoc, even if they could not outright gain control. Creating a more centralized government would inoculate the people against such contamination. From South Carolina, Charles Pinckney argued that the madness of the people had more ability to do damage in small societies. He told his listeners that they did not have to look any further than Shays's Rebellion to see just that. In small societies people were "always exposed to those convulsive tumults of infatuation and enthusiasm which overturn public order." If they enlarged the sphere of the national government, it would be less likely that "factious and designing men" could "infect the whole people."[26] If the stronger and more centralized government went into place, rational actors could step in at times of crisis and lead the people back to sanity and good government. If rationality did not work, in the new system, they would have the force of arms behind them. In number 28 of *The Federalist Papers*, Alexander Hamilton referred back to Shays's Rebellion, writing "that seditions and insurrections are, unhappily, maladies as inseparable from the body politic as tumors and eruptions from the natural body."[27] In this case, the cure was the power to raise a force for the common defense, something possible only with a stronger and more centralized government.

State by state, proponents of the Constitution convinced enough of the men in state conventions that theirs was the most rational solution. New Hampshire became the ninth state to ratify the Constitution on June 21, 1788 making the new government legal under its own benchmark. But while New Hampshire might have been the state that made the new government legal, neither Virginia nor New York had voted to ratify. Without these two states it would have been difficult, if not impossible, for the new government to function in a united fashion. Both states had powerful supporters for ratification but also powerful opponents who feared adopting an imperfect framework of government.

In Virginia, the two sides of the debate fought hard. The process of ratification demanded that states could only vote to ratify or reject the Constitution, "with no alterations and no middle ground."[28] This added fuel to the fire of division as some powerful political actors in that state felt that while they could accept many of the compromises as they appeared in the new framework of government, they could not accept it absent a bill of rights. Those who wished for ratification urged their fellow Virginians to accept the Constitution as it was and then work to add a bill of rights later. For Patrick Henry the risk was too great. In a speech evocative of the narratives of those claiming to be unjustly imprisoned for madness, Henry equated the strategy of ratifying first and amending second with voluntarily agreeing to be bound or shut in a dungeon with no guarantee of release. He asked, "Is there no danger when you go in, that the bolts of federal authority shall shut you in?" Henry knew he could not see the future but it was not unreasonable for him to fear that no rights would follow. After all, his generation had seen this in the mid-1760s with the rescinding of the Stamp Act followed immediately with the imposition of the Declaratory Act. Therefore, sane and rational men must refuse to ratify before a bill of rights was added to the Constitution.[29]

In the end, the arguments by Henry and other opponents of a constitution without a bill of rights did not win; the convention voted 89-79 in favor of the Constitution. Despite the fiery rhetoric in the Virginia convention, those opposed to ratification agreed to the decision and "declared themselves firmly attached to the Union" according to the *Pennsylvania Packet*.[30] On the very last day, Edmund Pendleton called on his fellow delegates "to forget the heat of discussion."[31] Only George Mason was maddened enough to call for an additional address to be written up and sent to their constituents, but according to historian Lorri Glover his address "was apparently so provocative" that the others in the group "all recoiled." There is no record left of what Mason said, but one eyewitness said his purposes were "to irritate, rather than quiet the public mind."[32] Despite Mason's attempt to infect the mind of the body politic one last time, the other men in the room stepped in as an antidote to his potential poison.

Now there were ten states, including powerful Virginia, signed onto the Constitution but New York still had not voted one way or the other. After New Hampshire's ratification, the delegates on both sides of the issue who were meeting in Poughkeepsie, New York continued to debate, but after Virginia's ratification, the proponents of the Constitution ceased their debate. In the streets and taverns, however, the people continued to take sides. The news of Virginia's ratification had arrived on July 3, affecting the planned Fourth of July celebrations throughout the state. In Albany, New York, the day ended with political opponents brawling against one another in the streets. Supporters of the Constitution even took their opponents prisoner before magistrates could finally restore order.[33] By the end of the month, however, men in convention had debated and compromised to the point of ratification by a close vote won only with the stipulation that, "in full confidence," a convention would be held to propose amendments. When the news of ratification arrived in New York City, however, the madness did not end. In the early morning hours of July 29, supporters of the Constitution attacked the print shop of Thomas Greenleaf, publisher of the *New-York Journal*, the one newspaper that had regularly published opposition to ratification. Greenleaf managed to escape through a back door and resume publishing his paper despite the destruction wreaked by the mob.[34]

The attack on Greenleaf and on other opponents to ratification signaled continued and persistent divisions in the country. Americans, although fearful of party rage, found themselves joining residual factions or creating and drifting toward newly formed factions. The Constitution did not remove the rage of party but created it in new ways. Even those who had worked toward ratification could find themselves with vastly different interpretations of the government they had helped to create. Some of the questions that Congress remained unable to solve under the Articles of Confederation proved to be persistent. In and of itself, the framework of government created by the Constitution did not offer a clear path forward. Politicians still scrabbled for compromise, crafted faulty solutions, and persisted on paths that continued to divide the country along ideological, geographical, and other fault lines.

On a national level these fault lines showed themselves from the beginning. The first Congress began to meet on March 4, 1789 before two of the state governments, North Carolina and Rhode Island, had agreed to ratify the Constitution, and it took until April 1 for the House of Representatives to have quorum. The Constitution had laid out a new framework of government but it is clear from the records of the House of Representatives that the framework was skeletal and that no one fully understood how to make it function. After all, it was one thing for men to agree to put words on the page in a particular order but it was entirely different when those men tried to put those words into action. The initial introductions, excitement, and cordiality gave way to occasional bouts of fiercely expressed hatred and deep-rooted suspicions of political opponents.

On April 1, the first order of business was the selection of the speaker of the house. On April 2, a committee was formed "to prepare and report such standing rules and orders of proceeding as may be proper to be observed in this House." On April 6, the House was informed that the Senate had also reached a quorum. The Legislative Branch could now begin the business of governing the nation, but the Constitution did not provide clear guidelines. Only on April 8, more than a month after the first delegates arrived, did James Madison rise to introduce a bill that would help the country recover "from the state of imbecility that heretofore prevented a performance of duty," and "to revive those principles of honor and honesty that have too long lain dormant."[35] The first effort, he suggested, should be a bill that laid a duty on rum and other distilled spirits, on wine, and on molasses. Thus they began a months' long debate that would be interrupted on a number of different occasions. The hope for a clear, national, and united path forward was left unfulfilled, a victim of different ideological standpoints and the very different needs and desires of the states.

The one South Carolina Congressman who was present for the first debates, Thomas Tudor Tucker, found the fact that North Carolina had not yet ratified the Constitution problematic. Like his more northerly colleagues, he believed the questions of revenue and imports was "of very great importance." However, on April 9, 1789, when he rose to address his colleagues, he was the only representative present from the lower south. Neither his fellow representatives from South Carolina nor the Georgia representatives had yet arrived. He did not believe the body should pass any bill without more men present "from that part of the Union which I have the honor to represent."[36] He understood that the different geographical regions would have very different ideas about how much tonnage duty should be laid on foreign shipping as they had very different economies. Should they not wait, at the very least, until the Georgians arrived to weigh in? Even once the more southerly delegates arrived, however, members of Congress could not agree on the language of what was to become the law of the land. Lacking precedent and guidance the debate maddeningly continued with little progress or yielding.

By June 8, still unable to agree on this important piece of legislation, Madison interrupted these proceedings. He felt that he was "bound in honor and duty" to address amendments to the Constitution. Virginia, New York, and other states had voted for ratification with the express stipulation that

Congress would address a bill of rights sooner rather than later. As the nation watched a Congress unable to legislate solutions for persistent problems, Americans continued to be restive. Madison believed that even a first move toward a bill of rights would act as medicine to troubled minds and prevent the outbreak of more serious illness in the body politic. Already Madison believed that he and the other members of Congress had erred by addressing the economy first. It would have been better, he stated, "to have made some propositions for amendments the first business we entered upon" even if they did not act on these propositions immediately. He feared that further delay would "inflame or prejudice the public mind" against any decisions Congress might make. Madison's fellow Virginia representative, Alexander White agreed that Congress should address a bill of rights "to tranquilize the public mind." If they did not do so, White continued, "it will irritate many of our constituents, which I do not wish to do." These Virginians did not invoke madness, but they certainly invoked the danger of distressing or irritating Americans' minds thereby provoking further protest or insurrection. A third Virginian, John Page, also raised the fear that those who wished for amendments would become impatient and the House would lose what little credit they had managed to build among their constituents. The people might "clamor for a new convention." Was it not worthwhile, then, to at least publish some proposed amendments so that those who wished for a bill of rights would understand their representatives were serious in honoring that wish?

The Virginians met with stiff resistance from Congressmen who believed that they needed to more clearly see what did not work in their new system before knowing what sort of amendments were necessary. Georgian James Jackson argued, "Our constitution, sir, is like a vessel just launched." Was it a good idea, therefore, to "employ workmen to tear off the planking and take asunder the frame?" He believed Congress should "not neglect the more important business which is now unfinished before them." If they could not generate revenue, their new government could not function. He understood that many of his fellow Americans wanted a bill of rights, but to Jackson it seemed "imprudent" to address merely theoretical problems, when the real problem of revenue stood right before them. Connecticut's Roger Sherman spoke out that he believed if the people did not want them to begin governing, "they might as well have rejected the constitution, as North Carolina has done, until the amendments took place." Delaware's John Vining added that "the most likely way to quiet the perturbation of the public mind, will be to pass salutary laws; to give permanency and stability to constitutional regulations, founded on principles of equity and adjusted by wisdom." The only way to provide medicine against the mobbing or madness of the people would be to complete the business already at hand, otherwise "we have done nothing to tranquillize that agitation which the adoption of the constitution threw some people into." To Vining, Madison's motion did nothing more than to "distract" the minds of his fellow Congressmen.[37]

Madison did not give up, however. In print, his next speech was impressive, calling on republicanism, liberty, and patriotism. He reminded his listeners, if they could hear him, that he "allude[d] in a particular manner to those two States that have not thought fit to throw themselves into the bosom of the Confederacy." If they did not do this one thing, they might lose "the great mass of people who opposed" the Constitution, who "disliked it because it did not contain effectual provisions against encroachments of particular rights." After setting the stage, he simply read the amendments he had proposed, putting these proposals into the record, a record that would be reprinted in newspapers throughout the country. He did not stop there, however. He continued that he had been against a bill of rights, but that in the time that elapsed between opening the doors and unbarring the windows in Philadelphia, and the sitting of the first Congress, he had grown to understand that many of the people wanted this barrier "against power in all forms and departments of Government." He ended his long speech by asserting that, at the very least they could not hurt and at the most it would win "the confidence of our fellow-citizens." Despite James Madison's argument, James Jackson remained unconvinced and used the example of Rhode Island. In that state, not yet a part of the union, "Their liberty is changed to licentiousness," and a bill of rights would not change that. He came back to his previous argument that they needed to stabilize the country's economy before they could do anything else. He told Madison that his fears about what could happen if amendments were not introduced were "a mere *ignis fatuus*," or delusion. After one day of debate, the proposals put forward by Madison were referred to a Committee of the whole and on the next day, the House once again took up the question of duties and revenue.

Madison's limited success in pushing forward amendments did little to satisfy North Carolina where the majority of the people feared a framework of government lacking a bill of rights. North Carolinians wanted to rest secure that their rights were protected but they saw no security when they read the debates of Congress. As the state held elections for delegates to a ratifying convention, the votes in the western counties went against established elites who might support ratification of a faulty constitution and supported the men who had emerged as political leaders in the aftermath of the war, some of whom who had little formal education but a good deal of appeal to others like them.

Many of the defeated men and their supporters were bitter. One of the issues most important to those who supported ratification was the recovery of runaway slaves. They believed a more centralized government would make the capture and return of their human property easier than it had been under the Articles of Confederation. They saw the election of men they deemed uneducated, ill-mannered, and ill-bred as an affront to both the protection of their property and to their status as men to whom deference was due. That lesser men were elected by the voters was further sign that their world was in danger and that they needed the checks on democracy provided by a national government. In some locales, this view held sway. For instance, the Grand Jury in Edenton published a memorial in which they wrote that the workings of the government under the Articles of Confederation had been in a "disordered and distracted state," and that the Constitution was a cure for the madness. They believed those who opposed the Constitution were mere "dupes of an insidious policy, working for our destruction."[38] The North Carolina supporters of the Constitution were so convinced that theirs was the only proper way to bring about law and order that they, ironically, turned to extralegal means to try to push through ratification, disrupting the good working of local governments and elections.

In Dobbs County, with less than a hundred ballots to be counted in the election for delegates to the convention in that state, it became clear that a man who opposed immediate ratification was going to win. Supporters of the more conservative Richard Caswell, who had twice served as governor and owned at least twenty slaves, responded with fury when it became clear that Caswell would be defeated. Instead of accepting the outcome, they knocked over all the candles, beat the sheriff unconscious, and stole the ballot box.[39] For men who argued that only a stronger and more centralized government would stop mob violence and mob rule, they served as their own worst example, using mob violence in order to get the result they desired. The very men who complained that the new actors on the political stage were uncouth and bent on overturning law and order showed their own tendencies toward licentiousness.

In July 1788, when North Carolina did hold a convention to consider the Constitution, the men who opposed ratification without the addition of a bill of rights did not see themselves as dupes working for destruction of government but as men determined to protect the liberty of the people. They brought to the convention "such rules or maxims as ought to be the fundamental principles of every free government" that the majority then voted to adopt.[40] Willie Jones, the leader of this opposition, gave one speech toward the end of the convention, stating his opinion that it would be better for North Carolina to "be eighteen years out of the Union than adopt it in its present defective form."[41] The majority agreed with this position and voted "neither to ratify nor reject the Constitution."[42] For the moment, North Carolina would remain separate from the states operating under the Constitution.

As the supporters of the Constitution left the convention, they redoubled their efforts to convince North Carolinians that theirs was the more rational position. After all, the framers of the Constitution were "respectable" men who had come to the process with "the utmost attention, moderation, and forbearance." While North Carolinians continued to express their doubts about the motives of men who had written a new framework of government behind closed doors, proponents of the Constitutions proposed that these men had worked in secret so as to have "the utmost freedom of discussion." They pointed to Virginia and New York as examples of states also attached to a bill of rights who knew that a government made up of good and virtuous men would not desert these goals and who, therefore, had voted for ratification. Instead of being suspicious of the motives of the framers, North Carolinians should be suspicious of those against ratification "who have taken so much pains to inflame you, condescending to use very little reason with a great deal of passion."[43] Did they really think they were smarter than the men in Pennsylvania, and Massachusetts, and all the other of the eleven states that had ratified? In the end, these arguments worked well enough. North Carolina held a second ratifying convention in November of 1789 resolving to "adopt and ratify" the Constitution, but including a Declaration of Rights and proposed Amendments to the Constitution.

Only tiny Rhode Island continued to hold out against ratification. In a letter addressed to the citizens of Rhode Island, the anonymous writer warned his readers that a stronger government was needed for questions of continued security. Without this protection, the citizens of Rhode Island would experience "cabals, mobs, riots, and tumults," ending in nothing but a civil war and a military government. Some of the citizens of Rhode Island certainly agreed with assessment, particularly the merchants who hated that state government's generous policies on paper money. Phocion addressed the people of Rhode Island, pleading with them to reject what he saw as lies "used to raise *innumerable visionary spectres without substance.*"[44] In other words, the opponents to the constitution frightened the people with ghost stories, harming their ability to reason. These arguments were not enough to persuade the opponents to the Constitution. In the end, it took an act from the new U.S. Congress that banned trade with Rhode Island until that state ratified the Constitution. To John Page of Virginia, this was marked with "a malevolence resembling that which Great Britain showed." In other words, their actions were like Parliament's dreaded Boston Port Act of 1774 that had helped lead to the American Revolution. The pressure from Congress to harm Rhode Island's economy as long as they refused to ratify the Constitution changed enough of the legislators' minds, however. On May 29, 1790, they voted to ratify by a narrow margin of 34 to 32. The problem of Rhode Island may have been taken care of and the more democratic impulses of the government restrained by the Constitution, but it remained difficult for the business of government to get done.

Fears of irrational actors in a rational state remained. Before North Carolina and Rhode Island had joined, members of the U.S. House of Representatives sought to understand the nature of the checks and balances within their new government. One clear example came when Congressmen debated whether the President should have the power to remove department heads from office. Theodore Sedgwick of Massachusetts asked, "Suppose, sir, a man becomes insane by the visitation of God, and is likely to run our affairs; are the hands of government to be confined from warding off the evil?" Sedgwick wanted the President to be able to act quickly to remove possible disease elements from government. Georgia Congressman James Jackson disagreed. He took the argument further, stating that it was possible that the President might suffer from "an absolute fit of lunacy," and continued that "although it was improbable that the majority of both houses of Congress may be in that situation, yet it is by no means impossible."[45] For Jackson, "madness is no treason, crime, or misdemeanor." According to the new Constitution, sold to the American people and ratified by the states, removal from office was only allowed in the cases of "Conviction of, Treason, Bribery, or other high Crimes and Misdemeanors," and *not* in cases of insanity.

For Jackson, the fact that a head of a department or a judge might go insane adding an element of madness to the body politic was less frightening than putting too much power in the hands of the President. After all, the President commanded the military. With the power of removing his department heads combined with the power of the military, he could establish "an arbitrary authority" relatively easily. Lest his listeners think *he* was the madman, Jackson said this was not "the mere chimeras of a heated brain," but a fear with both historical and present-day examples. Particularly because their government was so new, the members of the House of Representatives needed to be extremely cautious. The country would likely be fine under the Presidency of George Washington, but what about Presidents in the future? Should they not establish a precedent with an interpretation of the Constitution that would make it difficult for "a man with a Pandora's box in his breast" to take the country on the road to ruin. The power of removal was a power too great to be safely trusted in one man's hands. If individual actors holding seats of power went insane, they certainly could wreak havoc within their offices. If the system of checks and balances held, however, their madness could do little harm on a grand scale. The alternative was an authoritarian leader who had the power to subvert the liberties the Revolutionary generation revered and tried to protect in their new government.

While men in power on the national level figured out how the new government worked or did not work, on the ground the view was different. While the nation got on its feet economically, not all individuals were as lucky. From Braintree, Massachusetts, Richard Cranch wrote to James Elworthy, a nephew residing in London, catching him up on family news. Cranch wrote to him about his sorrow at deaths in their family, including Elworthy's sister Ebbet. He continued that, "Besides my Sorrow of Heart for the Loss of so many of my dear Relatives I have had the additional Affliction of seeing the children of my late aged and most worthy Sister left in very poor and destitute Circumstances." If Cranch could help financially he would, but "my Power to assist them much lessen'd by the additional publick Expenses and Debts accumulated in the late War which yet hang heavy on every member of the Community by reason of the great Taxes we are obliged to pay." Throughout the war, Shays's Rebellion, and the change in government, Cranch and many of his family members continued to struggle to make ends meet. He had served in the Massachusetts government but found "tho' high in Rank and Titles," that the offices he had held "were more expensive than profitable to me, as the Emoluments of Office here are very small."[46] Like other middling, struggling Americans, he could not afford to take an active role in the government, even if he were to be elected, unlike his better-off brother-in-law John Adams.

Richard Cranch's son William was more optimistic than his father. In December of 1791 he wrote to one of his sisters that Haverhill, where he was spending the winter, was "not the gay brilliant place it used to be." The British imports that had flooded American markets in the post-war years "very much impair'd our fortunes." He believed the worst of the economic crisis had passed however, and like other young Americans looked to the future. "There are many young people rising into affluence, who at [the time of the war] were not known," he wrote to one of his sisters.[47] Both Cranches were glad for a new country, often waxing eloquent about the differences between the "old" world and the "new," but continued economic hardship plagued the mental wellbeing of the elder while the younger could hope for a better future.

From the western reaches of Massachusetts, wealthy and prominent Theodore Sedgwick was pleased to be elected to the United States House of Representatives in 1789. An advocate for law and order, and a man who had faced down some of the insurrectionists in the recent Shays's Rebellion, he wanted the status that came with a position in the new Congress and was going to make the most of it. He loved his wife, Pamela, as is clear in their correspondence, but, like Patrick Henry in 1775, put his own career and position in society above that of his mad wife at home. Pamela was often very capable and clearly loved her children, writing warm and humorous updates about their loudness and naughtiness to her husband, but she also suffered from depression. All her intentions to be a good wife to her husband who was serving the cause of the new nation did not stop the mental illness that sometimes ruled her life. In February 1790, she wrote to her husband that she was jealous that he could not take more time away from his business to write to her. "Truly I am not so good as I should be nor will I make any great Pretentions to Public Spirit," she wrote. She continued, "I am very willing to leave that Virtue to the Fathers of our Infant Nation and let them Bustle and wrangle about the Interest of their country at their Leisure." She knew she should be "happy and as Great as an Empress," when she could "still a squalling Infant, and Settle a matter of Great Contention among a Company of unruly Boys," but she found it hard to come to peace with her husband's absence.[48]

Theodore Sedgwick acknowledged the difficulty of their separation, but believed it was his duty to serve in the government. "I am sorry my dearest love that you have cause to complain of my negligence in writing," he wrote, urging her to make peace with it because what he was doing was engaging in the great business of building up the new country. At that moment, Congress debated Alexander Hamilton's plan to assume state debts. Sedgwick wrote that unless Hamilton's plan went into effect, "the benefits which the friends of the Government expected from the adoption of the constitution would not be realized," and the body politic would remain in a state of confusion. He had to stay because there were powerful opponents working against the plan including James Madison. According to Sedgwick, Madison had become "an apostate from all his former principles." In his letter, Sedgwick explained that he did not know if Madison had become "a convert to antifederalism," whether he was courting popularity in order to become the next Virginia Senator, "or whether he means to put himself at the head of the discontented in America."[49] His wife's illnesses were important to him but not as important as the illness on a national level, an illness he believed he could help to cure.

Even women who did not have a mental illness found their husbands' absences sometimes trying to a breaking point; women discomfited with long absences asked their husbands to put aside the business of the public to tend to the business of family. This was amplified for women like Pamela Sedgwick. When she was healthy, she was sharp, writing insightfully about politics and encouraging her husband in his important work. When she was ill, her husband's absence pained her and she did not hesitate to let him know. On July 8, 1790 she wrote of her family's eagerness at his expected arrival. She asked him to think of her disappointment when she received a letter from her claiming he had to stay in New York to settle the question of where Congress would sit. She wondered about the wisdom of this, writing, "It must be [a] matter of surprise I think to almost every Person in the United States that Congress should make the matter of their Temporary Residence a Subject of so much consequence at this time." Was this the workings of a wise and rational government? The people "anticipated everything Great and Noble" from the conduct of members of Congress, "but Alas they are but Men and subject to all those Passions that Debase and Render [Human] Nature contemptible." She was angry both that passion rather than reason kept her husband from home and that it steered the ship of state off course. She asked her husband, "[D]o I write Treason," and imagined his reply, "I hear you say yes and that I am meddling with a subject I am Totally Ignorant of," but concluded that Theodore should "Suffer me to be a Little Angered with Congress for so long detaining my Husband from my Arms."[50] She then moved on in her letter another subject, first expressing her anger but then repressing it.

Theodore continued to believe his presence in Congress was absolutely necessary, that in his absence his political enemies might bring the body politic to distraction, but while he tried to build a rational state from the framework of the Constitution had provided, Pamela lost her rationality. At the end of 1791, pregnant with her last child, Charles, family members wrote distressing reports about Pamela's state to Theodore. He thought about returning home until a friend gave him the justification to avoid the trip. This friend had visited Pamela at home and wrote to Theodore, "Nothing but necessity ought to induce you to come home. *That necessity does not exist.*"[51] This reinforced Sedgwick's belief that the work of the nation was more vital than the work of the home. Pamela did not agree, writing to her husband, "I have lost my understanding." The family suffered "without a guide without a head." Her letter reflected her mental state and the conflict between her desire to have him home and her own belief in his importance. "I wish you at home," she wrote, followed immediately with, "for your sake I wish you not to come you must not come it would only make us both more wretched."[52] Like Sarah Henry before her, Pamela was confined during points in her life. Like Patrick Henry before him, Theodore would continue his political work while leaving his wife in the hands of friends, family members, and doctors.

Neither doctors nor politicians (as doctors to the body politic) can be successful without proper medicine and tools. This was truly the case in the case of slavery, which some Americans believed was one of the greatest causes of illness in their new republic. Politicians, even well-meaning politicians, could not be good doctors for they were denied the medicine and tools for a cure by state protections of human property and by the Constitution itself. During the debates over ratification, a small handful of Americans had raised the alarm about the Constitution's endorsement of slavery. Three writers from western Massachusetts—Consider Arms, Malichi Maynard, and Samuel Field—were particularly appalled by the passage in that document that allowed the continuation of the slave trade. Arms, Maynard, and Field believed that passage was not rational but was inconsistent with the ideas of liberty that Americans had fought so hard to put at the center of a new government. "*[G]reat men are not always wise*," they wrote. They questioned the wisdom of the man who "at the same time he is brandishing his sword, in the behalf of freedom for himself—is likewise tyrannizing over two or three hundred miserable Africans, as free born as himself." The Constitution was like the dream of a madman, "a curious piece of political mechanism," that despoiled the very idea of freedom.[53] These three men were exceptional in their public criticism of chattel slavery during the ratification debates although they were not alone. They recognized slavery as one of the illnesses in the body politic and that it was far from rational for white Americans to claim liberty while denying it to others and even less rational to embed this illness into the very fabric of the framework of government.

Debates over slavery led to series of threats of secession and civil war that rumbled through the nation for four score more years despite the efforts of some black and white Americans to end the institution. Black Americans fought against slavery and for equal access to employment, schooling, marriage, and the legal system for free people. Boston's Prince Hall, freed from slavery in 1770, pushed for access to public education and to an end of slavery. In 1788, Hall and other black freemasons petitioned the Massachusetts government after three free black men were abducted in Boston Harbor and sold into slavery in the French colony of Martinique. The petitioners understood that the abduction had been illegal, but as free black men they also understood that it could happen to any of them. After all, this had not been the first time free black people had been captured and sold into slavery. The petition asked, "What then are our lives and Lebeties worth if they may be taken a way in such a cruel & unjust manner as these"?[54] White Quakers and Boston clergy also petitioned. Governor John Hancock managed to get the three men returned home to great jubilation. On March 26, 1788, the General Court, passed an act "to prevent the Slave Trade, and for granting Relief to the Families of such unhappy Persons as may be Kidnapped or decoyed away from the Commonwealth." The very day after barring the slave trade, however, the General Court passed another law that prohibited black Americans, unless they carried citizenship certificates, from remaining in Massachusetts. If they could not produce a citizenship certificate, they would be imprisoned with the possibility of hard labor, whipping, and a warning out.[55] The question of what black lives and liberties were worth remained.

The answer to that question from the U.S. Congress was that black lives did not matter. Toward the end of his life, Benjamin Franklin became the president of the Pennsylvania Society for Promoting the Abolition of Slavery. In February 1790, less than a year after Congress began sitting under the Constitution, this society presented a memorial to Congress. Couched in the language of liberty and Christianity, the memorialists reminded Congress, "That mankind are all formed by the same Almighty

Being, alike objects of his care, and equally designed for the enjoyment of happiness . . . and the political creed of Americans fully coincides with the position."[56] As it would in the coming decades, even the presentation of the memorial sparked outrage for many of the southern delegates. South Carolinian Thomas Tucker believed even the hearing of the memorial was enough to push the slaves to revolt, in part because they were not mentally competent enough to fully consider it, or, as Tucker put it, "they could not reason on the subject, as more enlightened men would."[57] Did the petitioners want an end to slavery, Tucker asked. He then assured Congress, "This would never be submitted to the Southern States without a civil war." Other southern representatives agreed. South Carolina's William Smith said that just talking about the memorial was enough to "create great alarm."[58] From the very beginning of the nation, white men threatened war to protect a system of gross inequality.

The Virginians John Page and James Madison tried to reason with their colleagues from the deep south. Page even tried to imagine what he would feel if he were a slave. If he were a slave and heard that Congress refused to even consider a more humane slave trade, his mind would be impressed with "all the horrors of despair." In this mental state, it would be more likely for them to revolt against their masters. If Congress was at least willing to discuss the worst outrages involved in the slave trade, perhaps the slaves "would trust in their justice and humanity."[59] This last statement, of course, showed the limits to his imagination because only someone with no danger of becoming chattel could believe it was possible to create a kinder form of slave trade or, even if they could, that would somehow make people who had their freedom denied to them trust their enslavers. Madison did not bother with odd hypotheticals. Instead, he admitted that Congress could not abolish the slave trade until 1808 but perhaps they could limit the expansion of slavery. This was allowed in the Constitution according to his interpretation.

During the debate over the memorial, Pennsylvania's Thomas Scott took the opportunity to make an impassioned antislavery speech. He understood that the slave trade was part of the new framework of government, but called the slave trade "one of the most abominable things on earth."[60] Massachusetts's Elbridge Gerry agreed. More successfully than Page, he put himself into the shoes of the slaves, and said that whenever he thought about slavery he thought about how he would feel if "himself, his children, or friends were placed in the same deplorable circumstances."[61] Wasn't it madness to continue such an inhumane, immoral practice that went against the core values of the American people? According to Benjamin Rush, many of the diseases that slaves contended with were caused by their slavery. He did not go as far as to say, therefore, slavery would create a disease in the body politic, but he was a critic of slavery, telling his medical students that slavery was "as repugnant to the health, as it is to the morals, & general happiness of mankind."[62]

Others went further. The minister Jonathan Edwards claimed that the very fact that slavery "deprave[s] the morals of the people," made slavery also "extremely hurtful to the state." Slavery not only led to immorality, but it also damaged the economy. Subsequently, this opened the door for a more crime-ridden society as the less-well-off would turn to stealing or worse to make ends meet. Slavery also led to vices "such as intemperance, lewdness and prodigality." These vices did lead to mental incapacitation if not outright madness, or, as Edwards wrote, "they "enfeeble both the body and mind," and would continue to make Americans degenerate.[63] The body politic was endangered by this moral and economic evil.

As they would in the years to come, the men who refused to consider an end to slavery, called on economic necessity, biblical sanction, and racist arguments about blacks' inferiority to justify their continued use of chattel slavery. Agriculture in the South necessitated slave labor, the Constitution had guaranteed the continuation of slavery, and the Bible showed that slavery was part of the human condition. Georgia and the Carolinas would not have ratified the Constitution without a guarantee of slavery, and if other states tried to interfere with their right to property, they should expect a civil war. One center of the debate as well was the fear of the madness of slave insurrection, a fear that would soon be brought home to them with a large-scale slave revolt on the island of St. Domingue.

By 1791, there was an insurrection in St. Domingue that not only shook the French colony to its foundation, but also brought threats of madness and disorder to the American shores. The insurrection intensified in the years that followed, but even in its earliest forms, men sitting in Congress were very aware of the white refugees from St. Domingue that had escaped that island and fled to various points in the eastern Atlantic, including Philadelphia. Like their United States counterparts, these escapees published and consumed print materials, often times in both French and English. In 1791, the governor of St. Domingue sent deputies to seek military aid from the United States while villages and plantations burned. The white refugees who fled brought with them stories of the coordinated attacked of Boukman and other slave insurgents.

If some Americans found it irrational that slavery existed alongside their own rhetoric of liberty, they harbored very rational fears about the possibility of slave revolts. The insurrection in St. Domingue, like the insurrections and threat of insurrections before it, gave lie to their myths about well-treated slaves. In a pamphlet published in Philadelphia in 1792 entitled, *An Inquiry into the Causes of the Insurrection of the Negroes in the Island of St. Domingo* included the description of the gruesome execution Vincent Ogé, a free man of color who had revolted against continued restrictions against even free blacks. The pamphleteer asked, "If the cold-blooded sons of Europe, educated in the habits of improved society, and affecting to feel the precepts of a mild and merciful religion, can thus forget themselves, and insult their own nature, ought they to wonder that the African should imitate the pattern, and if possible improve upon their example?"[64] The slave insurrection was not madness, but was a rational response to the violence black men and women faced every day, whether they were free or slave.

In 1787, Benjamin Rush had been confident that the temple of tyranny had only two doors and that Americans could bolt shut both the door that opened onto monarchy and the one that opened onto "ignorance and licentiousness" with the implementation of a more powerful and centralized national government. What the challenges to slavery as well as the other continued problems of governance showed was that there were multiple doors in the temple of tyranny. As fast as one group of Americans pushed a door shut and bolted it, another group pushed one open. The Constitution had changed the form and direction of the national government but it did not prevent tyranny from insinuating itself into the body politic, creating mental or physical illnesses in the new republic. It was not clear that the new nation could survive.

NOTES

1. Thomas Paine, "The Last Crisis," April 19, 1783, in *The American Crisis* (London: R. Carlile, 1819), 187, https://google.com/books/edition/The_American_Crisis/.

2. Benjamin Rush, "Address to the People of the United States," *The American Museum*, January 1787, archive.csac.history.wisc.edu/Benjamin_Rush.pdf.

3. Noah Webster, "Remarks on the Manners, Government, and Debt of the United States," in *A Collection of Essays and Fugitiv [sic] Writings* (Boston: I. Thomas and T. Andrews, 1790), 71, https://books.google.com/books?isbn=3732647684.

4. Charlene Boyer Lewis, "Modern Gratitude: Patriarchy, Romance, and Recrimination in the Early Republic," *Journal of the Early Republic* 39 (Spring 2019): 28. Rosemarie Zagarri, *Revolutionary Backlash: Woman and Politics in the Early American Republic* (Philadelphia: University of Pennsylvania Press, 2008).

5. Mercy Otis Warren, "Primitive Simplicity," in *Poems, Dramatic and Miscellaneous* (Boston: I. Thomas and E.T. Andrews, 1790), 228, https://books.google.com/books/about/Poems_Dramatic_and_Miscellaneous.html.

6. Winslow C. Watson, ed., *Men and Times of the Revolution; Or, Memoirs of Elkanah Watson, Including His Journals of Travels in Europe and American from the Year 1777 to 1842, and His Correspondence with Public Men, and Reminiscences and Incidents of the American Revolution* (New York: Dana and Company, 1857), 287, https://www.loc.gov/item/03004951/.

7. *Memoirs of Elkanah Watson*, 288.
8. *Virginia Gazette and Alexandria Advertiser*, April 22, 1790. Quoted in Linda Kerber, *Women of the Republic: Intellect & Ideology in Revolutionary America* (New York: W. W. Norton & Company, 1980), 281.
9. "To James Madison from George Washington, November 5, 1786," *Founders Online*, National Archives, https://founders.archives.gov/documents/Madison/01-09-02-0070.
10. Abigail Adams to Elizabeth Smith Shaw, March 10, 1787, in Margaret A. Hogan et al., eds, *Adams Family Correspondence*, Vol. 8 (Cambridge: The Belknap Press of Harvard University Press, 2007), 4.
11. Eustace, *Passion Is the Gale*, 157.
12. William Livingston, "On Party Divisions," *American Museum*, October 1790.
13. Rufus King, Philadelphia, to Thomas Sedgwick, June 10, 1787. Sedgwick Family Papers, Massachusetts Historical Society.
14. Thomas Sedgwick, Boston, to Rufus King, June 18, 1787. Sedgwick Family Papers. Massachusetts Historical Society.
15. Proceedings of Commissioners to Remedy Defects of the Federal Government, https://avalon.law.yale.edu/18th_century/annapoli.asp.
16. Warren, *History of the Rise, Progress and Termination of the American Revolution*, Vol. II, 657.
17. Warren, *History of the Rise, Progress and Termination of the American Revolution*, 657.
18. Like Pauline Maier, I used the term "opponents" rather than Antifederalists. Antifederalist was a pejorative used against the opponents in order to discredit them. Those who opposed the Constitution often argued that they were the true federalists and that Madison, Hamilton, and the other framers had no claim to that word. See Maier's introduction to *Ratification: The People Debate the Constitution, 1787–1788* (New York: Simon and Schuster, 2010), particularly xiv–xv.
19. Samuel Bannister Harding, *The Contest over the Ratification of the Federal Constitution in the State of Massachusetts* (New York: Longmans, Green, and Company, 1896), 126.
20. Centinel, "To the People of Pennsylvania," in Herbert J. Storing, *The Complete Anti-Federalist*, Vol. 2 (Chicago: University of Chicago Press, 1981), 183.
21. Centinel, "To the People," 185.
22. Patrick Henry, June 9, 1788, in *Debates and Other Proceedings of the Convention of Virginia, Convened at Richmond, on Monday the Second Day of June, 1788, for the Purpose of Deliberating on the Constitution Recommended by the Grand Federal Convention* (Richmond: Enquirer-Press, 1805), 132, http://books.google.com/books/about/Debates_and_other_proceedings_of_the_Con.html.
23. It is unclear if Mercy Otis Warren was his target or not. Warren was adamantly opposed to ratification but published her opposition to the Constitution pseudonymously as "a Columbian Patriot." For over a century, the writing was erroneously attributed to a fellow Massachusetts resident Elbridge Gerry.
24. Francis Hopkinson, "The New Roof," *Pennsylvania Packet*, December 29, 1787, americainclass.org/sources/makingrevolution/constitution/text3/hopkinsonnewroof.pdf.

25. Quoted in Gordon S. Wood, "Interests and Disinterestedness in Making of the Constitution," in Richard Beeman, Stephen Botein, and Edward C. Carter II, eds, *Beyond Confederation: Origins of the Constitution and American National Identity* (Chapel Hill: University of North Carolina Press, 1987), 76.

26. Charles Pinckney, Speech in the Ratification Convention, May 14, 1788, https://archive.csac.history.wisc.edu/sc_pinckney.pdf.

27. Alexander Hamilton, The Federalist Papers: No. 28, https://avalon.law.yale.edu/18th_century/fed28.asp.

28. Lorri Glover, *The Fate of the Revolution: Virginians Debate the Constitution* (Baltimore: Johns Hopkins University Press, 2016), 29–30.

29. Patrick T. Conley and John P. Kaminski, eds, *The Bill of Rights and the States: The Colonial and Revolutionary Origins of American Liberties* (Madison, WI: Madison House, 1992), 33.

30. Quoted in Glover, *The Fate of the Revolution*, 144.

31. Glover, *The Fate of the Revolution*, 147.

32. Glover, *The Fate of the Revolution*, 148.

33. Maier, *Ratification*, 374.

34. Maier, *Ratification*, 398–399.

35. "Import and Tonnage Duties, [8 April] 1789," *Founders Online*, National Archives, https://founders.archives.gov/documents/Madison/01-12-02-0043.

36. Thomas Tucker, April 9, 1789, in *Annals of Congress*, https://memory.loc.gov.

37. The debate detailed on this page and the next is recorded in the *History of the Proceedings and Debates of the House of Representatives of the United States*, at *A Century of Lawmaking for a New Nation: U.S. Congressional Documents and Debates, 1774–1875*, https://memory.loc.gov/cgi-bin/ampage?collId=llac&fileName=001/llac001.db&recNum=51.

38. "Grand Jury to the Edenton District Court," in Donna Kelly and Lang Baradell, eds, *The Papers of James Iredell*, Vol. III (Raleigh: Office of Archives and History, 2003), 326, 327.

39. Thomas L. Howard, III, "The State that Said No: The Fight for Ratification of the Federal Constitution in North Carolina," *North Carolina Historical Review* 94 (January 2017): 16.

40. Quoted in Blackwell Pierce Robinson, "Willie Jones of Halifax: Part II," *North Carolina Historical Review* 18 (April 1941): 151.

41. Robinson, "Willie Jones of Halifax," 152.

42. Robinson, "Willie Jones of Halifax," 153.

43. A Citizen of North-Carolina, "To the People of the State of North Carolina," in *James Iredell*, 418–429.

44. Phocion, "To the People of the State of Rhode-Island," July 17, 1788, https://archive.csac.history.wisc.edu/ri_phocion.pdf. Italics in the original.

45. Jonathan Elliot, ed., *Debates in the Several State Conventions on the Adoption of the Federal Constitution as Recommended by the General Convention at Philadelphia in 1787. Together with the Journal of the Federal Convention, Luther Martin's Letter, Yates's Minutes, Congressional Opinions, Virginia and Kentucky Resolutions of '98-'99, and Other Illustrations of the Constitution*, Vol. 4 (Philadelphia: J.B. Lippincott & Co., 1866), 355, 372, https://memory.loc.gov/ammem/amlaw/lwed.html.

46. Richard Cranch to James Elworthy, February 14, 1791. Cranch-Bond Papers. Massachusetts Historical Society.
47. William Cranch to a sister, December 13, 1791, William Cranch Papers. Library of Congress.
48. Pamela Sedgwick to Theodore Sedgwick, February 26, 1790. Sedgwick Family Papers. Massachusetts Historical Society.
49. Theodore Sedgwick to Pamela Sedgwick, March 4, 1790. Sedgwick Family Papers. Massachusetts Historical Society.
50. Pamela Sedgwick to Theodore Sedgwick, July 8, 1790. Sedgwick Family Papers. Massachusetts Historical Society.
51. Quoted in Timothy Kenslea, *The Sedgwicks in Love: Courtship, Engagements, and Marriage in the Early Republic* (Boston: Northeastern University Press, 2006), 21.
52. Kenslea, *Sedgwicks in Love*, 21.
53. Consider Arms, Malichi Maynard, and Samuel Field, "Dissent to the Massachusetts," *Teaching American History,* https://teachingamericanhistory.org/library/document/consider-arms-malachi-maynard-and-samuel-field-dissent-to-the-massachusetts/.
54. Petition reprinted in Herbert Aptheker, ed., *A Documentary History of the Negro People in the United States*, Vol. 1 (New York: Citadel Press, 1969), 20.
55. Asahel Stearns and Lemuel Shaw, eds, *The General Laws of Massachusetts, from the Adoption of the Constitution, to February, 1822*, Vol. 1 (Boston: Wells & Lilly and Cummings & Hilliard, 1823), 324–325, ocm26871236-1822vol1.pdf.
56. In George Washington Williams, *History of the Negro Race in America from 1619 to 1880*, Vol. I (New York: G.P. Putnam's Sons, 1883), 432, http://www.gutenberg.org/ebooks/15735.
57. Benton, Thomas Hart, ed., *Abridgement of the Debates of Congress, from 1789 to 1856*, Vol. I (New York: D. Appleton & Company, 1857), 208, catalog.hathitrust.org/Record/008700946.
58. *Abridgement of the Debates of Congress*, 210.
59. *Abridgement of the Debates of Congress*, 210.
60. *Abridgement of the Debates of Congress*, 208.
61. *Abridgement of the Debates of Congress*, 211.
62. Quoted in Sarah Knott, "Benjamin Rush's Ferment: Enlightenment Medicine and Female Citizenship in Revolutionary America," in Sarah Knott and Barbara Taylor, eds, *Women, Gender and the Enlightenment* (New York: Palgrave Macmillan, 2005), 658.
63. Jonathan Edwards, *The Injustice and Impolicy of the Slave Trade, and of the Slavery of the Africans: Illustrated in a Sermon Preached before the Connecticut Society for the Promotion of Freedom, and for the Relief of Persons Unlawfully Holden in Bondage, at Their Annual Meeting in New-Haven, September 15, 1791* (Boston: Wells and Lilly: 1822), 11, 13. Evans Early American Imprint Collection.
64. *An Inquiry into the Causes of the Insurrection of the Negroes in the Island of St. Domingo* (London: J. Johnson, 1792), https://cdn.loc.gov/service/rbc/rbc0001/2019/2019preimp06338/2019preimp06338.pdf.

Chapter 8

Party Politics and Foreign Policy, 1792–1796

If the Constitution was supposed to ameliorate the dangers of irrational actors upsetting the rational state as its supporters had promised, the 1790s proved that assumption wrong. In the 1790s, politics divided Americans into two opposing—and often polar opposite—camps. Those who identified strongly as Federalist or Democratic Republican looked at one another suspiciously across that divide, believing those on the other side behaved irrationally and would harm their new republic. When writing the biography of her husband, Republican Dr. George Logan, Deborah Norris Logan described the times as filled with the "sparks of that inflammable and deleterious party spirit that mounted triumphant over every other consideration."[1] If the surviving print record is to be believed, she was not wrong in her assessment. Political differences provided fuel to fires of incivility, hardened political positions, and led to threats of civil war. The press reflected the political quarrels to a wider public, adding to American fears that their national experiment would not last. The expression of Oliver Wolcott, Sr.'s fear that "we are to calculate upon an early termination of our present system" was not unusual, and was repeated both publicly and privately among early national Americans.[2]

Many of the main political players in this drama are well known. President George Washington and his first Secretary of the Treasury, Alexander Hamilton became key figures for the Federalists. Although Hamilton and James Madison had worked in concert to craft and sell the U.S. Constitution, they were no longer on the same side. Madison now identified as Democratic Republican, but the main standard-bearer for that party was Thomas Jefferson. The divisions between Hamilton and Jefferson had existed from the beginning of the Washington administration, but those divisions became clearer and more sharply drawn during their tenure in that administration. Ordinary men, women, and children—the people out of doors—amplified the messages from party leaders and others. It was these ordinary people who translated the instability of the early republic into protests or mob actions and made the elite worry about the possibility of anarchy. The first American party system—a system of faction, sectionalism, and plenty of incivility—gained shape and form through this decade. As this chapter will show, foreign policy was one center of the growing party division; foreign policy created the conditions ripe for contagion and disease. Both sides employed disease metaphors, noting the possibility of both physical and mental illness in the body politic. Those who engaged with these metaphors and in the larger foreign policy debate did not see this as a simple philosophical debate but as a deep-rooted struggle for the future of the United States, indeed for the very continuation of their country. Because each side believed its vision presented the true path and the other side's vision led to ruin, the form of this political conflict was shaped both in word and in physical confrontation. This chapter will focus on some of those divides as well as the ways the language of madness wove its way through all of it.

As shown in previous chapters, the use of disease metaphors reflects back to us the ways Americans saw government and society as an actual physical body. They believed that the life cycle of a government followed the life cycle of a human being, and they believed that irrationality was contagious and could spread as rapidly as diseases like yellow fever. In 1812, looking back over the age of revolutions, Dr. Benjamin Rush translated this into medical terms. In his *Medical Inquiries and Observations, Upon the Diseases of the Mind*, he wrote about the physical and mental dangers that accompanied revolutions, particularly when "accompanied with injustice, cruelty, and the loss of property and friends" or when they challenged "ancient and deep-seated principles and habits."[3] He believed these revolutions and disruptions led to increased insanity. French doctors agreed. As Laure Murat has shown in *The Man Who Thought He Was Napoleon: Toward a Political History of Madness*, doctors "spoke first of 'political monomania,' followed by *morbus democraticus* (democratic disease), and finally 'revolutionary neurosis,' or *paranoia reformatia*."[4] Murat asks us not to dismiss these diagnoses as silly, but to understand that psychiatrists paid "serious attention . . . to the correlation between madness and ideology." Rush took it seriously as did the French revolutionary, Dr. Volney. Rush wrote that Volney had revealed there were three times as many cases of madness in Paris in the year 1795, as there were before the commencement of the French Revolution.

It was not only psychiatrists or other doctors who paid serious attention to this correlation, Americans with no medical training whatsoever agreed. Oliver Wolcott, Sr. wrote to his son in 1793 that it was evident to him "that there are a set of men in Congress, who from pride, ignorance, ambitions or interest, or all of them, mean to make a steady exertion materially to derange the present system of government."[5] The Wolcotts alternatively called this set of men, "Jacobins" or "antifederalists." Infected by the ideology that arose during the war in France, their goal was to derange the body politic, to confuse the American people, and to substitute (in the Wolcotts's minds) the good beginning and proper order of the United States with a version of government that would result in leveling, anarchy, and a destruction of the new country. While these fears had dogged Americans throughout the era of the American Revolution, Americans' relationship to France had altered the equation and raised the fears in new ways.

By the 1790s, it was the incendiary quality of the French Revolution as well as the European war that emerged in that decade that would infect people on both sides of the Atlantic. Americans and Europeans were connected after all. As historian Rachel Hope Cleves showed, "Early national citizens viewed themselves as participants in a transnational community, drawn together by sinews of trade, migration, and information."[6] Although American responses to foreign revolutions and wars reflected their own understanding of themselves as Americans, they were aware of those connections and believed that what happened in other parts of the world did have a direct impact on their communities and nation.[7] Those same sinews of trade, migration, and information could transmit contagion. John Jay and Rufus King advised in 1793 that if Americans kept good watch, they would remain uncontaminated, but it was possible to become "seduced, infected, and inflamed, by foreign influence."[8] To Jay, King, and others, foreign influence was a poison, one that Americans did not seem capable of avoiding despite the rational heads that advised them against becoming pulled into another country's affairs. The spirit of revolution coming from France was enticing, particularly for a people born out of revolution. Conservative Chauncey Goodrich wrote: "It is natural to expect the Sans Culottish spirit should in a degree infect people and contaminate public measure."[9] There was something very compelling about that spirit, even if it posed a threat.

In 1789, when news of the commencement of the French Revolution reached American shores, many Americans celebrated. They believed that the French would continue the work begun by the American Revolution. In addition, Americans were very aware that the success of the American war for independence would have been more difficult—if not impossible—without the support of the French government. The 1778 Treaty of Amity and Commerce had pledged perpetual peace and friendship between France under King Louis and the new United States. The French, who had been enemies to British North American colonists through most of the period of settlement, had become friends and allies, had helped the United States emerge as a legitimate nation on the world stage.

While many celebrated the coming of the French Revolution, others expressed caution. President Washington wrote to Gouverneur Morris in France praying "that the revolution in France may terminate in the permanent honor and happiness of her government and people," but cautioning that this was but the "first paroxysm," that "the revolution is of too great a magnitude to be effected in so short a space, and with the loss of so little blood."[10] Although Washington hoped for a good outcome, a few, like John Adams, were gloomy. Adams wrote to his cousin Sam Adams, asking, "Will the struggle in Europe, be anything more than a change of impostors and impositions?"[11] The gloom is understandable. Washington, Adams, and others were aware that their colonial history had created the American Revolution in a particular shape that might not be replicable. British colonies in North America had been embroiled in imperial politics but were also an ocean apart from the centers of imperial power. The French, on the other hand, were living and breathing in the center. They were not trying to create a new nation from 3,000 miles distant, they were doing it from within. They had less room to maneuver than their American counterparts had.

Despite the doomsday attitude from Adams, other Americans celebrated without reservation. In the era of the American Revolution, many Americans had hoped that the ideals of a government based on the consent of the governed and committed to the safety and happiness of its people would spread. They claimed these principles as "an 'American fever' which was 'shaking to the foundations the thrones of enlightened Europe.'"[12] The fact that these principles were now being put in place by the people of France was the fulfillment of a secular version of a city upon a hill: the Americans had built a new government and now others would take their example and form republican governments throughout the world. Americans proudly signaled their support for the French Revolution by adding French cockades to their wardrobes and by reading dispatches about the war. They believed the American fever was not a deleterious one. It was catching, yes, but would spread liberty and good government along its disease routes.

While the American people celebrated the French Revolution, the business of Congress remained largely unaffected in the first years of that war. One has to go searching for the French Revolution in the records of Congress. It was not entirely absent, but in order to see it, one has to look very carefully. Congress did confirm William Short as *chargé d'affaires* to replace Jefferson (on Jefferson's recommendation) in France. France did come into the debate over duties on imports and was alluded to in debates over the assumption of debt. In a debate over public credit, France was held up as a negative example. The meaning of the French Revolution or its relationship to U.S. foreign policy, however, was absent from Congressional debate. Still focused on building a republic to stand the test of time, the members of Congress turned their attention to matters other than the war in France.

The contagion of war may not have reached the floor of Congress in the early years of the revolution, but it certainly had infected the print sphere. Federalist commentators believed that the newspapers and pamphlets spread the contagion of anarchy and licentiousness through the mail and other transportation routes. By 1791, party newspapers had been established. For the Federalists, John Fenno had begun publishing the *Gazette of the United States* "for the purpose of disseminating favorable sentiments of the federal Constitution and the Administration" in 1789.[13] Made uneasy by this voice for the Federalists, in 1791 Jefferson and Madison began to provide financial support to Philip Freneau so that he could begin printing an opposition paper that would denounce the "doctrines of monarchy, aristocracy, & the exclusion of the influence of the people" that the Democratic Republicans believed were at work in the Washington administration.[14] The voice of faction and party hostility found home on the printed page.

How Americans viewed this contagion had everything to do with where you stood politically. Disgusted by some of the turns her country had taken, Mercy Otis Warren wrote to Catharine Graham, her English friend and fellow historian, that even former American patriots now seemed "to be at war with every Democratic principle," to the extent of becoming "advocates for Monarchy and all the trappings of Royalty." She hated that these Americans, many of whom held positions of power, believed "that the mass of people have not the capacity nor the right to choose their own master."[15] For Warren, these Federalists worked to delude the minds of the people. They were not doctors to the body politic, but deceivers who strove to plant false ideas into the minds of the people in order to mislead them. Her former allies and friends had followed a path of power, rushing to imitate some of the worst abuses of the British system that had so oppressed them.

The printed page reflected the changing views of Americans about the French Revolution. The adulation of Americans for the French Revolution became less universal as the nature of the revolution changed. In July 1792, William Short wrote to Jefferson from the Hague about "those mad and corrupted people in France who under the name of liberty have destroyed their own government, and disgusted all the real supporters of the constitution." These madmen violated liberty "daily," and "with impunity;" their actions had led to "universal anarchy" and "no succour from the protecting arm of the law against mobs and factions which have assumed despotic power."[16] Eleven days later, Short wrote to Jefferson again, this time that the system had "concentrated all power in the hands of the most mad, wicked and atrocious assembly that ever was collected in any country."[17] When Short viewed the changes that had occurred in France in 1792, he did not see the glories of republicanism taking hold and the rights of man everywhere exalted. Instead he saw men in power who had lost their minds leading to a breakdown of society that was rapidly being replaced not by liberty but by despotic rule.

After the news arrived of the September Massacres, where upwards of 1,300 prisoners were summarily executed, other Americans also saw madness in the actions of the French. Even these grisly executions did not end all Americans' support for the French cause, however. Jefferson wrote back to Short on January 3, 1793, that he deplored the fact that "many guilty persons fell without the forms of trial, and with them some innocent." Nonetheless, he still believed that, "The liberty of the whole earth was depending on the issue of the contest." He then asked Short if there "was ever such a prize won with so little innocent blood?"[18] Although the violence was unsettling, in the end, Jefferson believed, history would bear out the guilt of many of the actors and the righteousness of the action. Even after the massacres, when he looked at France he saw the hope for a better, republican future modeled after the American example.

While Jefferson continued to praise the French cause, others either backed away from their support or became cautious, distancing themselves from the bloodshed and anarchy of that war. In a piece published in the *American Museum*, Cato worried: "It becomes every reflecting man in the united states, to ask himself these serious questions—are there not among us too many of a character exactly similar to the men, who have plunged the affairs of France into the extreme of disorder and jeopardy in which they are now involved?" Employing a disease metaphor, he continued, "Are there not men among us . . . who seem to have no other object then to keep the community in an unsettled, convulsed and feverish state?" He concluded that, "The present is a very momentous crisis in the affairs of the United States—factious men are unusually active and noisy—they prove, by the violence of their efforts, the violence of the disease."[19] As Americans had hoped that their revolution would be reflected in movements in other parts of the world, men like Cato now worried that the madness of the French Revolution would infect American society and government. Would it be possible to continue to build a rational state when so many had caught the disease of the French brand of revolution and its attendant irrationality?

When King Louis was arrested, Americans waited for news. Writing as Pacificus, Alexander Hamilton asked, "can it be consistent with our justice or our humanity, to partake in the angry and vindictive passions which are endeavoured to be excited against the unfortunate monarch?"[20] When the news reached the United States of the January 21, 1793 execution of the king, many expressed horror and dismay. The memory of the American Revolution and French aid was tied up with the memory of the king. The toasts they had drunk in taverns during the American Revolution had included those to Louis

XVI King of France. For men like Chauncey Goodrich, the execution was "a wanton act of barbarity," one that "threaten[ed] the success of Republicanism in France."[21] For Americans who saw themselves as "friends to order," the French Revolution had become something very different from the American Revolution; the French had descended into madness and that madness was spreading across the Atlantic to the new United States.

The differences between the American and French Revolutions was a theme that Americans came back to repeatedly throughout the rest of the eighteenth century. In a 1793 Fourth of July oration, John Quincy Adams proclaimed that the American Revolution had borne "a character different from that of any other civil contest, that had ever arisen among men." In his version, the American Revolution involved "the elementary principles of government," it was "a question of right between the sovereign and the subject." It had not been without bloodshed and sacrifice, of course, but it bore no resemblance to what was happening in France. In France, the events "have let slip the dogs of war, to prey upon the vitals of humanity; which have poured the torrent of destruction over the fairest harvests of European fertility; which have unbound the pinions of desolation, and sent her forth to scatter pestilence and death among the nations."[22] In a February 1795 Thanksgiving sermon, David Osgood proclaimed that Americans had renounced tyranny "without any great struggle, or violent commotion." While there had been "much blood," in the end the war was settled through "free debate and mature deliberation" rather than through the frenzy and madness of military conflict.[23] By the turn of the century this had become a standard narrative. The American Revolution had been born out of rationality rather than radicalism. Assiduously, these men and others worked to convert Americans to this understanding. Americans were exceptional in that they had kept their heads—metaphorically and literally—during a war that had the potential to make them insane.

More than the violence and bloodshed in France itself, it was the French declaration of war against Great Britain on February 1, 1793 that drew the lines between political parties in the United States even more distinctly. The divisions over the war between France and Britain were marked by name calling, finger pointing, and increased fears of frenzy, anarchy, and madness. When the news of the declaration of war reached the United States in April, George Washington called his cabinet to meet in Philadelphia to devise a strategy of neutrality, posing a list of questions, starting with these three: "Shall a proclamation issue for the purpose of preventing interferences of the Citizens of the United States in the War between France & Great Britain &ca? Shall it contain a declaration of Neutrality or not? What shall it contain?"[24] Washington and other Federalists saw an increased potential for confusion in an expanding war, one that would move beyond the realms of Europe and reach across the Atlantic into the western hemisphere.

Even before he attended the meeting, Jefferson had become suspicious. The day before they gathered, he noted in his diary that "it was palpable from the style" of the questions that "they were not the President's, that they were raised upon a prepared chain of argument, in short that the language was Hamilton's."[25] Jefferson believed Hamilton's approach to foreign policy was wrong and was jealous of the influence Hamilton exerted over the President. Unlike Hamilton, he hated Great Britain and loved France. Jefferson and Hamilton, sworn political enemies, became key figures in party machinations. However, in April 1793, regardless of Jefferson's suspicions and the existing animosity between him and Hamilton, they and the other cabinet members managed to work together to craft a statement. On April 22, Washington proclaimed publicly that the United States "should with sincerity and good faith adopt and pursue a conduct friendly and impartial toward the belligerent powers." The United States would try to stay out of the conflict and they hoped the warring nations would respect their neutrality.

In November, when both chambers of Congress returned from a long recess, they accepted the proclamation without public debate. The Senate responded with "hearty approbation," believing it "a measure well timed and wise."[26] The House praised President Washington for "the vigilance with which you have guarded against an interruption of that blessing [of peace], by your Proclamation."[27] While contention was already part and parcel of the life of Congress, in this case the lack of debate in Congress reflected a fairly unanimous response to the diplomatic gaffes by the French minister to the United States, Edmund Genet, and the uneasiness about foreign interventions in American actions. After all, one of the benefits of the new United States was that the Atlantic was supposed to be a barrier from active foreign interference.

Shortly before the declaration of impartiality on the part of the United States, the enthusiastic and enthusiastically received French minister Genet had appeared on the scene. Within a month, he had caused a diplomatic scandal by overstepping the bounds of propriety and legality, using American ports for his cause and trying to recruit American people. In a special message to Congress in December 1793, Washington noted that Genet had "breathed nothing of the friendly spirit of the nation which sent them," and that he had tried "to involve us in war abroad and discord and anarchy at home."[28] Despite the fact that many Democratic Republicans continued to support the French war in Europe, lawmakers could not put themselves behind a French minister who had actively tried to involve American citizens in a European war. Written retrospectively, and therefore to be taken with a grain of salt, Deborah Norris Logan commented that she heard "Jefferson remonstrate with Genet on the rashness and impropriety of his conduct, and insist upon the inviolability of those eternal principles of justice to other nations and respect for their rights."[29] If Norris's account was accurate, even the French-loving Jefferson believed Genet had gone too far.

While government officials felt they had no course of action other than promoting non-intervention in the European war, ordinary citizens were not so constrained. Democratic-Republican societies began to form promising to further what they called, "The right secured to us by the late glorious struggle for liberty, and guaranteed by the constitution of our country." They wrote constitutions and proudly proclaimed their attachment to the French cause. When accused of breaking the President's proclamation "by constantly and publicly rejoicing at every success of the French," the Democratic Society of Chittenden County in Vermont wrote, "The facts in this accusation we firmly believe many of the Societies have more or less committed; and with a degree of pleasure bordering on ecstasy." After all, as the Democratic Society of Pennsylvania wrote, the cause of France was the cause of "*Liberty*, [and] the sacred *Rights of Man*;" furthermore they could not stay neutral in a war "between a nation fighting for the dearest, the undeniable, the invaluable Rights of Human Nature, and another nation or nations wickedly, but hitherto (we thank God) vainly, endeavoring to oppose her in such a virtuous, such a glorious struggle."[30] The President might have desired neutrality but members of these societies tied themselves to the cause of France, seeing in the French Revolution a cause for all of mankind.

To their opponents, these clubs added to the threat of contagion and madness. Christopher Gore, writing as Manlius, claimed that these clubs were a threat to mental stability designed "to deceive and delude the people from their true interests." Their end goal, according to Gore, "was to involve the country in war; to assume the reins of government and tyrannize over people."[31] Jedidiah Morris scoffed that the men who joined these clubs saw themselves as the protectors of the rights of man and laughed that they thought of themselves as a check on rational and good government. Their opponents saw the clubs as a sign that madness that had swept through France could take hold in America. In France, George Cabot explained, "We have seen the expression of the general will of a great society silenced, the legal representatives of the people butchered; and a band of murderers ruling in their stead with rods of iron." He then asked, "Will not this, or something like it, be the wretched fate of our country?" He concluded, "*The Anarchists are up and doing.*"[32] If these so-called anarchists had their way, the United States would have a very short history.

By the mid-1790s, Federalists believed anarchists were up and doing in the western regions of the United States. Westerners protested against the new federal excise tax on whiskey, erecting liberty poles and using force and intimidation against the tax collectors. While the protestors believed their actions were wholly consistent with their own recent American history, Federalists disagreed. "Harrisburgh was quickly infected," Federalist Alexander Graydon wrote, noting that he and some others were "untouched by the contagion."[33] Noah Webster believed the actions in the west were serious enough to overturn the workings of "the mildest and most rational government," replacing it with harsh and irrational anarchy. The contagion of the French Revolution had jumped the ocean and landed in western Pennsylvania. In his later memoir, Graydon wrote that the western insurrection (as it was called at the time) had been "cherished . . . by the French minister as a favorable circumstance toward the predominance of the Gallic interest."[34] Graydon and others worried that the French would use the instability in the early United States to once again gain a foothold in North America. He recalled that, before Washington headed a militia to put the insurrection down, the tax protestors flew a French flag at the Harrisburgh courthouse, a clear symptom of the French madness that infected the protestors.

Washington did not speak of the western insurrection as being of French design. He did, however, believe the insurrectionists were guided by passions which "produced symptoms of riot and violence." For Washington, it was not the French but "certain self-created societies," the Democratic-Republican clubs, that had fanned the flames of opposition to the government. Others agreed with Washington, and worried about the leveling spirit that accompanied the democracy espoused by the rebels. This was seen not just in the letters of men in power; it wove its way into broader culture and society. Helena Wells published a series of letters regarding female education that dated back to 1794. In the first letter to a student she raised the specter of democracy. Wells had written, "In the present rage for levelling distinctions, it has become fashionable to descant on the pride of those who boast a long train of ancestors." However, Wells disliked the "rage" or madness of "levelling distinctions," and as she continued her letter, she wrote against men of self-made wealth whom she found too "supercilious," too "puffed up with [their] own importance."[35] In Wells's opinion, these self-made men were not to be celebrated, but were to be shunned because their embrace of the madness of democracy and leveling wreaked havoc. All good Americans, including young women, should guard themselves against these dangers.

If Americans worried about the dangers of the spread of French influence at home, the threat level increased as the war in Europe expanded. Inexorably, Americans found themselves drawn into the conflict despite Washington's proclamation that the United States would remain impartial. In late 1793, Americans at home learned about the extent of the depredations against American seamen and merchants trading in the French West Indies. Shortly after Genet's appearance on the American stage, Great Britain began to seize American merchant ships and on November 6, 1793 issued an Order in Council which claimed any American ships going to or coming from the

French West Indies were subject to confiscation.[36] What should the United States do in light of these depredations and the clear refusal by Great Britain to honor American sovereignty? The debates over a response took up much of the time of the Third Congress. On January 13, 1794, Representative William Smith of South Carolina acknowledged "that this country is at present in a very delicate crisis, and one requiring dispassionate reflection, cool and mature deliberation."[37] Even translated into print the debates seem far from dispassionate reflection; however, after a week of heated debate, members of the House voted 51-47 to postpone a decision about a response until the March session. On April 21, the House finally resolved that "after the first day of November next, all commercial intercourse between the citizens of the United States and the subjects of the King of Great Britain . . . shall be prohibited."

The prospect of cutting off trade with Great Britain frightened many Americans. Judith Sargant Murray believed that this step had been taken by a faction that "that introduced its cloven foot among us." For those who worried about the influence of the French and an American descent into disorder and anarchy, this step worried them. Murray believed that this faction, "drawing the sword of discord" would plunge that sword "in the vitals of that infant constitution," perhaps giving the nation a fatal blow. Raising the alarm, she asked, "Is not the idea of murdering in the very cradle so promising an offspring, a conception which can have received a form only in the maddening pericranium of hell-born anarchy?"[38] Faction, born in madness, could destroy the constitution and everything it stood for: rationality, mental well-being, and liberty. "Liberty has been compared to an informed, elevated, and well regulated mind; her movements are authorized by reason." Faction led to licentiousness, which she personified as a mad drunkard, "intoxicated by the inebriating draught, and having renounced his understanding." This mad drunkard "would invert the order of nature," and "annihilate every distinction."[39] The world was being turned upside down again, but this time Americans were not replacing a corrupted British system with a virtuous American one. Instead some Americans corrupted the virtuous American system leaving the wreckage of the republic behind.

While Congress debated the solution to the attacks on American shipping, President Washington sent John Jay to London to negotiate. The end result was a Treaty of Amity, Commerce, and Navigation with Britain, or, as it was more often called, the Jay Treaty or Jay's Treaty. Jay signed the treaty on November 19, 1794, and the treaty arrived in the United States in March of the following year after Congress had adjourned.[40] Washington called the Senate into a special session on June 8, explaining that "matters touching the public good required that the Senate should be convened." Once convened Senators would "receive and deliberate on such communications as he shall then make to them." Most of the debate in the Senate focused on the slaves who had run to the British during the war, but in the end the Senate resolved simply to ask the President to "renew, by friendly negotiation . . . the claims of the American citizens, to compensation for the negroes and other property" who had run to British lines during the war. In the end the Senate ratified the treaty on the condition that there would be more negotiation regarding the United States trade with the British West Indies.

Virginia Senator Steven Mason passed along his copy of the treaty, which was still supposed to be secret, to Democratic Republican printer, Benjamin Franklin Bache. Bache printed the treaty in pamphlet form. Although information had been leaking out about the treaty almost from the beginning, this printing confirmed many Americans' fears and unleashed a storm of criticism; the anger was "like that against a mad dog," according to Washington.[41] In Portsmouth, New Hampshire, a handbill proclaimed that, "The Senate have bargained away your *Blood-Bought* privileges for less than mess of pottage." The writer claimed, however, that there was still hope. Although the Senate had voted for ratification, the President had not yet signed the treaty. Therefore readers were instructed to "Repair to the State-House; Remonstrate with coolness, but spirit, against his signing the Treaty which will be the Death Warrant of your Trade, & entail beggary on us and our posterity forever!"[42] In Charleston, South Carolina, a "Gentleman" wrote into the *Aurora*: "There is creeping into your Constitution an insidious Serpent, whose venom, once infused, will exterminate every remaining Spark of Gratitude and National Faith! Attend! your rights are invaded!"[43] Calls to action and active protests against the treaty were repeated throughout the United States.

In Boston, Federalists looked around and saw that their town was, as Fisher Ames wrote, "in a very inflammatory state." The men working to convene a town hall meeting—Ames called them Jacobins—were spreading a dangerous disease, "So many feel dislike of the treaty, and so few dare oppose the popular feeling, that I apprehend not only mischievous proceedings in town-meeting, but also that the contagion will spread, especially southward." Rufus King regretted that Bostonians had held a meeting. If they had "remained silent . . . the country would have escaped that Fever into which it is likely to be thrown."[44] Ames and King feared that this Jacobin fever would weaken the new United States. For Ames, "The prejudices and passions of the multitude are scarcely more deadly to public order than the theories of our philosophers."[45] The French-identified men and those infected with the fever of sedition were not simply "half-witted," but were seditious to the extreme. Their actions were a threat to both the body and mind of the body politic.

In *The Foresters: An American Tale,* a political satire published the following year, Jeremy Belknap made fun of the opponents of the treaty for their response, while insinuating that they were under the influence, or perhaps the pay, of the French revolutionaries. As soon as the treaty was printed, "and even before the instrument was executed," he wrote, "those choice spirits whom Teneg had instructed, as aforesaid, in the use of the bird-call, set all the chickens a crying ja, ja, ja—treaty, treaty, treaty."[46] Teneg, of course, was Genet, just cleverly (or not) with the letters in reverse order. The chickens were not just chickens, but were "Mother Carey's chickens," a reference to the printer Matthew Carey, who had been a supporter of the Federalists until alarmed by the Jay Treaty. Their call, "ja, ja, ja," or in other places in the text, "jaco, jaco, jaco," noted the chickens as Jacobins, or Democratic-Republicans, in case Belknap's readers had any doubt.[47]

For the men and women who objected to Jay's Treaty, the contagion was a love of Britain and aristocracy. "What dotage!—what lunacy!. . . A government, which, in its now existing executive form . . . has been discovered to possess, and actually exercised, an uncontrollable power, subversive of our dearest, inalienable rights."[48] Those opposed to the treaty would do what they could to stop the spread of that disease and keep, instead, the true meaning of the American Revolution in place. According to Phineas Hedges, speaking to a Republican Society in Montgomery, New York, "The violent tide of the passions in favor of despotism, requires the most vigilant caution." If they were not careful, the "the minions of despotism" would "regain an empire in our hearts."[49] Others, like South Carolinian Richard Beresford, tussled in print with those who used words like Jacobins, deceivers, or antifederalists to describe the treaty objectors. Instead, Beresford wrote, many who opposed the treaty were veterans of the American Revolution who were alarmed by the connection with Great Britain. These men were not delusional nor mad; they were sane and rational and yet had been "branded with every mark of contumely and disgrace." Like his political opponents, Beresford worried about the future of the country, but it was the Federalists who worried him. He asked, "When men, whose heads had whitened with the cares of government, and the toils of war—whose hearts remained still spotless and unsophisticated with the foppery of courts, the corruptions of speculation, or the fever of ambition; when such citizens as these, are censured as the deluders of the people, to whom, beside, shall we apply for counsel and consolation?"[50] For Beresford the true patriots were those who resisted both Britain itself and the modes and culture of Britain that stood in the way of developing an un-British United States.[51]

In towns throughout the United States, Americans gathered to craft responses to the treaty and to urge Washington to reject it. Although Federalists sometimes charged their opponents with not actually having read the treaty, being simply "aided by that spirit of irritation which exists against Great Britain," it was clear from the detailed and often line-by-line responses sent to Washington that many in these large gatherings had read the treaty closely.⁵² Typical of their responses was one from citizens in New York City urging Washington "to withhold his assent" by refusing to sign the treaty. Among other things, they believed that, because the House of Representatives had not weighed in, that the treaty violated the Constitution. They concluded with condemnation, painting the treaty, "As hazarding [the country's] internal peace, and prosperity—and as derogatory from her sovereignty, and Independence."⁵³ In a country where many still feared the dangers of concentrated power, at the very least *all* of Congress had to be consulted before such a weighty decision was made.

In an anti-Jay Treaty rally in New York, Alexander Hamilton, one of the architects of the treaty, tried to speak at the public gathering in favor of the treaty. Or, as he wrote, he tried: "to moderate the violence of these views, and to promote a spirit favourable to a fair discussion of the treaty." In some accounts of this event, the crowd responded with a volley of rocks. Hamilton simply wrote: "The leaders . . . resisted all discussion, and their followers, by their clamours and vociferations, rendered it impracticable, notwithstanding the wish of a manifest majority of the citizens convened upon the occasion."⁵⁴ Washington's second Secretary of the Treasury, Oliver Wolcott, Jr., described an anti-Jay Treaty rally in Philadelphia in a letter to the President. He wrote that the leaders read a memorial against the treaty before they threw a copy of the treaty to the crowd "who placed it upon a pole." The protestors preceded first to the French minister's house, and then to the houses of other supporters of the treaty, burning a copy of the treaty in front of each house "with huzzas and acclamations." When they reached the house of U.S. Senator William Bingham, who had voted in favor of the treaty, they also broke some of his windows. Wolcott downplayed both the size and the impact of this protest to the President, assuring Washington that the French minister had played no part and that citizens of the city as a whole "are temperate, and that they feel entire confidence in the President, and will support his decision."⁵⁵ However, in a letter to his father, Wolcott was more despairing. The government must stay rational to function, but, "Faction, dependence, pride, and turbulence, are too general characteristics of the different states." He feared that the American experiment had lost "that sobriety and order upon which this government is predicated."⁵⁶

For a moment, Federalists saw a Jacobin frenzy take hold in cities and towns. George Cabot believed that it represented an "insanity which is epidemic in this quarter." He worried that, "Faction, and especially the faction of great towns always the most powerful, will be too strong for our mild and feeble government."⁵⁷ As the nation divided, Washington stepped in. He wrote letters to the various petitioners including the Boston Selectmen. In that letter, he asserted that he did have the power to make treaties with the advice and consent of the Senate, that, "It was doubtless supposed that these two branches of government would combine, without passion, (and with the best means of information), those facts and principles upon which the success of our foreign relations will always depend: that they ought not to substitute for their own conviction the opinions of others."[58] Finally, on August 18, despite some misgivings, President Washington signed the Treaty. This gave brief comfort to some of his Federalist supporters, and by late summer and early fall of that year these supporters could proclaim to one another, "if all remains right and sound at the head, there is little danger of contaminating the mass . . . at the present."[59]

When others looked around, however, they still saw the madness of factionalism and licentiousness and the potential for serious sectional division. From her viewpoint in Massachusetts, Abigail Adams wrote to one of her sons that, "The late Treaty between Great Britain and the United states, has excited all the Malovelence and awakened all the animosity of the Democratick Societies throughout the United States." Like others, she attributed much of the madness to French influence, continuing, "Boys and the Rabble are the only Actors in these Scenes, but the fowl Stock from which they originate may be traced beyond the American shore."[60] And in Maryland, anticipating the debate that was to come in the House of Representatives, William Vans Murray wrote to Wolcott, Jr., that he saw "the temper of the Southern States swelling into gall and mischief. This will vent itself in violent declamatory speeches in Congress."[61] Murray was correct that the matter had not been put to rest.

When Congress reconvened on November 3, 1795, it was not immediately clear what steps, if any, the House of Representatives would take in response to being left out of the treaty negotiations. Washington, clearly, hoped that the matter of the treaty was settled. In his state of the union address, he kept his commentary on the treaty to one short paragraph, informing the House that the Senate had made a minor revision and that he gave sanction to the treaty with that revision. He had not yet heard back from Great Britain regarding the West Indian trade, but as soon as he had word "the subject will without delay be placed before Congress." Since the work of the treaty was more or less over, barring an unexpected response from Great Britain, he suggested to the House that they tackle a system of public credit and the expenses that had come from putting down the insurrection in Pennsylvania. The House had other ideas, however. Once they had the state of the union in hand, they turned their attention to responding to the President's message. Almost all of November's business was taken up in this manner.

Virginia Representative William Giles wrote about the lack of action of the House's response to the treaty in a letter to Jefferson on December 20, 1795. He told Jefferson that the Democratic Republicans in the House had decided to divorce their disapproval of the treaty from their response to the state of the union, and that any declaration from the House "should be a distinct, solemn and independent act." He was not sure this was the best strategy. He feared that the longer they waited, the more the pro-treaty forces could muster their strength. Support for the treaty would grow "not on account of the daily discovery of intrinsic merit; but on account of the astonishing exertions and artifices employed to give it efficacy." He continued that the friends of the administration were good at raising alarm, "Foreign war—Internal disorganization—'nefarious and detestable conspiracies'—French influence—Disunion of states—bribery &c. &c. have been sounded in the public ear, until the public mind seems to be distracted. If this be not the reign of terror, it is at least, the reign of alarm, and its effect hitherto has exceeded all rational calculation."[62] In that list of alarms, he effectively summarized the Federalist tactics of raising fear in the minds of the American public by painting anything other than full support of the administration as leading down the road to ruin.

Not until March 1796, did the House begin a debate on the Jay Treaty. The debate focused on whether or not the House had the right to refuse to assent to a treaty which required action by the House, particularly appropriation of money and the regulation of commerce. New York Representative Edward Livingston believed that "the late British Treaty" raised "important and constitutional questions," and called for a resolution that the President to provide the instructions given to Minister John Jay before he had gone to London to negotiate.[63] At this point, Wolcott, Sr., wrote to his son: "I had no apprehension that our system of government would be so soon threatened as it is at present." He worried that "disorganization may be expected to follow, and the states who precipitate the event will, I believe, be left to themselves, and will be gratified by becoming provinces of France."[64] The nefarious design of France was to disorder its pretended ally enough to allow the French to reassert themselves in North America.

In mid-April, the debate continued. On one side, there were men like Massachusetts Samuel Lyman who told the body that although he had first opposed the treaty because it appeared "some of its stipulations were too favorable for Britain, and too disadvantageous to us," the more he studied it, the more he supported it.[65] On the other side were those like Virginian William Giles who spent what must have been hours going through each of the articles of the treaty before concluding that "he conscientiously believed the Treaty to be a bad one," that "it contained the most complete evidence of British interference in our internal affairs, and had laid the foundation for the further extension of British influence."[66] Secretary of the Treasury, Wolcott, Jr., who could only watch and worry about these debates, believed French money had influenced Democratic Republican actions. "I believe there never was a public body deserved less the public confidence; who were more ignorant, vain and incompetent, than the majority of the present House of Representatives," He wrote to his father. In his mind, "The whole session has been a disgraceful squabble for power, and a display of unworthy passions. He blamed Representative Albert Gallatin for his leadership of the opposition, a man Wolcott believed was, "directed by foreign politics and influence."[67]

Even before this debate, Gallatin had become a lightning rod for party differences. In 1793, he had been chosen by the Pennsylvania legislature as a U.S. Senator, but in February 1794 he was removed from the Senate by a 14-12 vote. Although 13 of the 14 who voted to remove him were strongly Federalist, they claimed it was not their ideology that made them vote the way they did, but their belief that Gallatin was not a citizen of Pennsylvania. Shunted from the Senate, Gallatin returned to Pennsylvania where the voters elected him to serve in the House of Representatives where he became one of the most outspoken members of the House against the Jay Treaty. Starting in March, Gallatin argued that if the members of the House disagreed with the treaty they could, in effect, make it null and void by not passing appropriations or legislation that would allow the treaty to function. For, "if a treaty embraces objects within the sphere of the general powers delegated to the Federal Government, but which have been exclusively and specially granted to a particular branch of Government . . . [it] does not become the law of the land until it has obtained the sanction of that branch."[68] In the end, the House took a safer route and simply voted asked for a copy of the instructions to Minister John Jay as well as any other relevant documents before they could make any decisions regarding appropriations. George Washington declined the measure, citing his belief that treaty-making lay solely with the executive branch and the Senate and that the asked-for intelligence could harm future diplomatic missions.

The House debated whether or not they would approve the funding needed for the Jay Treaty to function. If the opponents of the Jay Treaty had prevailed, this would have been a way to stop the close connection to Great Britain, a move they saw as a patriotic duty. For Federalists like Wolcott, Sr., however, this move would be madness. Writing to his son about the debates in the House, he remarked that, "Derangement of every kind seems to be" the object of the Democratic Republicans in that body.[69] To Wolcott, they were not good Americans, but simply men bent on infecting the nation with the contagion of mental illness.

In the House, after more than a month of debate, Representatives voted in a way indicative both of the division in the House of Representatives and of the general citizenry. They voted on three different questions and were split on the first two. The first call was, "For declaring the Treaty highly objectionable," and the second simply, "For declaring the Treaty objectionable." In the first case, the vote was split 48-48 and the second 49-49. In both cases, the Federalist Speaker of the House, Jonathan Dayton of New Jersey broke the tie in the negative. In the official notes on these votes, it is clear that the numbers don't tell the whole story. Those voting against the language that the treaty was objectionable came to their vote from different standpoints. Some were outright in favor of the treaty. Others feared that calling the treaty objectionable "would be injurious," presumably to the republic. Lastly, some were "so opposed to the Treaty, as to object to all compromise." The last vote was "For carrying into effect the Treaty." Despite the best efforts by Gallatin and others, the vote carried in the affirmative, 51-48, with the note reading that some believed the treaty was a good one but others voted for it because it was "best to execute it under existing circumstances."[70] Despite the action by the House, objections to the treaty did not die away immediately. By May, Mercy Otis Warren wrote to her son James that she hoped he had protected himself from "the violence of party which rages with so much virulence not only in your town but in almost every other place."[71] When she looked at the treaty and Congress's actions, she saw differences that could not be bridged and bad policy that created conditions that were dangerous to the safety of the American people. For Democratic Republican printer James Callender, the ratification was proof "that nations are sometimes actuated by a degree of madness;" in this case, it was the United States that acted on irrational rather than on rational principles.[72]

With the treaty now in full effect and funded, Federalists briefly believed that the contagion of anarchy that they feared had been contained. However, Washington's retirement, considered and rumored since 1792, now became a reality. Wolcott, Sr. fretted about it to his son during the House debates over the Jay Treaty, writing, "I think it will be most for his honour at any event not to quit the helm during a storm. I am certain that it will be utterly inconsistent with our safety."[73] On September 19, however, Washington made it official, publishing an address in the *American Daily Advertiser* that he and others had been working on, in one form or another, since the end of his first administration. In his address, he asked Americans to "discountenance irregular oppositions to [the government's] acknowledged authority" and to refrain from sectionalism. Shortly after it was published Wolcott, Sr. wrote to his son again, this time in even more alarming tones. In Wolcott's mind, Washington's retirement "will probably, within no distant period, ascertain whether our present system and union can be preserved." He believed it would not be for, "It may exist a few years, but the violent symptoms which have attacked it so early, evince to my mind that it will be of short duration." He then came back to the effects of irrationality on the rational state he and his generation had tried to create, "We have not the least evidence that this is the age of reason." Despite their best efforts, it seemed, they could not overcome "ignorance and vice" nor "baseness."[74]

In the House of Representatives, the Federalists wrote an adulatory response to Washington's address and tried to get that response approved by the rest of that body. The Democratic Republicans spent days fighting back. They believed that the Federalist praises were overblown. For instance, Edward Livingston of New York said that he "believed the United States did not enjoy . . . tranquil prosperity; on the contrary, he thought this was a time of great calamity in the country, and he thought that it was owing, principally, to the measures of the Government." Isaac Parker from Maine thought "the last four years Administration had convinced many, as well as himself, that the Administration was not the most enlightened." Washington's opponents came back to what they saw as his failures: the treaty with Great Britain, a military response to the tax protestors in western Pennsylvania, and other policies. They believed Washington had been corrupted by power and had become aristocratical. Publisher William Duane made no bones about it (although he did write under a pseudonym, Jasper Dwight). In a widely published letter to George Washington, he wrote: "You are lost, Sir, in the treacherous mazes of passion; you have given way to the jealousy of irritated feelings, before reflection could soften the violence of your choler." In dozens of pages, Duane dissected Washington's Farewell Address, pointing out what was, to Duane's mind, the "political diseases" and the "loathings of a sick mind" that it exposed.[75]

The passions of those opposed to Washington, both in and out of Congress, were worrisome as he exited from the political stage. In a letter, Fisher Ames brought his thinking back to the problems of trying to create a rational state, writing, "I have long seen with terror that our destiny is committed to our prudence, which I have ever believed to be weaker than our prejudice and passion." If prudence could not overrule passion, the country might just be doomed. As the door opened to the first contested presidential election, Ames worried, "Yet as the seekers of popularity are corrupters of the multitude, the malady is endemical and incurable." Democracy, rule by the mob, anarchy, and the popularity of figures like Thomas Jefferson who stood for all of those things and more in Ames's mind, meant that a nation founded on the principle of consent of the governed would devolve into corruption and disease. In 1787, Alexander Hamilton had hoped that the government under the constitution would work to alleviate the "seditions and insurrections" that "are, unhappily, maladies as inseparable from the body politic as tumors and eruptions from the natural body." Instead, for those who wanted a government that suppressed the more democratic impulses of the people, it seemed that, in less than a decade, as if the Constitution could not protect them from these or other maladies.

Two decades after independence had been declared in the midst of the folly and madness of war, the United States still faced an uncertain future. The first generation of American citizens had dreamed first of a union and then of a more perfect union but were unable to fulfill those dreams. Differences between subjects and then citizens ran too deep to allow the creation of the rational social contract that had seemed a possibility between the break from British rule and the messy reality of governing a vast and unequal nation. Throughout the first decades of this experiment, Americans had hoped for sanity and rationality but refused to see sanity and rationality as negotiated social constructs. Instead, they became fixed on defining the sane and rational as those who believed as they did, who defined the legacy of the American Revolution as they had, and dismissed their opponents as lunatics. In our world, politicians and pundits love to call on the mythic founding generation as an example without understanding that the founding generation was equally divided, equally irrational, and equally dismissive of their opponents. Today we pick and choose among a small sample of those in the founding era to make our arguments, often spinning tales of a perfectly functioning and golden era when, instead, the lessons of the past should be that creating enemies also creates irrational violence, and that in no era in American history have political actors embraced their opponents or believed those opponents had ideas equally valid.

NOTES

1. Deborah Norris Logan, *Memoir of Dr. George Logan of Stenton: With Selections from His Correspondence* (Philadelphia: Historical Society of Pennsylvania, 1899), 58.

2. Oliver Wolcott, Sr. to Oliver Wolcott, Jr., April 25, 1796. In George Gibbs, ed., *Memoirs of the Administrations of Washington and John Adams Edited from the Papers of Oliver Wolcott, Secretary of the Treasury*, Vol. I (New York: Burt Franklin, 1846; reprint 1971), 332.

3. Benjamin Rush, *Medical Inquiries and Observations* (Philadelphia: Thomas Dobson, 1794), 68.

4. Laure Murat, *The Man Who Thought He Was Napoleon: Toward a Political History of Madness*, trans. Deke Dusinberre (Chicago: The University of Chicago Press, 2014), 148.

5. Oliver Wolcott, Sr. to Oliver Wolcott, Jr. 25 March 1793 in Gibbs, ed., *Memoirs*, 91.

6. Rachel Hope Cleves, *The Reign of Terror in America: Visions of Violence from Anti-Jacobinism to Antislavery* (New York: Cambridge University Press, 2009), 3.

7. Stanley Elkins and Eric McKitrick, *The Age of Federalism* (New York: Oxford University Press, 1993), 309.

8. "For the Daily Advertiser," 2 December 1793, in *Historical Magazine, and Notes and Queries, Concerning the Antiquities, History and Biography of America*, 833.

9. Chauncey Goodrich to Oliver Wolcott, Jr., 10 March 1794, in Gibbs, ed., *Memoirs*, 131. John Jay and Rufus King, "To the Public," in the *Daily Advertizer*, New York, *Supplement ... Monday evening, December 2.* New York, 17893. https://www.loc.gov/item/rbpe.11201 10e/.

10. Quoted in Charles Gayarre, *Aubert Dubayet: or, The Two Sister Republics* (Carlisle, MA: Applewood Books, 1882), 162.

11. John Adams to Samuel Adams, September 12, 1790, reprinted in William Holt Starr, *The Repository*, Vol. I (New London, CT: W.H. Starr & Company, 1858): 236, https://books.google.com/books/about/The_Repository.html.

12. Quoted in Davis R. Dewey, "News of the French Revolution in America," *New England Magazine* 1 (September 1889): 87.

13. Elkins and McKitrick, *The Age of Federalism*, 284.

14. Elkins and McKitrick, *The Ae of Federalism*, 240.

15. Mercy Otis Warren to Catharine Sawbridge Macaulay Graham, May 31, 1791, in Richards and Harris, eds, *Mercy Otis Warren*, 231.

16. "To Thomas Jefferson from William Short, 20 July 1792," *Founders Online*, National Archives, last modified June 13, 2018, http://founders.archives.gov/documents/Jefferson/01-24-02-0227.

17. William Short to Thomas Jefferson, July 31, 1792 in John Catanzariti, ed., *The Papers of Thomas Jefferson*, Vol. 24 (Princeton: Princeton University Press, 1990), 271.

18. Quoted in Elkins and McKitrick, *The Age of Federalism*, 316–317.

19. Cato, "French Revolution," *The American Museum, or, Universal Magazine* 12, no. 5, American Periodicals.

20. Alexander Hamilton, *Letters of Pacificus: Written in Justification of the President's Proclamation of Neutrality* (Philadelphia: Samuel H. Smith, 1793), 48, Evans Early American Imprint Collection.

21. Chauncey Goodrich to Oliver Wolcott, Jr., 24 March 1793, in Gibbs, ed., *Memoirs*, 90.

22. John Quincy Adams, *An Oration, Pronounced July 4th, 1793, at the Request of the Inhabitants of the Town of Boston; in Commemoration of the Anniversary of American Independence* (Boston: Benjamin Edes & Son, 1793), 17–19, Evans Early American Imprint Collection.

23. David Osgood, *A Discourse, Delivered February 19, 1795. The Day Set Apart by the President for a General Thanksgiving through the United States*, 1795, 11–12, https://books.google.com/books?id=Vu5CAQAAMAAJ.

24. "From George Washington to the Cabinet, 18 April 1793," *Founders Online*, National Archives, last modified June 13, 2018, http://founders.archives.gov/documents/Washington/05-12-02-0358.

25. "Thomas Jefferson's Notes on a Cabinet Meeting, 6 May 1793," Founders Online, National Archives, last modified June 13, 2018, http://founders.archives.gov/documents/Washington/05-12-02-0426.

26. Benton, ed., *Abridgment of the Debates of Congress*, 444.

27. *Journal of the Senate of the United States of America*, December 9, 1793, memory.loc.gov.

28. George Washington, "Special Message," December 5, 1793, Gerhard Peters and John T. Woolley, eds, *The American Presidency Project*, https://www.presidency.ucsb.edu/node202898.

29. *Memoir of Dr. George Logan*, 53–54.

30. Resolutions of the Democratic Society of the County of Chittenden, January 8, 1795. In Philip S. Foner, ed., *The Democratic-Republican Societies, 1790–1800: A Documentary Sourcebook of Constitutions, Declaration, Addresses, Resolutions, and Toasts* (Westport, CT: Greenwood Press, 1976), 311. "Address to the Republican Citizens of the United States," May 23, 1794, In Foner, *Democratic-Republican Societies*, 175.

31. Christopher Gore, *Manlius: With Notes and References* (1794). Evans Early American Imprint Collection.

32. George Cabot to Theophilus Parsons, August 12, 1794. In Charles Warren, *Jacobin and Junto, or, Early American Politics as Viewed in the Diary of Dr. Nathaniel Ames, 1758–1822* (Cambridge: Harvard University Press, 1931), 51.

33. Alexander Graydon, *Memoirs of a Life, Chiefly Passed in Pennsylvania, within the Last Sixty Years; with Occasional Remarks upon the General Occurrences, Character and Spirit of That Eventful Period* (Harrisburgh: John Wyeth, 1811), 342, https://catalog.hathitrust.org/Record/000364765.

34. Graydon, *Memoirs*, 343.

35. Helena Wells, Letters on subjects of importance to the happiness of young females, addressed by a governess to her pupils, chiefly while they were under her immediate tuition: To which are added, some practical lessons on the improprieties of language, and errors in pronunciation, which frequently occur in common conversation, 2nd ed. (London: Sabine & Son, 1807), 7.

36. Elkins and McKittrick, *The Age of Federalism*, 389. Gordon E. Sherman, "Orders in Council and the Law of the Sea," *American Journal of International Law* 16 (July 1922): 400–419, https://www.jstor.org/stable/pdf/2188177.pdf.

37. William Smith, 13 January 1794, in John C. Rives, ed., *Abridgement of the Debates of Congress, from 1789 to 1856*, Vol. 1 (New York: D. Appleton and Company, 1857), 464, https://books.google.com/books?id=H1gUAAAAYAAJ.

38. Judith Sargent Murray, "Sketch on the Present Situation of America, 1794," in Sharon M. Harris, ed., *Selected Writings of Judith Sargent Murray* (New York: Oxford University Press, 1995), 53–54.

39. Murray, "Sketch," 57.

40. James Roger Sharp, *American Politics in the Early Republic: The New Nation in Crisis* (New Haven: Yale University Press, 1993), 117.

41. Quoted in Robert C. Byrd, *The Senate, 1789–1989: Addresses on the History of the United States Senate*, Vol. 1 (Washington: U.S. Government Printing Office, 1988), 31.

42. Quoted in John Bach McMaster, *A History of the People of the United States: From the Revolution to the Civil War*, Vol. II (New York: D. Appleton and Company, 1915), 226.

43. Quoted in McMaster, *A History of the People of the United States*, 224.
44. Rufus King to Christopher Gore, July 24, 1795 in Charles R. King, ed., *The Life and Correspondence of Rufus King: Comprising His Letters, Private and Official, His Public Documents and His Speeches* (New York: G.P. Putnam's Sons, 1895), 16–17.
45. Fisher Ames to Oliver Wolcott, Jr., July 9, 1795, in Gibbs, ed., 210.
46. Jeremy Belknap, *The Foresters, an American Tale: Being a Sequel to the History of John Bull the Clothier. In a Series of Letters to a Friend* (Boston: I. Thomas and E.T. Andrews, 1796), 233, Early American Imprint Collection.
47. Belknap, *The Foresters*.
48. Letter addressed to "Messeurs Freneau and Paine" published in the *City Gazette*, South Carolina in Foner, ed., *Democratic-Republican Societies*, 400.
49. Phineas Hedges, An Oration, Delivered before the Republican Society, of Ulster County, and Other Citizens, Convened at the House of Daniel Smith, in the Town of Montgomery, for the Purpose of Celebrating the Anniversary of American Independence, the 4th of July, 1795 (Goshen, NY: David M. Westcott, 1795), 14, Evans Early American Imprint Collection.
50. Richard Beresford, S*ketches of French and English Politicks in America, in May, 1797. By a Member of the Old Congress* (Philadelphia: W.P. Young, 1797), 54–55.
51. One of the best monographs on the attempts to "unbecome" British is Yokota, *Unbecoming British*.
52. Benjamin Goodhue to Oliver Wolcott, Jr., August 1, 1795, in Gibbs, ed., *Memoirs*, 221.
53. "To George Washington from New York Citizens, 20 July 1795," *Founders Online*, National Archives, last modified June 13, 2018, http://founders.archives.gov/documents/Washington/05-18-02-0274.
54. Alexander Hamilton, "The Defence No 1," *The Papers of Alexander Hamilton*, Vol. 18, January 1795–July 1795, ed. Harold C. Syrett (New York: Columbia University Press, 1973), 485.
55. Oliver Wolcott, Jr. to George Washington, July 26, 1795, in Gibbs, ed., *Memoirs*, 217–218.
56. Oliver Wolcott, Jr. to Oliver Wolcott, Sr., August 10, 1795, in Gibbs, ed., *Memoirs*, 224.
57. George Cabot to Rufus King, July 25, 1795, in Warren, *Jacobin and Junto*, 61.
58. George Washington, *George Washington Papers*, Series 2, Letterbooks 1754 to 1799: Letterbook 40, October 2, 1794. 1794. Manuscript/Mixed Material. https://www.loc.gov/item/mgw2.040/.
59. Christopher Gore to Rufus King, September 13, 1795 in King, ed., *The Life and Correspondence of Rufus King*, 31.
60. Abigail Adams to Thomas Boylston Adams, September 17, 1795, *Founders Online*, https://founders.archives.gov/documents/Adams/04-11-02-0012.
61. William Vans Murray to Oliver Wolcott, Jr., October 2, 1795, in Gibbs, ed., *Memoirs*, 249.
62. William Branch Giles to Thomas Jefferson, December 20, 1795. *Founders Online*, https://founders.archives.gov/documents/Jefferson/01-28-02-0434.

63. *Abridgement of the Debates of Congress*, 639.
64. Oliver Wolcott Sr. to Oliver Wolcott Jr., March 21, 1796 in Gibbs, ed., *Memoirs*, 323.
65. *Abridgement of the Debates of Congress*, 707.
66. *Abridgement of the Debates of Congress*, 717.
67. Oliver Wolcott Jr. to Oliver Wolcott Sr., April 18, 1796, in Gibbs, ed., *Memoirs*, 327.
68. *Abridgement of the Debates of Congress*, 644.
69. Oliver Wolcott, Sr. to Oliver Wolcott, Jr., February 15, 1796, in Gibbs, ed., *Memoirs,* 300.
70. *Abridgement of the Debates of Congress*, 754.
71. Richards and Harris, eds, *Mercy Otis Warren*, 242.
72. James Callender, *The History of the United States for 1796; Including a Variety of Interesting Particulars Relative to the Federal Government Previous to That Period* (Philadelphia: Snowden & McCorkle, 1797), 231, Evans Early American Imprint Collection.
73. Oliver Wolcott Sr. to Oliver Wolcott Jr., April 25, 1796, in Gibbs, ed., *Memoirs,* 332.
74. Oliver Wolcott Sr. to Oliver Wolcott Jr., October 3, 1796 in Gibbs, ed. *Memoirs*, 335–336.
75. William Duane, *A Letter to George Washington, President of the United States: Containing Strictures on His Address of the Seventeenth of September, 1796, Notifying His Relinquishment of the Presidential Office* (Philadelphia: Benjamin Franklin Bache, 1796), Evans Early American Imprint Collection.

Epilogue

As George Washington's administration came to a close, he pled with the nation not to dissolve into faction. Washington's plea for unity was likely sincere; he believed in the words that had been crafted for him. He had honor, he tried to live according to his principles. He was a man who had given away military power in 1783 in order to give the new republic the best chance possible to survive as a civilian government rather than a military one. But, it is easy for those in power to believe that they are not the ones promulgating faction and to blame others whom they denigrate by calling self-created societies, Jacobins, political enemies, lunatics, or other pejorative terms. Of course the policies of the Washington administration had been part of what had created faction. As wagerers in the creation of new political systems, Washington and his supporters dismissed alternative interpretations of the legacies of the American Revolution as erroneous or dangerous. Despite the fact that Washington is still painted in our social memory as the father of our country, the political household he headed was not always a happy one. Others in the household chafed at continued inequalities, offered democratic alternatives, and pushed the boundaries of what was possible or imagined. Washington's administration did not bring disparate elements together in a cohesive whole. What continued after Washington's retirement and death was the push and pull of a society split by evolving definitions of equality and the desire of some to keep others down. Men in power remained corruptible and the people out of doors continued to distrust those who held office and, through their actions, to let them know how completely dissatisfied they remained.

In the early years of the nation's existence, Americans were not able to solve the problem of irrational actors in governments that needed rational ones. The problem of irrational actors did not go away; instead medical experts believed that the society and state Americans had created increased rather than decreased the possibilities of madness. Because of this, Americans continued to attempt to address the problems posed by mad men and women in society but also the problems posed by a mentally ill body politic.

On a personal level, insanity continued to bring grief, sorrow, and concern, and to exact a financial toll on individuals. After David Heath lost his mind and was chained in his father's house, Heath's wife had to take on boarders to try to keep her family financially solvent. Heath's "poor wife seemed very unhappy," Deborah Norris Logan wrote in her diary, "and deeply regretted the fatal propensity which had robbed them of all comfort—she has had a toilsome life this summer, for they had had sometimes upwards of an hundred Boarders besides their servants, to provide for."[1] A caregiver for Jane Mecom's insane son, Peter, demanded five dollars a week, a sum Mecom could not afford. In 1778, she tried to get Peter placed in an Alms House and, when that failed, wrote a letter to her brother asking him for financial assistance. Peter died shortly thereafter.[2]

At the ends of their rope, and without adequate care facilities, the solutions were often dire. People confined their loved ones in cellars, pens, straightjackets, or chains. In his *Observations on the Deranged Manifestations of the Mind, or Insanity*, Spurzheim described "the poor insane," who, instead of receiving adequate care "lie on straw and dirt, exposed to all vicissitudes of season and weather, reduced to the mercy of the turnkey, and less attended to than a horse or a wild beast." He reasoned this went against the dictates of a good society and asked: "is not less the duty of a Christian to relieve the sufferings of his countrymen and fellow-citizens"?[3] By 1832, a committee reported to the New Hampshire House of Representatives that more than half of the reported insane were classified as paupers. The report detailed some of the gross abuses, sometimes leading to death, that these men and women faced because their families became unwilling or unable to care for them. According to the report, even the most caring of family members or friends found themselves taxed to the limit both financially and emotionally, forcing a caregiver to become a "jailor" rather than a "friend."[4]

From the colonial era and into the early republic, financial hardship figured into the arguments made by supporters of medical care for the mentally ill. In 1761, in a report on the progress being made toward building the Pennsylvania Hospital, the managers highlighted the effects of poverty not just on individuals, but on family and society. If poor people "cannot labour, they cannot live, without the help of the more fortunate." Their own insanity, or the insanity of family members, could keep them from needed income. The managers asked how a poor man could support his family if afflicted by "any distemper." They continued: "should any sudden hurt happen to him, which should render him incapable" of work, or "should his duty to his aged and diseased parents, or his fatherly tenderness for an afflicted child, engross his attention and care," he would no longer be able to fulfill his financial obligations. Then "how great the calamity for the family! How pressing their wants! How moving their distresses!"[5] Reformers seeking funds to build asylums made this assertion well into the nineteenth century, emphasizing the breakdown of family and society when the insane were left without care or treatment, and appealing to the duty of Americans as both Christians and members of a commonwealth to intervene.

Reformers believed their appeals for intervention particularly compelling because, according to many, the insane were not to blame for their own behavior. In a pamphlet on robbery, piracy, murder, dueling, and suicide, Thomas Baldwin wrote: "An insane person is not a moral agent, consequently not accountable for what he does. Such are to be pitied, and ought to be watched and taken care of by their friends."[6] Many agreed with Baldwin; American towns had long been making provisions for those not able to take care of themselves. As early as 1676 a town in Pennsylvania had made provisions for the care of Erik Vorelissen who had "turned quyt madd." Because his father was "a poore man" the town raised taxes to build a house in which to take care of Vorelissen. In Massachusetts, in the same year, a statute was passed to see to "distracted persons in some tounes, that are unruly."[7] The managers of the Pennsylvania Hospital contended that "the good particular men may do separately in relieving the sick, is small, compared with what they may do collectively; or by a joint endeavor and interest."[8] Intent on building workable communities, reformers wanted to provide treatment for those outside the bounds of acceptable behavior in order to make them, again, good productive citizens, as a step toward building a more productive and healthier society.

The advocates for the Pennsylvania Hospital wanted to relieve the sick, but lawmakers emphasized communities rather than individuals. In 1798, Massachusetts passed a regulatory act that read as follows: "That when it shall be made to appear to any two justices . . . that any person . . . is lunatick and so furiously mad as to render it dangerous to the peace or the safety of the good people for such lunatick person to go at large; the said justices shall have full power . . . to commit such person to the house of correction, there to be detained till he or she be restored to his right mind, or otherwise delivered by due course of law."[9] The stress was on protecting "the safety of the good people" from the "furiously mad." For the insane, this law provided incarceration rather than care. As legislators encountered lunatics and saw the ways such madmen and women could disrupt the workings of society, they responded with legal attempts to remove those disruptions. Care for the mad figured into the equation but was secondary to protecting the community and working toward order and stability.

Although the new legislation demanded that lunatics be committed to a prison, the law was not always followed. In addition, like Peter Mecom had been, the insane were sometimes turned away from the existing institutions of hospitals or almshouses. Private diaries and letters are filled with references to people otherwise confined. Wealthy John Macpherson was both confined in a straightjacket and locked into a building on his own property. Benny Mecom was cared for in a private house. David Heath was "obliged to be confined with a chain in one of the Rooms at his Fathers house."[10] Sarah Shelton Henry was locked into a basement room. Those lucky enough to belong to families with means might receive medical care or other attention during their confinement and might be restored to reason. Often, however, only minimal care was provided and lunatics could live out the rest of their lives chained or in straightjackets, locked into rooms, and without a physician's visit to provide the latest in medical care.

In the United States, the building of asylums went in fits and starts in the first decades of the nation, but concerned citizens continued to raise money and to petition legislatures. They hoped the care would restore people to reason, returning them as active participants in the social compact. In a lecture to the Massachusetts Humane Society in 1802, Eliphalet Porter told his audience that the insane, and particularly the suicidal insane might be "restored . . . to light and the comforts of reason, and to a capacity for those of virtue and religion."[11] The evidence they used supported these goals as they recited the curative practices of famous mad doctors and, as asylums were built, the success that came from those efforts. The McLean Asylum for the Insane was opened in Charlestown, Massachusetts in 1818 and in the next half century most other states had set up institutions modeled in some way or another upon McLean.

The new hospitals and asylums being built provided an avenue on which reformers could focus their attention, but lunatics continued their erratic path into the nineteenth century. One of the great historians of medicine, Charles E. Rosenberg, argued that "in our culture a disease does not exist as a social phenomenon until we agree that it does—until it is named." Eighteenth- and nineteenth-century Americans agreed that mental illness did exist as a social phenomenon in both the body and the body politic. Insanity infected individuals making it impossible for them to engage in the social and political experiment of the new United States in a rational way. At the same time some of the very building blocks for the character of the nation—striving, competition, liberty, choice—created conditions that could also lead to the nation's downfall. As Americans tried to legislate for stability and to create working political and social institutions, they named insanity as a threat to the social order. The specter of the lunatic remained.

A quarter of a century after the Continental Congress had declared independence, Americans remained convinced that crisis and instability had a good chance to unhinge the republic, plummeting the nation into anarchy or tyranny.

The crises that marked society and government in between Washington's retirement and the turn to a new century gave no comfort to Americans as they watched political divisions deepen over the undeclared naval war with France, the passage of the Alien and Sedition Acts, and the hotly contested election of 1800. As Joanne B. Freeman has noted, in this era, "National crises occurred almost annually, and though not all of them percolated down to the realm of local politics with equal intensity, it took only the slightest spark to ignite and uproar of outraged entitlement and revolutionary fervor among populace and politicians alike."[12] The language of madness used so frequently in the 1770s and 1780s remained salient and circulating and speakers and writers continued to express a desire for stability. The war an increasingly distant memory, Americans continued to see threat everywhere they looked.

During the heated election of 1800, Americans saw a crisis with the potential for civil war and disunion. When the election was finally settled on February 17, 1801 with the 36th ballot in the House of Representatives, not all Americans breathed a sigh of relief. Like those who had come before him, in 1801 the lawyer Epaphras Bull invoked the humoral theory of medicine in his Fourth of July oration. During the recent election there had been "nothing heard but the horrid din of overheated partizans and the spiteful venom of audacious faction." In order to get beyond the excess of heat and the illness it brought, he called on his listeners to "let not the spirit of party drive you to madness."[13] Individuals and the nation teetered on the brink of insanity but the cause was not yet lost, according to Bull. It was still possible to balance the humors and restore the nation to good health.

As war continued to rage in Europe, if Americans could not tame their propensity for party rage, the devastation of the French Revolution would be wrought on the United States. White Americans celebrated the liberty and independence that was the legacy of the American Revolution but they continued to worry that liberty presented danger to their own mental health as well as the health of the nation. In Concord, Massachusetts, Judge Samuel Phillips Prescott Fay opined that "liberty is the native soil of faction" and that liberty "furnishes arms for our own destruction." Only "the good sense and discernment of the people" could guarantee the future success of the nation.[14] Individuals needed to avoid the pitfalls of excessive liberty and the insanity that accompanied it to keep the body politic mentally healthy and fully functioning.

The spirit of party, liberty, or other phenomena that led to excessive passions could drive an individual or the nation mad. Many Americans continued to believe that Americans shared a propensity to "run into . . . lunacy & dissipations of every kind," and after other measures had been taken throughout the nation to address the problem of lunacy, lawmakers did not put a sanity test for office in place.[15] This fact came to the forefront in 1804 with the impeachment and removal from office of Federalist Judge John Pickering.

Pickering had been a well-respected community leader who had helped write the New Hampshire constitution and had been appointed as the Chief Justice of the New Hampshire Superior Court in 1790. However, he was also an alcoholic and by 1795 had begun to demonstrate signs of mental illness. At that point, however, he was not removed from office but simply reassigned to the less-demanding United States District Court, a position in which he was confirmed by the U.S. Senate. By 1800, his mental deterioration was clear to everyone who observed him in court. Federalists wanted to keep him in office so that the Jefferson administration would not appoint a Republican successor and Republicans wanted him out, not just because he was a lunatic but because they wanted to dismantle the Federalist-dominated judiciary. Short of Pickering tendering his resignation, however, there was no clear path to removal from office. As Senator William Cocke stated, there was "no law that makes derangement criminal."[16] Nonetheless, Republicans began impeachment hearings without being able to square insanity with the insistence of the Constitution that removal from office was contingent only on "Conviction of, Treason, Bribery, or other high Crimes and Misdemeanors." They decided that his "constant and habitual intoxication," including appearing drunk in court was enough and proceeded with the process of impeachment all while leaving the question of his insanity aside. As Congressman Jackson said, "Insanity is here a bar to all proceedings on an Impeachment," and worried that considering Pickering's mental health or illness would mean they could not "get rid of the Judge."[17] The Republicans could all agree that they did not want an insane Federalist judge in office and then ignored the finer points of constitutional principle to remove him. It was not the first or last time political parties played more of a role in decisions about federal justices than qualifications or fitness for office.

The problem remained for although someone who is insane, temporarily or permanently, certainly poses a danger to the body politic, the American legal system has never found a way to address the problem. In 1905, Senator Augustus Bacon of Georgia proposed an amendment to the Constitution that would have allowed removal from office "on account of immorality, imbecility, maladministration, misfeasance or malfeasance in office" but it never made it out of Congress.[18] In 1967, the Twenty-Fifth Amendment to the U.S. Constitution was adopted, which does include a section that allows the vice president, together with a majority of other stipulated leaders, to present a written declaration that "the President is unable to discharge the powers and duties of his office," but the process is unwieldy, unlikely to result in removal, and makes no stipulation for other federal offices. There is still no clear way to remove someone who evinces mental illness beyond trying to convince him or her to step aside.

When I started this project in 2011, all of this seemed like an intellectual problem, but since the election of Donald Trump in November of 2016, the politicking, the debates, and the fear of unstable or lunatic leadership from the mid to late eighteenth century that compose the evidence for this book seems increasingly relevant. On February 13, 2017, thirty-three physicians signed a letter to the *New York Times* that stated, "We believe that the grave emotional instability indicated by Mr. Trump's speech and actions makes him incapable of serving safely as president." Even a quick glance at social media or political buttons and bumper stickers shows us that these doctors are not the only ones who worried about President Trump and the future of our republic. Americans' current level of concern about the mental health of the man serving in the White House goes beyond what many of us have seen in our lifetimes but, as this book shows, it is a concern with a long history.

The founding generation confronted the question of what to do about irrational actors, but could not come up with a clear answer. In a social compact, physical and mental impairment of an individual can injure the body politic. Nevertheless, in a government committed to opposing tyrannical rule, political motivations behind desire for removal have to be closely examined. Determining where the line rests between just and unjust removal from office is an uncomfortable calculus. It was uncomfortable for many of the men who assumed the first mantles of power in the new United States. It is uncomfortable for those of us now who worry about the future of our nation as we wobble on our current course.

The world is a very different place than it was in the early republic, but we find ourselves grappling with some of the same questions the founding generation did. The government that was adopted in 1787 has been amended and revised, but still, at its core, is a social compact based on the necessity of rational actors. Our historical record is strewn with irrational leaders, but we still have no mechanism for dealing with irrationality: despite Pickering's removal, irrationality is still not an impeachable offense. Thus, there is no Constitutional answer to the dangers posed by someone who, according to the same doctors quoted above, exhibits traits that "distort reality to suit [his] psychological state, attacking facts and those who convey them." But, perhaps we can find some small comfort in looking back and uncovering partisanship, pettiness, egotistical behavior, and irrationality in the early republic. At the time of this book's publication, the republic survives despite the fact that sometimes (often?) those in positions of power have not been motivated not by love of country, but by "[a]mbition, avarice, personal animosity, [and] party opposition." The historical record is filled with Americans who have been convinced, as I am now, that a head of state can be a dangerous demagogue; nevertheless, we have persisted. With our distance, it is easy to contextualize the past; perhaps, now, we can more fully understand the fears of those who lived in that past.

NOTES

1. Logan Diary, volume 3, June 14, 1817 to December 31, 1818. Historical Society of Pennsylvania.
2. Jill Lepore, *Book of Ages: The Life and Opinions of Jane Franklin* (New York: Alfred A. Knopf, 2014), 188–189.
3. Spurzheim, *Observations on the Deranged Manifestations of the Mind, or Insanity*, 160.
4. *Report of the Select Committee to the House of Representatives upon the Subject of Building an Insane Hospital* (Concord, NH: Hill and Barton, 1832), New Hampshire Historical Society.
5. *Some Account of the Pennsylvania Hospital*, 113–114.
6. Thomas Baldwin, *The Danger of Living without the Fear of God. A Discourse on Robbery, Piracy, and Murder. In which Duelling and Suicide Are Particularly Considered* (Boston: James Loring, 1819).
7. Albert Deutsch, *The Mentally Ill in America: A History of Their Care and Treatment from Colonial Times*. 2nd ed. (New York: Columbia University Press, 1949), 42–43.
8. *Some Account of the Pennsylvania Hospital*, 33.
9. "An Act in Addition to an Act entitled 'An Act of Suppressing Rogues,' Vagabonds, Common Beggars and Other Idle, Disorderly and Lewd Persons," quoted in Henry M. Hurd, ed., *The Institutional Care of the Insane in the United States and Canada*, Vol. II (New York: Arno Press, 1973), 584.
10. Logan Diary, volume 3, June 14, 1817 to December 31, 1818, Historical Society of Pennsylvania.
11. Quoted in Richard Bell, *We Shall Be No More: Suicide and Self-Government in the Newly United States* (Cambridge: Harvard University Press, 2012), 106.
12. Joanne B. Freeman, "The Election of 1800: A Study in the Logic of Political Change," *Yale Law Journal* 108, no. 8 (June 1999): 1966–1967.
13. Epaphras W. Bull, *An Oration, Delivered at Danbury on the Fourth of July, 1801. In Commemoration of Our National Independence* (Danbury, CT: Nichols & Rowe, 1801), 14.
14. Samuel P. P. Fay, *An Oration, Delivered at Concord, on the Anniversary of American Independence, July 4th, 1801* (Cambridge: William Hilliard, 1801), 17.
15. Quotation appeared first in Chapter 6: William Samuel Johnson to Benjamin Gale, 2 February 1785. *Letters to Delegates of Congress, 1774–1789*. https://archive.org/stream/lettersofdelegat22smit/lettersofdelegat22smit_djvu.txt.
16. Lynn W. Turner, "The Impeachment of John Pickering," *American Historical Review* 54 (April 1949): 494, https://www.jstor.org/stable/1843004. Despite the fact that there was not a law that made derangement criminal, Pickering was removed from office on a party-line vote.
17. Quoted in Turner, "The Impeachment of John Pickering," 499.
18. *Congressional Record-Senate*, 3474, https://www.govinfo.gov/content/pkg/GPO-CRECB-1905-pt4-v39/pdf/GPO-CRECB-1905-pt4-v39-5-1.pdf.
19. Lance Dodes and Joseph Schacter, letter to the editor, *New York Times*, February 13, 2017.

Bibliography

PRIMARY SOURCES—ARCHIVAL COLLECTIONS

Amory Family Papers, 1697–1894, Personal papers, 1725–1890. Ms. N-2024. Box 1. Massachusetts Historical Society, Boston, Massachusetts.

Deborah Norris Logan. Diary, 1816–1817. Collection #0379. Volume III. Historical Society of Pennsylvania, Philadelphia, Pennsylvania.

Diary of Anna Rawle. Transcript of diary. Collection AM. 13745. Rebecca Shoemaker Papers. Historical Society of Pennsylvania, Philadelphia, Pennsylvania.

Diary of Experience Wight Richardson. Transcription on microfilm. P-289. Massachusetts Historical Society, Boston, Massachusetts.

Fisher, Joseph Francis. Letter to Robert Walker. September 8, 1775. Collection 1858. Series 1, Box 1. Joseph Francis Fisher Papers. Historical Society of Pennsylvania, Philadelphia, Pennsylvania.

Henry Laurens Papers, Collection 356. Historical Society of Pennsylvania, Philadelphia, Pennsylvania.

Henry Strachey Papers, 1768–1802. 647098902. William L. Clements Library, Ann Arbor, Michigan.

Hooper, William. Letter to Mary Hooper, November 7, 1774. James Murray Robinson Family Papers. Ms. N-801, box 1, folder 1. Massachusetts Historical Society, Boston, Massachusetts.

Nathanael Greene Papers, 1762-1852. 759179083. William L. Clements Library, Ann Arbor, Michigan.

Newell, Timothy. A journal kept during the time Boston was shut in 1775, manuscript transcription. Ms. S-259. Massachusetts Historical Society, Boston, Massachusetts.

Park Holland. Diary. Holland Family Papers, 1774–1849. Ms. N-1418. Massachusetts Historical Society, Boston, Massachusetts.

Rea, Sampson. Letter to Samuel Phillips Savage, November 21, 1786. Lemuel Shaw Papers. P-206, reel 19. Massachusetts Historical Society, Boston, Massachusetts.

Robert Treat Paine Papers. Microfilm reel 5. Ms. N-641. Massachusetts Historical Society, Boston, Massachusetts.
Sedgwick Family Papers, 1717–1946. Ms. N-851. Massachusetts Historical Society, Boston, Massachusetts.
Shays' Rebellion Collection, 1784–1787. 844726307. William L. Clements Library, Ann Arbor, Michigan.
Sparkhawk, John. Letter to Joseph Whipple, June 11, 1776. Charles Lowell Collection, 1657–1853. Ms. N-1587. Massachusetts Historical Society, Boston, Massachusetts.
Thomas McKean Papers, Collection 405. Historical Society of Pennsylvania, Philadelphia, Pennsylvania.
William Knox Paper, 1757–1811. 829745903. William L. Clements Library, Ann Arbor, Michigan.
Strachey, Henry. Papers.

PRINT SOURCES

Abbot, W. W. ed. *The Papers of George Washington. Confederation Series.* Vol. 4. Charlottesville: University Press of Virginia, 1995.
The Acts and Resolves, Public and Private, of the Province of the Massachusetts Bay. Vol. IV. Boston: Wright & Potter, 1890. catalog.hathitrust.org/Record/008374362.
Adair, Douglass, and John A. Schutz, eds. *Peter Oliver's Origin & Progress of the American Rebellion.* Stanford: Stanford University Press, 1961.
Adams, Charles Francis, ed. *The Works of John Adams, Second President of the United States.* Boston: Little, Brown, and Company, 1854.
Adams, John Quincy. *An Oration, Pronounced July 4th, 1793, at the Request of the Inhabitants of the Town of Boston; in Commemoration of the Anniversary of American Independence.* Boston: Benjamin Edes Son, 1793. Evans Early American Imprint Collection.
"The Address and Petition of the Officers of the United States." *A Century of Lawmaking for a New Nation: U.S. Congressional Documents and Debates, 1774–1875.* memory.loc.gov/ammem/amlaw/lawhome.html.
Allen, James. "Diary of James Allen, Esq., or Philadelphia, Counsellor-at-Law, 1770–1778. *Pennsylvania Magazine of History and Biography* 9, no. 2 (July 1885): 176–196. https://www.jstor.org/stable/20084701.
American Archives: Consisting of a Collection of Authentick Records, State Papers, Debates, and Letters and Other Notices of Publish Affairs, the Whole Forming a Documentary History of the Origin and Progress of the North American Colonies; of the Causes and Accomplishment of the American Revolution; and of the Constitution of Government for the United States, to the Final Ratification Thereof. Vol. 1. Washington: M. St. Clair Clarke and Peter Force, 1833. https://books.google.com/books/about/American_Archives.html.
Anderson, Alexander. *An Inaugural Dissertation on Chronic Mania.* New York: T. and J. Swords, 1796. Urn:oclc:record:1046641738.

Aptheker, Herbert, ed. *A Documentary History of the Negro People in the United States*. Vol. 1. New York: Citadel press, 1969.
Apthorp, East. *The Felicity of the Times. A Sermon Preached at Christ-Church, Cambridge, on Thursday, XI August, MDCCLXIII. Being a Day of Thanksgiving for the General Peace*. Boston: Green and Russell, 1763. Evans Early American Imprint Collection.
Archer, John. *Every Man His Own Doctor*. London, 1673. https://books.google.com/books?id=I83Mzl0q2qMC.
Arms, Consider, Malachi Maynard, and Samuel Filed. "Dissent to the Massachusetts." *Teaching American History*. https://teachingamericanhistory.org/library/document/consider-arms-malachi-maynard-and-samuel-field-dissent-to-the-massachusetts/.
Arnold, Thomas. *Observations on the Nature, Kinds, Causes, and Prevention of Insanity, Lunacy, or Madness*. Vol. I. Leicester: G. Ireland, 1782. https://archive.org/details/b21440712_0001.
"Articles, Lawes, and Orders, Divine, Politique, and Martiall for the Colony in Virginia." Virtual Jamestown. http://www.virtualjamestown.org/exist/cocoon/jamestown/laws/J1056.
Austin, Jonathan L. *An Oration, Delivered July 4, 1786, at the Request of the Inhabitants of the Town of Boston, in Celebration of the Anniversary of American Independence*. Boston: Peter Edes, 1786. Early American Imprint Collection.
Bailyn, Bernard. *The Ideological Origins of the American Revolution*. Enlarged edition. Cambridge: Belknap Press of Harvard University Press, 1992.
———. *The Ordeal of Thomas Hutchinson*. Cambridge: The Belknap Press of Harvard University Press, 1974.
Baldwin, Thomas. *The Danger of Living without the Fear of God. A Discourse on Robbery, Piracy, and Murder. In which Duelling and Suicide are Particularly Considered*. Boston: James Loring, 1819.
Barnard, Thomas. *A Sermon Preached before His Excellency Francis Bernard, Esq; Governor and Commander in Chief, the Honourable His Majesty's Council, and the Honourable House of Representatives, of the Province of the Massachusetts-Bay in New-England, May 25th, 1763. Being the Anniversary for the Election of His Majesty's Council for Said Province*. Boston: Richard Draper, 1763. Evans Early American Imprint Collection.
Battie, William. *A Treatise on Madness*. London: J. Whiston and B. White, 1763. doi: 10.1136/bmj.39297.741644.94.
Beeman, Richard, Stephen Botein, and Edward C. Carter II, eds. *Beyond Confederation: Origins of the Constitution and American National Identity*. Chapel Hill: University of North Carolina Press, 1987.
Belknap, Jeremy. *The Foresters, an American Tale: Being a Sequel to the History of John Bull the Clothier. In a Series of Letters to a Friend*. Boston; I. Thomas and E.T. Andrews, 1792. Evans Early American Imprint Collection.
Bell, Richard. *We Shall Be No More: Suicide and Self-Government in the Newly United States*. Cambridge: Harvard University Press, 2012.
Benton, Thomas Hart, ed. *Abridgement of the Debates of Congress, from 1789 to 1856*. Vol. 1. New York: D. Appleton & Company, 1857. catalog.hathitrust.org/Record/08700946.

Beresford, Richard. *Sketches of French and English Politicks in America, in May, 1797. By a Member of the Old Congress.* Philadelphia: W.P. Young, 1797.

Blake, John B. "The Inoculation Controversy in Boston: 1721–1722." *The New England Quarterly* 25, no. 4 (1952): 489–506. doi:10.2307/362582.

Bouton, Nathaniel, ed., *Documents and Records Relating to the State of New-Hampshire during the Period of the American Revolution, from 1776 to 1783.* Vol VIII. Concord: Edward A. Jenks, 1874. https://catalog.hathitrust.org/Record/10 1782272.

Bowler, R. Arthur. *Logistics and the Failure of the British Army in America, 1775–1783.* Princeton: Princeton University Press, 1975.

Bradford, Alden, ed. *Speeches of the Governors of Massachusetts, 1765–-1775. The Answers of the House of Representatives Thereto with Their Resolutions and Addresses for that Period.* New York: Da Capo Press, 1971.

Broadwater, Jeff, and Troy L. Kickler. *North Carolina's Revolutionary founders.* Chapel Hill: University of North Carolina Press, 2019.

Brooke, John L. *The Heart of the Commonwealth: Society and Political Culture in Worcester County, Massachusetts, 1713–1861.* New York: Cambridge University Press, 1979.

Brown, Charles Brockden. *Alcuin: A Dialogue.* New York: T & J Swords, 1798. Evans Early American Imprint Collection.

Brown, Richard D., ed. *Major Problems in the Era of the American Revolution, 1760–1791.* Boston: Houghton Mifflin, 2000.

Bruce, La Marr Jurelle. "Mad Is a Place; or, the Slave Ship Tows the Ship of Fools." *American Quarterly* 69, no. 2 (June 2017): 303–308.

Buchan, William. *Domestic Medicine: Or a Treatise on the Prevention and Cure of Diseases, by Regimen and Simple Medicine. To Which Is Added, Characteristic Symptoms of Diseases, from the Nosology of the Late Celebrated Dr. Cullen of Edinburgh.* Newcastle: K. Anderson, 1812. xxii, https://collections.nlm.nih.gov/bookviewer?PID=nlm:nlmuid-0217316-bk.

Bull, Epaphras W. *An Oration, Delivered at Danbury on the Fourth of July, 1801. In Commemoration of Our National Independence.* Danbury, CT: Nichols & Rowe, 1801.

Burnett, Edward C., ed. *Letters of Members of the Continental Congress.* Vol. 1. Washington: Carnegie Institution of Washington, 1921. http://books.google.com/books?id=4AmKAAAAMAAJ.

Burnham, John C. *Health Care in America: A History.* Baltimore: Johns Hopkins University Press, 2015.

Butterfield, Lyman H., ed. *The Adams Papers, Adams Family Correspondence.* Vol. 1. Cambridge: Harvard University Press, 1963.

Byrd, Robert C. *The Senate, 1789–1989: Addresses on the History of the United States Senate.* Vol. 1. Washington, DC: U.S. Government Printing Office, 1988.

Callender, James. *The History of the United States for 1796; Including a Variety of Interesting Particulars Relative to the Federal Government Previous to that Period.* Philadelphia: Snowden & McCorkle, 1797. Evans Early American Imprint Collection.

Calloway, Colin G. "Indians, Europeans, and the New World of Disease and Healing." In *Major Problems in the History of American Medicine and Public Health*, edited by John Harley Warner and Janet A. Tighe, 41–48. Boston: Houghton Mifflin, 2001.

A Candid Examination of the Address of the Minority of the Council of Censors to the People of Pennsylvania. Philadelphia, 1784. https://catalog.hathitrust.org/Record/010446583.

Catanzariti, John, ed. *The Papers of Thomas Jefferson*. Vol. 24. Princeton: Princeton University Press, 1990.

Chakravarti, Paromita. "Natural Fools and the Historiography of Renaissance Folly." *Renaissance Studies* 25, no. 2 (April 2011): 208–227. https://doi.org/10.1111/j.1477-4658.2010.00674.x.

Chandler, Thomas Bradbury. *What Think Ye of the Congress Now? Or, An Inquiry, How Far Americans are Bound to Abide by and Execute the Decisions of, the Late Congress*. New York: James Rivington, 1775. Evans Early American Imprint Collection.

Channing, Edward. *A History of the United States*. Vol. III. New York: Macmillan Company, 1912.

Channing, Edward, and Archibald Cary Coolidge, eds. *The Barrington-Bernard Correspondence and Illustrative Matter, 1760–1770. Drawn from the "Papers of Sir Francis Bernard" (Sometime Governor of Massachusetts-Bay*. Cambridge: Oxford University Press, 1912.

Chase, George Wingate. *The History of Haverhill, Massachusetts*. Haverhill: New England History Press and the Haverhill Historical Society, 1983.

Clark, J. C. D. *Thomas Paine: Britain, America, and France in the Age of Enlightenment and Revolution*. New York: Oxford University Press, 2020.

Cleves, Rachel Hope. *The Reign of Terror in America: Visions of Violence from Anti-Jacobinism to Antislavery*. New York: Cambridge University Press, 2009.

Commager, Henry Steele, and Richard B. Morris, eds. *The Spirit of 'Seventy-Six: The Story of the American Revolution as Told by Participants*. New York: Harper & Row, 1958.

Colley, Linda. *Captives*. New York: Pantheon Books, 2002.

Conley, Patrick T., and John P. Kaminski, eds. *The Bill of Rights and the States: The Colonial and Revolutionary Origins of American Liberties*. Madison, WI: Madison House, 1992.

Copy of Letters Sent to Great-Britain, by His Excellency Thomas Hutchinson, the Hon. Andrew Oliver, and Several Other Persons, Born and Educated aAmong Us. Which Original Letters Have Been Returned to America, and Laid before the Honorble [sic] House of Representatives of This Province. Boston: Edes and Gill, 1773. Evans Early American Imprint Collection.

Cutbrush, Edward. *An Inaugural Dissertation on Insanity: Submitted to the Examination of the Rev. John Ewing, S.T.P. Provost; The Trustees and Medical Professors of the University of Pennsylvania; for the Degree of Doctor of Medicine, On the Nineteenth Day of May, A.D. MDCCXCIV*. Philadelphia: Zachariah Pouslon, Jr., 1794. https://archive.org/details/2548037R.nlm.nih.gov.

Dalrymple, John. *The Rights of Great Britain Asserted against the Claims of America: Being an Answer to the Declaration of the General Congress*. Philadelphia: R. Bell, 1776. Evans Early American Imprint Collection.

Darwin, Erasmus. *Zoonomia; Or, the Laws of Organic Life. In Three Parts*. Boston: Thomas and Andrews, 1803.

Deutsch, Albert. *The Mentally Ill in America: A History of Their Care and Treatment from Colonial Times*. 2nd ed. New York: Columbia University Press, 1949.

Dewey, Davis R. "News of the French Revolution in America." *New England Magazine* 7, no. 1 (September 1889).

"Dialogue on Civil Liberty, Delivered at a Public Exhibition in Nassau-Hall. Jan. 1776." *The Pennsylvania Magazine* 2 (April 1776).

Diary of John Adams. *Adams Family Papers: An Electronic Archive*. https://www.masshist.org/digitaladams/archive/diary/.

Dickinson, Harry T., ed. *British Pamphlets on the American Revolution, 1763–1785*. Vol. 3. London: Pickering & Chatto, 2007.

Dickinson, John. "The Liberty Song." *Dickinson College Archives and Special Collections*. http://archives.dickinson.edu/sundries/liberty-son-1768.

Digital Paxton: Digital Collection, Critical Edition, and Teaching Platform. http://digitalpaxton.org.

Dodd, W. F. "The First State Constitutional Conventions, 1776–1783." *American Political Science Review* 2, no. 4 (November 1908): 545–561. https://www.jstor.org/stable/1944479.

Duane, William. *A Letter to George Washington, President of the United States: Containing Strictures on His Address of the Seventeenth of September, 1796, Notifying His Relinquishment of the Presidential Office*. Philadelphia: Benjamin Franklin Bache, 1796. Evans Early American Imprint Collection.

———. *Letters to Benjamin Franklin, from His Family and Friends, 1751–1790*. New York: C. Benjamin Richardson, 1859. https://catalog.hathitrust.org/Record/006255147.

Dunbar, John R., ed. *The Paxton Papers*. The Hague: Martinus Nijhoff, 1957.

Edwards, Jonathan. *The Injustice and Impolicy of the Slave Trade, and of the Slavery of the Africans: Illustrated in a Sermon Preached before the Connecticut Society for the Promotion of Freedom, and for the Relief of Persons Unlawfully Holden in Bondage, at Their Annual Meeting in New-Haven, September 15, 1791*. Boston: Wells and Lilly, 1822. Evans Early American Imprint Collection.

Elkins, Stanley, and Eric McKitrick. *The Age of Federalism*. New York: Oxford University Press, 1993.

Elliott, Jonathan, ed. *Debates in the Several State Conventions on the Adoption of the Federal Constitution as Recommended by the General Convention at Philadelphia in 1787. Together with the Journal of the Federal Convention, Luther Martin's Letter, Yates's Minutes, Congressional Opinions, Virginia and Kentucky Resolutions of '98-'99, and Other Illustrations of the Constitution*. Vol. 4. Philadelphia: J.B. Lippincott & Co., 1866. https://memory.loc.gov/ammem/amlaw/lwed.html.

Eustace, Nicole. "Emotions and Political Change." In *Doing Emotions History*, edited by Susan J. Matt and Peter N. Sterns, 104–183. Champaign: University of Illinois Press, 2014.

———. *Passion Is the Gale: Emotion, Power, and the Coming of the American Revolution.* Chapel Hill: University of North Carolina Press, 2008.

Fay, Samuel P. P. *An Oration: Delivered at Concord, on the Anniversary of American Independence, July 4th, 1801.* Cambridge: William Hilliard, 1801.

Fenn, Elizabeth A., and Peter Wood. *Natives and Newcomers: The Way We Lived in North Carolina before 1770.* Chapel Hill: University of North Carolina Press, 1983.

Ferguson, Robert A. *The American Enlightenment, 1750–1820.* Cambridge: Harvard University Press, 1994.

Finley, Samuel. *The Madness of Mankind, Represented in a Sermon Preached in the New Presbyterian Church in Philadelphia, on the 9th of June 1754.* Library Company of Philadelphia.

Fitch, William Edward. *Some Neglected History of North Carolina, Being an Account of the Revolution of the Regulators and the Battle of Alamance, the First Battle of the American Revolution.* New York: 1914. https://archive.org/details/somenegl ectedhis00fitcuoft.

Foner, Eric. *Tom Paine and Revolutionary America.* New York: Oxford University Press, 1976.

Foner, Philip S., ed. *The Democratic-Republican Societies, 1790–1800: A Documentary Sourcebook of Constitutions, Declarations, Addresses, Resolutions, and Toasts.* Westport, CT: Greenwood Press, 1976.

Fontana, Alan, and Robert Rosenheck. "Traumatic War Stressors and Psychiatric Symptoms among World War II, Korean, and Vietnam War Veterans." *Psychology and Aging* 9, no. 1 (1994): 27–33. doi:10.1037//0882-7974.9.1.27.

Ford, Paul Leicester, ed. *The Writings of John Dickinson.* Vol. 1. Philadelphia: Historical Society of Pennsylvania, 1895. https://books.google.com/books?id=2 -kzAQAAMAAJ.

Ford, Timothy. "Diary of Timothy Ford, 1785–1786." *South Carolina Historical and Genealogical Magazine* 13, no. 3 (July 1912): 132–147. https://www.jstor.org/sta ble/pdf/27575338.pdf.

Foucault, Michel. *History of Madness.* Edited by Jean Khalfa. Translated by Jonathan Murphy and Jean Khalfa. New York: Routledge, 2006.

Freeman, Joanne B. "The Election of 1800: A Study in the Logic of Political Change." *Yale Law Journal* 108, no. 8 (June 1999): 1959–1994.

Friends, Society of. *The Testimony of the People Called Quakers, Given Forth by a Meeting ... Held at Philadelphia the Twenty-Fourth Day of the First Month, and Subsequent Documents, 1776 to 1777.* Philadelphia: John Dunlap, 1777. https:// www.loc.gov/item/2006566657/.

Gayarre, Charles. *Aubert Dubayet: Or, the Two Sister Republics.* Carlisle, MA: Applewood Books, 1882.

Gibbs, George, ed. *Memoirs of the Administrations of Washington and John Adams Edited from the Papers of Oliver Wolcott, Secretary of the Treasury.* Vol. 1. New York: Burt Franklin, 1846; reprint 1971.

Gilpin, Thomas, and Joseph Meredith Toner Collection. *Exiles in Virginia: With Observations on the Conduct of the Society of Friends during the Revolutionary*

War, Comprising the Official Papers of the Government Relating to That Period. Philadelphia, 1848. https://lccn.loc.gov/06042550.

Glenn, Myra C. "Troubled Manhood in the Early Republic: The Life and Autobiography of Sailor Horace Lane." *Journal of the Early Republic* 26, no. 1 (Spring 2006): 59–93.

Glover, Lorri. *The Fate of the Revolution: Virginians Debate the Constitution.* Baltimore: Johns Hopkins University Press, 2016.

Gordon, Scott Paul. "Patriots and Neighbors: Pennsylvania Moravians in the American Revolution." *Journal of Moravian History* 12, no. 2 (Fall 2012): 111–142. https://www.jstor.org/stable/10.325/jmorahist.12.2.0111.

Gore, Christopher. *Manlius: With Notes and References.* Boston: Benjamin Russell, 1794. Evans Early American Imprint Collection.

Gould, Eliga. *Among the Powers of the Earth: The American Revolution and the Making of a New World Empire.* Cambridge: Harvard University Press, 2010.

Graydon, Alexander. *Memoirs of a Life, Chiefly Passed in Pennsylvania, within the Last Sixty Years; with Occasional Remarks upon the General Occurrences, Character and Spirit of That Eventful Period.* Harrisburg: John Wyeth, 1811. https://catalog.hathitrust.org/Record/000364765.

Greene, Jack P., ed. *The Diary of Colonel Landon Carter of Sabine Hall, 1752-1778.* Vol. II. Charlottesville: University Press of Virginia, 1965.

Gregory, Anthony. "'Formed for Empire': The Continental Congress Responds to the Carlisle Peace Commission." *Journal of the Early Republic* 38, no. 4 (Winter 2018): 643–672.

Griffith, William, ed. *Historical Notes of the American Colonies and Revolution, from 1754–1775.* Burlington, NJ: Joseph L. Powell, 1843. https://www.google.com/books/edition/Historical_Notes_of_the_American_Colonie.

Grosvenor, Benjamin. *Health: An Essay on Its Nature, Value, Uncertainty, Preservation and Best Improvement.* Boston: D. and J. Kneeland, 1761. http://resource.nlm.nih.gov/2555049R.

Grotius. *Pills for the Delegates: Or the Chairman Chastised, in a Series of Letters, Addressed to Peyton Randolph, Esq.; on His Conduct, as President of the General Congress: Held at the City of Philadelphia, September 5, 1774.* New York: James Rivington, 1775. Evans Early American Imprint Collection.

Hamilton, Alexander. *Letters of Pacificus: Written in Justification of the President's Proclamation of Neutrality.* Philadelphia: Samuel H. Smith, 1793. Evans Early American Imprint Collection.

Harding, Samuel Bannister. *The Contest over the Ratification of the Federal Constitution in the State of Massachusetts.* New York: Longmans, Green, and Company, 1896.

Harris, Sharon M. ed. *Selected Writings of Judith Sargent Murray.* New York: Oxford University Press, 1995.

Haslam, John. *Illustrations of Madness.* Edited by Roy Porter. London: Routledge, 1988.

Haywood, Eliza. *The Distress'd Orphan, Or Love in a Mad-House.* Reprint Edition. New York: AMS Press, Inc., 1995. First published in 1726.

Hazard, Samuel, ed. *Hazard's Register of Pennsylvania, Devoted to the Preservation of Facts and Documents, and Every Kind of Useful Information Respecting the States of Pennsylvania.* Volume XII. Philadelphia: William F. Gedes. https://books.google.com/books?id=t30UAAAAYAAJ&ppis.

Hedges, Phineas. *An Oration, Delivered before the Republican Society, of Ulster County, and Other Citizens, Convened at the House of Daniel Smith, in the Town of Montgomery, for the Purpose of Celebrating the Anniversary of American Independence, the 4th of July, 1795.* Goshen, NY: David M. Westcott, 1795. Evans Early American Imprint Collection.

Henderson, Richard. *An Account of Mob Violence Witnessed in the Courts of New Bern.* Adams Matthews Colonial America Database.

Hichborn, Benjamin. *An Oration, Delivered July 5th, 1784 at the Request of the Inhabitants of the Town of Boston; in Celebration of the Anniversary of American Independence.* Boston: John Gill, 1784. Evans Early American Imprint Collection.

Historical Magazine, and Notes and Queries, Concerning the Antiquities, History and Biography of America. Vol. 5. Morrisania, NY: Henry B. Dawson, 1869. https://archive.org/details/historicalmagazi1869morr/page/n19.

The History of the War in America, between Great Britain and Her Colonies from Its Commencement to the End of the Year 1778. Vol. II. Dublin: The Company of Booksellers, 1778. https://www.google.com/books/edition/The_History_of_the_War_in_America_Betwee.

Hogan, Margaret A., et al., eds. *Adams Family Correspondence.* Vol. 8. Cambridge: The Belknap Press of Harvard University Press, 2007.

Hogarth, Rana A. *Medicalizing Blackness: Making Racial Difference in the Atlantic World, 1780–1840.* Chapel Hill: University of North Carolina Press, 2017.

Holland, Brenna. "Mad Speculation and Mary Girard: Gender, Capitalism, and the Cultural Economy of Madness in the Revolutionary Atlantic." *Journal of the Early Republic* 29, no. 4 (Winter 2019): 647–675. https://muse.jhu.edu/article/740242.

Holstein, James A. *Court-Ordered Insanity: Interpretative Practice and Involuntary Commitment.* New York: Aldine de Gruyter, 1993.

Hopkinson, Francis. "The New Roof." *Pennsylvania Packet.* http://americainclass.org/sources/makingrevolution/constitution/text3/hopkinsonnewroof.pdf.

Horrocks, James. *Upon the Peace. A Sermon. Preach'd at the Church of Petsworth, in the County of Gloucester, on August the 25th, the Day Appointed by Authority for the Observation of that Solemnity.* Williamsburg: Joseph Royle, 1763. Evans Early American Imprint Collection.

Hosmer, James Kendall. *The Life of Thomas Hutchinson: Royal Governor of the Province of Massachusetts Bay.* Boston: Houghton, Mifflin and Company, 1896. https://books.google.com/books?id=KloYAAAAIAAJ.

Howard, Thomas L. "The State that Said No: The Fight for Ratification of the Federal Constitution in North Carolina." *North Carolina Historical Review* 94, no. 1 (January 2017): 1–58.

Hurd, Henry M. *The Institutional Care of the Insane in the United States and Canada.* Vol. II. New York: Arno Press, 1973.

Hulton, Ann. *Letter of a Loyalist Lady: Being the Letters of Ann Hulton, Sister of Henry Hulton, Commissioner of Customs in Boston, 1767–1776.* Cambridge: Harvard University Press, 1927.

Huw, David. *Trade, Politics, and Revolution: South Carolina and Britain's Atlantic Commerce, 1730-1739.* Columbia: University of South Carolina Press, 2018.

Inglis, Charles. *The Christian Soldier's Duty Briefly Delineated: In a Sermon Preached at King's Bridge, September 7, 1777, before the American Corps Newly Raised for His Majesty's Service.* New York: H. Gaine, 1777. Library Company of Philadelphia.

Ingram, Allan, ed. *Voices of Madness: Four Pamphlets, 1683–1796.* Thrupp: Sutton Publishing Limited, 1997.

An Inquiry into the Causes of the Insurrection of the Negroes in the Island of St. Domingo. London: J. Johnson, 1792. https://cdn.loc.gov/service/rbc/rbc001/2019/2019preimp06338/2019preimp06338.pdf.

Isaac, Rhys. *The Transformation of Virginia, 1740–1790.* New York: W. W. Norton & Company, 1982.

Jensen, Merrill, ed. *English Historical Documents: American Colonial Documents to 1776.* New York: Oxford University Press, 1964.

Jimenez, Mary Ann. "Madness in Early American History: Insanity in Massachusetts from 1700 to 1830." *Journal of Social History* 20, no. 1 (Autumn 1986): 25–44.

Kelly, Donna, and Lang Baradell, eds. *The Papers of James Iredell.* Vol. III. Raleigh: Office of Archives and History, 2003.

Kenslea, Timothy. *The Sedgwicks in Love: Courtship, Engagements, and Marriage in the Early Republic.* Boston: Northeastern University Press, 2006.

Kerber, Linda. *Women of the Republic: Intellect & Ideology in Revolutionary America.* New York: W. W. Norton & Company, 1980.

Ketchum, Richard M. *Divided Loyalties: How the American Revolution Came to New York.* New York: Henry Holt and Company, 2002.

King, Charles, ed. *The Life and Correspondence of Rufus King: Comprising His Letters, Private and Official, His Public Documents and His Speeches.* New York: G. P. Putnam's Sons, 1895.

Knott, Sarah, and Barbara Taylor, eds. *Women, Gender and the Enlightenment.* New York: Palgrave Macmillan, 2005.

Langdon, Samuel. *Government Corrupted by Vice, and Recovered by Righteousness. A Sermon Preached before the Honorable Congress of the Colony of the Massachusetts-Bay in New England, Assembled at Watertown, on Wednesday the 31st of May, 1775. Being the Anniversary Fixed by Charter for the Election of the Counsellors.* Watertown: Benjamin Edes, 1775. Evans Early American Imprint Collection.

Leach, John. "A Journal Kept by John Leach during His Confinement by the British, in Boston Gaol, in 1775." *New England Historical and Genealogical Register* 19 (1865): 255–263. https://books.google.com/books/about/New_England_Historical_and_Genealogical.html.

Lee, Francis Hazley, ed. "Early Revolutionary Letters of Peter Stretch, a Philadelphia Whig Merchant." *Pennsylvania Magazine of History and Biography* 36, no. 3 (1912): 324–328. https://www.jstor.org/stable/20085604.

Leonard, Daniel. "Massachusettensis." Boston: Mill and Hicks, 1775. https://oll.libertyfund.org/titles/leonard-massachusettensis.

Lepore, Jill. *Book of Ages: The Life and Opinions of Jane Franklin*. New York: Alfred A. Knopf, 2014.

Lewis, Charlene Boyer. "Modern Gratitude: Patriarchy, Romance, and Recrimination in the Early Republic." *Journal of the Early Republic* 39, no. 1 (Spring 2019): 27–56. 10.1353/jer.2019.0004.

Lewis, Joseph. "The Diary of Joseph Lewis." *Proceedings of the New Jersey Historical Society* 60, no. 1 (January 1942): 58–66.

Lincoln, William, ed. *The Journals of Each Provincial Congress of Massachusetts in 1774 and 1775, and of the Committee of Safety*. Boston: Dutton and Wentworth, 1838. https://google.com/books.edition/The_Journals_of_Each_Provincial_Congress.

Linebaugh, Peter, and Marcus Rediker, "The Many-Headed Hydra: Sailors, Slaves, and the Atlantic Working Class in the Eighteenth Century." *Journal of Historical Sociology* 3, no. 3 (September 1990): 225–252. https://doi.org/10.1111/j.1467-6443.1990.tb00149.x.

Lint, Gregg L., et al., eds. *The Adams Papers, Papers of John Adams*. Vol. 15. Cambridge: Harvard University Press, 2010.

Logan, Deborah Norris. *Memoir of Dr. George Logan of Stenton: With Selections from His Correspondence*. Philadelphia: Historical Society of Pennsylvania, 1899.

Logan, George. *A Letter to the Citizens of Pennsylvania*. Philadelphia: Patterson & Cochran, 1800.

Loring, Thomas, ed. *Proceedings of the Safety Committee: for the Town of Wilmington, NC from 1774 to 1776, Printed from the Original Record*. Raleigh, 1844. https://books.google.com/books?id=gHItAAAAYAAJ.

Lowenthal, David. *The Past is a Foreign Country*. New York: Cambridge University Press, 1985.

Mackay, Charles. *Memoirs of Extraordinary Popular Delusions and the Madness of Crowds*. London: National Illustrated Library, 1852. http://www.gutenberg.org/files/24518/24518-h/24518-h-htm.

Macpherson, John. *Macpherson's Letters, &c*. Philadelphia, 1770. http://opac.newsbank.com/select/evans/11713.

Maier, Pauline. *From Resistance to Revolution: Colonial Radicals and the Development of American Opposition to Britain, 1765–1776*. New York: W. W. Norton & Company, 1972.

———. *Ratification: The People Debate the Constitution, 1787–1788*. New York: Simon and Schuster, 2010.

Martin, Joseph Plumb. *A Narrative of a Revolutionary Soldier*. New York: Signet Classic, 2001.

McCord, David J., ed. *The Statutes at Large of South Carolina*. Vol. 7. Columbia, SC: A.S. Johnston, 1840. https://hdl.handle.net/2027/hvd.32044013334099.

McMaster, John Bach. *A History of the People of the United States: From the Revolution to the Civil War*. Vol. II. New York: D. Appleton and Company, 1915.

M'Kean, Thomas. *The Inaugural Address of Thomas M'Kean*. Lancaster, PA: Dickson, 1800.

McRuer, Robert. "Disability Nationalism in Crip Times." *Journal of Literary & Cultural Disability Studies* 4, no. 2 (2010): 163–178. https://www.muse.jhu.edu/article/390397.

Messer, Peter C. "'A Species of Treason & Not the Least Dangerous Kind': The Treason Trials of Abraham Carlisle and John Roberts." *Pennsylvania Magazine of History and Biography*. 123, no. 4 (October 1999): 303–332. https://www.jstor.org/stable/20093317.

Miller, Perry, ed. *The Complete Writings of Roger Williams*. Vol. 7. New York; Russell & Russell, Inc., 1963.

Monro, John. *Remarks of Dr. Battie's Treatise on Madness*. London: John Clarke, 1768. catalog.hathitrust/org/Record/009290937.

Moody, James. *Lieut. James Moody's Narrative of His Exertions and Sufferings in the Cause of Government, since the Year 1776; Authenticated by Proper Certificates*. 2nd ed. London: Richardson and Urquhart, 1783.

Moore, Frank, ed. *The Diary of the Revolution: A Centennial Volume Embracing the Current Events in our Country's History from 1775 to 1781 as Described by American, British, and Tory Contemporaries, Compiled from the Journals, Documents, Private Records, Correspondence, etc. of That Period, Forming and Interesting, Impartial, and Valuable Collection of Revolutionary Literature*. Hartford: J.B. Burr Publishing Company, 1876. https://books.google.com/books?id+UWIFAAAAQAAJ.

Morgan, Edmund S. *American Slavery, American Freedom*. New York: W. W. Norton & Company, 1975.

———. *The Birth of the Republic, 1763–89*. Revised edition. Chicago: University of Chicago Press, 1977.

———. *Prologue to Revolution: Sources and Documents on the Stamp Act Crisis, 1764–1766*. Chapel Hill: University of North Carolina Press, 1959.

Morgan, Edmund S., and Helen M. Morgan. *The Stamp Act Crisis: Prologue to Revolution*. Chapel Hill: University of North Carolina Press, 1953.

Morton, Thomas G., and Frank Woodbury. *The History of the Pennsylvania Hospital 1751–1895*. Facsimile ed. New York: Arno Press, 1973.

Murat, Laure. *The Man Who Thought He Was Napoleon: Toward a Political History of Madness*. Translated by Deke Dusinberre. Chicago: The University of Chicago Press, 2014.

Nelson, Craig. *Thomas Paine: Enlightenment, Revolution, and the Birth of Modern Nations*. New York: Penguin Books, 2006.

Niles, Hezekiah, ed. *Republication of the Principles and Acts of the Revolution in America*. New York: A.S. Barnes & Co., 1876. http://books.google.com/books?isbn=5881459903.

North, Louise V., Janet M. Edge, and Landa M. Freeman, eds. *In the Words of Women: The Revolutionary War and the Birth of the Nation, 1765–1799*. Lanham, MD: Lexington Books, 2011.

Oaks, Robert F. "Philadelphians in Exile: The Problem of Loyalty during the American Revolution." *Pennsylvania Magazine of History and Biography.* 96, no. 3 (July 1972): 298–319. https://www.jstor.org/stable/20090650.
Oliver, Peter. *Origin and Progress of the American Rebellion, 1781.* americainclass. org/sources/makingrevolution/rebellion/text2/oliverloyalistsviolence.pdf.
Osgood, David. *A Discourse, Delivered February 19, 1795. The Day Set Apart by the President for a General Thanksgiving through the United States.* Boston: Samuel Hall, 1795. https://books.google.com/books?id+Vu5CAQAAMAAJ.
Paine, Thomas, "The Last Crisis." In *The American Crisis*, 187–193. London: R. Carlile, 1819. https://books.google.com/books/edition/The_American_Crisis/.
Pargeter, William. *Observations on Maniacal Disorders.* Reading, 1792. https://archive.org/details/b21522388/page/n151.
Parry-Jones, William Ll. *The Trade in Lunacy: A Study of Private Madhouses in England in the Eighteen and Nineteenth Centuries.* London: Routledge and Kegan Paul, 1972.
Pierce, Edward L., ed. *The Diary of John Rowe, A Boston Merchant, 1764–1779.* Cambridge: John Wilson and Son, 1895). https://catalog.hathitrust.org/Record/00 1262059.
Pinel, Philippe. *A Treatise on Insanity, in which Are Contained the Principles of New and More Practical Nosology of Maniacal Disorders Than Has Yet Been Offered to the Public.* Sheffield: W. Todd, 1806. https://books.google.com/books?id=E 4FIAAAAYAAJ.
Porter, Roy. "Reason, Madness, and the French Revolution." *Studies in Eighteenth-Century Culture* 20 (1991): 55–79. 10.1353/sec.2010.0299.
Pownall, Thomas and John Almon, eds. *The Remembrancer; or, Impartial Repository of Public Events, for the Year 1778, and Beginning of 1779.* London: J. Almon, 1779. catalog.hathitrust.org/Record/000641873.
Price, Richard. *Observations on the Importance of the American Revolution, and the Means of Making It a Benefit to the World.* Boston: Powars and Willis, 1784. Evans Early American Imprints Collection.
Raphael, Ray. *Founders: The People Who Brought You a Nation.* New York: The New Press, 2009.
Ray, Isaac. *A Treatise on the Medical Jurisprudence of Insanity.* London: G. Henderson, 1839. https://books.google.com/books?id=sFwqJ0hFrvgC.
Reed, William B., ed. *Life and Correspondence of Joseph Reed.* Vol. 1. Philadelphia: Lindsay and Blakiston, 1847. https://catalog.hathitrust.org/Record/000364985.
Report of the Select Committee to the House of Representatives upon the Subject of Building an Insane Hospital. Concord, NH: Hill and Barton, 1832. New Hampshire Historical Society.
Richards, Jeffrey H., and Sharon M. Harris, eds. *Mercy Otis Warren: Selected Letters.* Athens: University of Georgia Press, 2009.
Riley, Stephen T. "Dr. William Whiting and Shays' Rebellion." *Proceedings of the American Antiquarian Society* 66 (October 1956): 119–166. https://www.americanantiquarian.org/proceedings/44539282.pdf.

Robertson, David, ed. *Debates and Other Proceedings of the Convention of Virginia, Convened at Richmond, on Monday the Second Day of June, 1788, for the Purpose of Deliberating on the Constitution Recommended by the General Federal Convention*. Richmond: Enquirer-Press, 1805.https://books.google.com/books/about/Debates_and_other_proceedings_of_the_Con.html.

Robinson, Blackwell Pierce. "Willie Jones of Halifax: Part II." *North Carolina Historical Review* 18, no. 2 (April 1941): 133–170. https://www.jstor.org/stable/23516615.

Rogal, Samuel J. "Pills for the Poor: John Wesley's *Primitive Physic*." *Yale Journal of Biology and Medicine* 51 (1978): 81–90. https://www.ncbi.nlm.nih.gov/pmc/articles/PMC2595647/.

Rogers, James E. Thorold, ed. *A Complete Collection of the Protests of the Lords with Historical Introductions*. Vol. II. Oxford: Clarendon Press, 1875. https://books.google.com/books/about/A_Complete_Collection_of_the_Protests_of.html.

Rothman, David J. *The Discovery of the Asylum: Social Order and Disorder in the New Republic*. Boston: Little, Brown and Company, 1971.

Rush, Benjamin. "Address to the People of the United States." *The American Museum*. January 1787. archive.csac.history.wisc.edu/Benjamin_Rush.pdf.

———. *Medical Inquiries and Observations*. Philadelphia: Prichard & Hall, 1789. Evans Early American Imprint Collection.

———. *Observations on the Duties of a Physician, and the Methods of Improving Medicine. Accommodated to the Present State of Society and Manners in the United States*. Philadelphia: Prichard & Hall, 1789. Evans Early American Imprint Collection.

Ryerson, Richard Alan, et al., *Adams Family Correspondence*. Vol. 6. Cambridge: The Belknap Press of Harvard University Press, 1993.

Samuelson, Richard A. "The Constitutional Sanity of James Otis: Resistance Leader and Loyal Subject." *The Review of Politics* 61, no 3. (Summer 1999): 493–523. https://www.jstor.org/stable/1408465.

Saunders, William L., ed. *The Colonial Records of North Carolina*. Vol. IX. Raleigh: Josephus Daniels, 1890. https://books.google.com/books/about/The_Colonial_Records_of_North_Carolina.html.

Schaw, Janet. *Journal of a Lady of Quality; Being the Narrative of a Journey from Scotland to the West Indies, North Carolina, and Portugal, in the Years 1774 to 1776*. Edited by Evangeline Walker Andrews. New Haven: Yale University Press, 1921. https://docsouth.unc.edu/nc/schaw/schaw.html.

Scherr, Arthur. *John Adams, Slavery, and Race: Ideas, Politics, and Diplomacy in an Age of Crisis*. Santa Barbara, CA: Praeger, 2018.

Schmidt, Fredrika Teute, and Barbara Ripel Wilhelm, eds. "Early Proslavery Petitions in Virginia." *William and Mary Quarterly* 30, no. 1 (January 1973): 133–146. https://www.jstor.org/stable/1923706.

Seabury, Samuel. *Free Thoughts, on the Proceedings of the Continental Congress, Held at Philadelphia Sept. 5, 1774*. http://anglicanhistory.org/usa/seabury/farmer/01.html.

———. *A View of the controversy between Great-Britain and Her Colonies: Including a Mode of Determining Their Present Disputes, Finally and Effecually*

[sic]; and of Preventing all Future Contentions. New York: James Rivington, 1774. http://anglicanhistory.org/seabury/farmer/03.html.

Sharp, James Roger. *American Politics in the Early Republic: The New Nation in Crisis.* New Haven: Yale University Press, 1993.

Sherman, Gordon E. "Orders in Council and the Law of the Sea." *American Journal of International Law* 16, no 3 (July 1922): 400–419. https://www.jstor.org/stable/pdf/2188177.pdf.

Shy, John. *A People Numerous and Armed: Reflections on the Military Struggle for American Independence.* Ann Arbor: University of Michigan Press, 1976.

Shy, John, ed. *Winding Down: The Revolutionary War Letters of Lieutenant Benjamin Gilbert of Massachusetts, 1780–1783 from His Original Manuscript Letterbook in the William L. Clements Library, Ann Arbor, Michigan.* Ann Arbor: The University of Michigan Press, 1989.

Siege of Boston: Eyewitness Accounts from the Collection of the Massachusetts Historical Society. https://www.mashist.org/online/siege/.

Sipe, C. Hale. *The Indian Wars of Pennsylvania: An Account of the Indian Events, in Pennsylvania, of the French and Indian War, Pontiac's War, Lord Dunmore's War, the Revolutionary War and the Indian Uprising from 1789 to 1795.* Harrisburg: The Telegraph press, 1929. https://archive.org/details/indianwarsofpenn00sipe.

Skemp, Sheila L. *Benjamin and William Franklin: Father and Son, Patriot and Loyalist.* Boston: Bedford St. Martin's, 1994.

Smith, J. E. A. *The History of Pittsfield, (Berkshire County,) Massachusetts from the Year 1734 to the Year 1800.* Boston: Lee and Shepard, 1869. https://books.google.com/books/about/The_History_of_Pittsfield_Berkshire_Coun.html.

Smith, Leonard. "'The Keeper Must Himself be Kept': Visitation and the Lunatic Asylum in England, 1750–1850." *Clio Medica* 86 (2009): 199–222.

Smith, Paul H. ed. *Letters of Delegates to Congress: 1774–1789.August 1774–August 1775.* Washington: Library of Congress, 1976.

Some Account of the Pennsylvania Hospital. Philadelphia: Office of the United States Gazette, 1817. http://resource.nlm.nih.gov/2554043R.

"Some Extracts from the Papers of General Persifor Frazer." *Pennsylvania Magazine of History and Biography* 31, no. 2 (1907). https://www.jstor.org/stable/20085377.

Sprague, Jenks S. "Observations on Various Subjects in Forensic Medicine." *Transactions of the Medical Society of the State of New-York, during Its Annual Session, Held at Albany, February 5, 1850.* Albany: Weed, Parsons & Co., 1850. https://hdl.handle.net/2027/mdp.39015076629271.

Spurzheim, J. G. *Observations on the Deranged Manifestations of the Mind, or Insanity.* First American Edition. Boston: Marsh, Capen & Lyon, 1833. Library Company of Philadelphia.

Starr, Paul. *The Social Transformation of American Medicine: The Rise of a Sovereign Profession and the Making of a Vast Industry.* New York: Basic Books, 1982.

Stearns, Asahel, and Lemuel Shaw, eds. *The General Laws of Massachusetts, from the Adoption of the Constitution, to February 1822.* Vol. 1. Boston: Wells & Lilly and Cummings & Hilliard, 1823. ocm26871236-1822vol1.pdf.

Storing, Herbert J., ed. *The Complete Anti-Federalist*. Vol. 2. Chicago: University of Chicago Press, 1981.

Syrett, Harold C., ed. *The Papers of Alexander Hamilton*. Vol. 18. New York: Columbia University Press, 1973.

Szasz. Thomas S. *The Age of Madness: The History of Involuntary Mental Hospitalization*. Lanham, MD: Jason Aronson, Inc., 1974.

———. *The Manufacture of Madness: A Comparative Study of the Inquisition and the Mental Health Movement*. Syracuse: Syracuse University Press, 1970.

Szatmary, David P. *Shays' Rebellion: The Making of an Agrarian Insurrection*. Amherst: University of Massachusetts Press, 1980.

Taylor, Robert J., ed. *The Adams Papers, Papers of John Adams*. Vols 3 and 4. Cambridge: Harvard University Press, 1979.

Tiedemann, Joseph S. "A Revolution Foiled: Queens County, New York, 1775–1776. *Journal of American History* 75, no. 2 (September 1988): 417–444. https://www.jstor.org/stable/1887865.

"To the Honourable House of Representatives of the Province of Pennsylvania, The Petition of Sundry Inhabitants of the Said Province." In *The History of the Pennsylvania Hospital, 1751–1895*, edited by Thomas G. Morton, 8–10. Philadelphia: Times Printing House, 1895. https://books.google.com/books?id=W85XAAAAMAAJ.

Trenchard, John, and Thomas Gordon. *Cato's Letters, or Essays on Liberty, Civil and Religious, and Other Important Subjects*. Four volumes in Two, edited and annotated by Ronald Hamow. Indianapolis: Liberty Fund, 1995. https://oll.libertyfund.org/titles/1237#Trenchard_0226-01_777.

The Trial of the British Soldiers, of the 29th Regiment of Food, for the Murder of Crispus Attucks, Samuel Gray, Samuel Maverick, James Caldwell, and Patrick Carr, on Monday Evening, March 5, 1770, before the Honorable Benjamin Lynde, John Cushing, Peter Oliver, and Edmund Trowbridge, Esquires. Boston: William Emmons, 1824. https://www.loc.gov/law/help/rare-books/pdf/john_adams_1824_version.pdf.

Turner, Lynn W. "The Impeachment of John Pickering." *American Historical Review* 54, no. 3 (April 1949): 485–507. https://www.jstor.org/stable/1843004.

Unger, Harlow Giles. *Lion of Liberty: Patrick Henry and the Call to a New Nation*. Philadelphia: De Capo Press, 2010.

Wallace, Tara Goshall. "'About savages and the awfulness of America': corruptions in Humphry Clinker." *Eighteenth Century Fiction* 18, no. 2 (Winter 2005–2006): 229–250. http://muse.jhu.edu/article/200591.

Walker, Corey D. B. *A Noble Fight: African American Freemasonry and the Struggle for Democracy in America*. Champaign: University of Illinois Press, 2008.

Walmsley, Andrew Stephen. *Thomas Hutchinson and the Origins of the American Revolution*. New York: New York University Press, 1999.

Warren, Charles. *Jacobin and Junto, or, Early American Politics as Viewed in the Diary of Dr. Nathaniel Ames, 1758–1822*. Cambridge: Harvard University Press, 1931.

Warren, Mercy Otis, *History of the Rise, Progress and Termination of the American Revolution by Mrs. Mercy Otis Warren*. Two Volumes. Edited by Lester H. Cohen. Indianapolis: Liberty Fund, 1994.

———. *Poems, Dramatic and Miscellaneous*. Boston: I Thomas and E. T. Andrews, 1790s. https://books.google.com/books/about/Poems_Dramatic_and_Miscellaneous.html.

Washington, George. *A Circular Letter, from His Excellency George Washington, Commander in Chief of the Armies of the United States of America; Addressed to the Governors of the Several States, on His Resigning the Command of the Army, and Retiring from Public Business*. Philadelphia: Robert Smith, Jr., 1783. Evans Early American Imprint Collection.

Watson, Winslow C., ed. *Men and Times of the Revolution; or, Memoirs of Elkanah Watson, Including His Journals of Travels in Europe and America from the Year 1777 to 1842, and His Correspondence with Public Men, and Reminiscences and Incidents of the American Revolution*. New York: Dana and Company, 1857. https://www.loc.gov/item/03004951/.

Webster, Noah. "The Devil Is in You." *Worcester Magazine* 2 (November 1786).

———. "Remarks on the Manners, Government, and Debt of the United States." In *A Collection of Essays and Fugitive Writing*, 81–118. In *A Collection of Essays and Fugitiv [sic] Writings*. Boston: I. Thomas and T. Andrews, 1790. https://books.google.com/books?isbn=3732647684.

Wells, Helena. *Letters on Subjects of Importance to the Happiness of Young Females, Addressed by a Governess to Her Pupils, Chiefly While They Were under Her Immediate tuition: To which Are Added, Some Practical Lessons on the Improprieties of Language, and Errors in Pronunciation, which Frequently Occur in Common Conversation*. 2nd ed. London: Sabine & Son, 1807.

Wheatley, Phillis. "Liberty and Peace, a Poem." Boston: Warden and Russell, 1784. Evans Early American Imprint Collection.

Whidbee, Paige L. "The Quaker Exiles: The Cause of Every Inhabitant." *Pennsylvania History: A Journal of Mid-Atlantic Studies* 83, no. 1 (2016): 28–57.

Whitaker, Robert. *Mad in America: Bad Science, Bad Medicine, and the Enduring Mistreatment of the Mentally Ill*. Cambridge, MA: Perseus Publishing, 2002.

White, George, ed., *Historical Collections of Georgia: Containing the Most Interesting Facts, Traditions, Biographical Sketches, Compiled from Original Records and Official Documents*. New York: Pudney & Russell, 1855. https://books.google.com/books?id=oWIGNjgAlpkC.

Willcox, William B., ed. *The Papers of Benjamin Franklin*. Vol. 22. New Haven: Yale University Press, 1982.

Williams, George Washington. *History of the Negro Race in America from 1619 to 1880*. Vol. 1. New York: G.P. Putnam's Sons, 1883. http://www.gutenberg.org/ebooks/15735.

Winlick, John R. "The Moravians and the American Revolution: An Overview." *Transactions of the Moravian Historical Society*. 23, no 1 (1977): 1–16. https://www.jstor.org/stable/41179398.

Whittenburg, James P. "Planters, Merchants, and Lawyers: Social Change and the Origins of the North Carolina Regulation." *William and Mary Quarterly* 34, no. 2 (April 1977): 215–238.

Wood, Gordon S. *The Radicalism of the American Revolution*. New York: Random House, 1992.

Yokota, Kariann Akemi. *Unbecoming British: How Revolutionary America Became a Postcolonial Nation.* New York: Oxford University Press, 2011.

York, Neil Longley, ed. *Henry Hulton and the American Revolution: An Outsider's Inside View.* Boston: The Colonial Society of Massachusetts, 2010.

Young, Alfred F., Gary B. Nash, and Ray Raphael, eds. *Revolutionary Founders: Rebels, Radicals, and Reformers in the Making of the Nation.* New York: Vintage Books, 2001.

Zagarri, Rosemarie. *Revolutionary Backlash: Women and Politics in the Early American Republic.* Philadelphia: University of Pennsylvania Press, 2008.

———. *A Woman's Dilemma: Mercy Otis Warren and the American Revolution.* Wheeling, IL: Harlan Davidson, Inc., 1995.

Index

Page references for figures are italicized.

Adams, Abigail, 125–26, 139–40, 161, 162, 176, 185–86, 225
Adams, John, 31–32, 100, 119, 141, 145, 148, 153, 163, 176, 214
Adams, John Quincy, 217
Adams, Samuel, 65, 108–9
Air Loom, 26, 90
Alcuin, 19
Allen, James, 93–95, 152–53
American Board of Customs Commissioners, 32
American Political Society, 108
Ames, Fisher, 222, 229
Anarchia, 8
anarchy, 8, 48, 58, 66, 79, 80, 82, 86, 124, 136, 142, 143, 152–54, 164, 170–72, 175, 177, 179, 184, 185, 189, 212, 213, 215–18, 220, 221, 228, 229, 238
Anderson, Alexander, 8, 20, 32
Annapolis Convention, 187–88
antislavery, 202–6
Archer, John, 8
Arms, Consider, 202–3
Armstrong, John, 165–66
Articles of Confederation, 131, 155, 162, 187–89, 191, 193, 197

Association. *See* Continental Association
asylums, 7–8, 21, 23, 237–38
attacks on American shipping, 218–22

Bache, Benjamin Franklin, 222
balls, 92
Barnes, Christian, 63
Barrington, William, 58
Battie, William, 7, 111
Bayard, John, 97
Beatty, Erkuries, 128
Bedlam. *See* Bethlem Hospital
Beebe, Abner, 137
Belcher, William, 30
Belknap, Jeremy, 222–23
Bernard, Francis, 53, 58–61, 63
Bethlem Hospital, 7, 25–26, 29, 32, 59, 67, 127, 141
Bigelow, Timothy, 108
bill of rights, debate over, 192–96
Birkbeck, George, 26
bleeding, 4, 7, 33, 107–8, 111, 114, 145, 175
Boston Massacre, 66–67, 138, 141; trial, 67
Boston Tea Party, 72, 142

262 *Index*

Bowdoin, James, 172–73, 175–77
Brigham, Amariah, 8, 32
Brown, Charles Brockden, 19
Bruckshaw, Samuel, 30, 37
Buchan, William, 6, 58
Buford, Abraha, 129–30
Bulloch, Archibald, 88
Bunker Hill, Battle of, 147
Burgoyne, John, 120

Cadwalader, Thomas, 38
Cain, Elizabeth, 124–25
Cain, Sarah, 124–25
Canada, 39, 146, 149
captivity narratives, 23, 24, 30, 38–39
Carlisle Peace Commission, 125–27
Carter, Landon, 151–52
Cartwright, Samuel, 36
Cassell, Richard, 97, 144
Cato's Letters, 18
Chandler, Thomas Bradbury, 84
checks and balances, 11, 199
civilians, effect of war on, 121, 124–25, 128–29
Clarke, Charity, 63
Clutterbuck, Henry, 26
Clymer Margaret, 35–36
Coercive Acts, 72, 78, 82, 89, 143, 172
committees of correspondence, 52, 83, 90
Common Sense, 150–52, 170
Confederation Congress. *See* Continental Congress
Connecticut, 82, 86, 137, 141–43
Connolly, John, 23, 83
Constitution, United States: opposition to, 189–93; opposition to, North Carolina, 195–98; opposition to, Rhode Island, 193, 196, 198; ratification, 188–93
Constitutional Convention, 188
Continental Association, 78–79, 87, 90, 92–93, 129, 142–43, 144; resistance to, 82–88

Continental Congress, 34, 78, 94, 99, 114–15, 125–27, 131, 138, 141, 144–50, 155, 162–63, 165
Conway, Henry, 60
Cornwallis, Charles, 101, 130–31
court closures, 68, 154, 167–68, 171–73, 177, 179
Cranch, Mary, 80
Cranch, Richard, 199–200
Cranch, William, 200
Cressener, George, 4, 107–8
Crozier, John, 111
Cruden, Alexander, 23–24, 28–30, 37, 38
Cutbrush, Edward, 4, 21

Dalrymple, John, 148–49
Darwin, Erasmus, 2
Dawes, William, 108–9
deception, 90–91, 126, 215, 219, 223
Declaration of Independence, 41, 94, 100, 152, 155, 163
Declaration of the Causes and Necessity of Taking Up Arms, 148–49
Declaratory Act, 61, 66, 70, 192
Defoe, Daniel, 22
democracy, fear of, 59, 184, 186–87, 197, 220, 229
Democratic Republican Party/ Democratic Republicans, 211, 215, 218, 222, 227–29
Democratic Republican societies, 219, 220, 223–24
diagnosis, 2, 18, 22, 23–26, 35, 38, 62, 63, 70
Dickinson, John, 34, 37–41, 55, 62, 145, 146, 166
disease metaphors, 2, 55, 61, 62, 79, 107, 111, 141, 144–46, 191–92, 212, 214, 216
Döer, Conrad, 36–37
Döer, Mary Elizabeth, 36–37
Drapetomania, 36
Dunlap, Alexander, 123
Dunmore's Proclamation, 149

economic depression, post war, 161, 167–68, 170, 172, 177
Edes, Peter, 140–41
Edwards, Jonathan, 205
Elder, John, 48–50
election of 1800, 239
Elliot, Andrew, 138
Ellis, Henry, 112
enslaved people, 5, 9, 34–36, 149; Black Adam, 35–36; corpse of, 69
Ettwein, Joseph, 97
Evelyn, W. G., 110–11
extralegal actions, 77–78, 81, 88, 93, 146, 197

Fanning, Edmund, 68–69
Fauquier, Francis, 20, 54–55
Federalist Party/Federalists, 211, 215, 217, 219–20, 222, 223–29, 239–40
Fenno, John, 215
Field, Samuel, 202–3
Finley, Samuel, 118
Fisher, Joshua, 97–98
Fisher, Sarah Logan, 99
Fitz-Geffrey, Charles, 23
folk remedies, 4–6
Ford, Timothy, 163, 168–70
Foucault, Michel, 21, 30
Fourth of July Orations, 163, 170–71, 217, 239
Franklin, Benjamin, 49–50, 57, 61, 64, 77, 95–96, 145, 188–89, 203
Franklin, Deborah, 57–58
Franklin, William, 142–43, 147
Frazer, Persifor, 119
French Revolution, 213–19
Freneau, Philip, 215
frenzy, 2, 4, 8, 54, 57–59, 78, 94, 117, 118, 143, 149, 151, 161, 170, 174, 217, 224

Gage, Thomas, 86, 90, 107–8, 111, 113, 136–43, 147, 172
Gale, Henry, 179
Gallatin, Albert, 227–28

Galloway, Joseph, 57, 77–78
Garrick, Edward, 66
Garth, Charles, 52–53
Gates, Horatio, 96–97
Genet, Edmund, 218–20, 223
George III, 60–61, 84, 86, 88, 98, 113, 124, 127, 136, 138, 148
Georgia, 88–90, 126, 146, 194, 205
Gerry, Elbridge, 204
Gilbert, Benjamin, 129
Gill, Sarah, 63
Golden Hill, Battle of, 65
Gordon, Thomas, 18
Graydon, Alexander, 220
Greene, Nathanael, 121–23
Grenville, William, 52–53
Griffits, Hannah, 62–63
Grimke, John, 167–69
Grosvenor, Benjamin, 54

habeas corpus, 28, 100, 175, 178
Hall, Moses, 129–130
Hall, Prince, 175–76, 203
Hamilton, Alexander, 162, 165, 191–92, 201, 211, 216–18, 224, 229
Hancock, John, 108–9, 203
Haslam, John, 26–27, 53
Hathway, Daniel, 121, 123
Hawley, Joseph, 119
Haw River, Battle of, 130
Haywood, Eliza, 27–28
Hazen, Moses, 121
Hedge, Barnabas, 71
Henderson, Richard, 68
Henry, Patrick, 34–35, 190, 192, 200, 202
Henry, Sarah Shelton, 34–35, 238
Hessians, 116, 123–24, 130
Hewes, Joseph, 97, 144, 149
history, as a cautionary tale, 11, 18, 162
Holland, Park, 120–21, 179
Hooper, Jr., William, 81, 144
Hooper, Sr., William, 81
Hopkinson, Francis, 190–91
Horrocks, James, 47, 66, 80

Horsmanden, Daniel, 141
Houston, William, 56
Houstoun, John, 88
Howe, Richard, 114
Howe, William, 116
Hughes, John, 57–58
Hulton, Ann, 63, 85, 137
Hulton, Henry, 141–42
humoral theory, 7, 53, 54, 59, 60, 72, 239
Hunt, Isaac, 87–88
Husband, Herman, 68
Hutchinson, Thomas, 32, 33, 66, 71–72

illness metaphor. *See* disease metaphors
Indians, 5, 38–39, 48–51, 53, 88, 127–28, 146
Inglis, Charles, 117–18, 122, 151
Iredell, James, 81, 187

Jackson, James, 196, 199
Jackson, Richard, 53
Jacobin/Jacobitism, 61, 213, 222–24, 235
Jamestown, 17–18
Jay, John, 213, 221–22, 226
Jay Treaty, 221–28; debate in the House of Representatives, 225–28; opposition to, 222–25
Jefferson, Thomas, 124, 211, 214–16, 218–19, 225, 229, 240
Johnson, Samuel, 113
Johnston, Samuel, 97
join or die, 79, 94
Jones, Noble, 88
Jones, Willie, 197–98

King, Rufus, 170, 187, 191, 213, 222
Kip's Bay, Battle of, 119–20, 129
Knox, Henry, 114, 191

Langdon, Samuel, 143–44
Lee, Charles, 96–97
Lee, Richard Henry, 70
Lexington and Concord, Battles of, 93–110, 135, 137–38, 143, 145, 163

liberty poles, 64–65, 79, 108, 167, 219
"Liberty Triumphant", *91*
Lillie, Theophilus, 62, 71
Lincoln, Benjamin, 175, 177
Logan, Deborah Norris, 211, 218–19, 236
Logan, George, 3, 211
Long Island, Battle of, 115–16, 119
Louis XVI, arrest and execution, 216–17
Loyalist Association. *See* Ruggles Covenant
loyalists, 79, 85, 86, 94–99, 115, 117, 122, 126, 128–29, 176, 178
lunatic, 3–4, 19–21, 24–27, 30, 33, 35, 36, 53, 82, 85, 95, 111, 118, 121, 130, 136, 141, 149, 151, 162, 166, 188, 190–91, 230, 235, 237–38, 240–41
Lunenburg County petitions, 169

Macaulay, Catharine, 63
Macpherson, John, 37–41, 48, 62, 71, 77, 99
Macpherson, Peggy, 38–40
madhouse, 22–31, 63, 92, 127, 141
Madhouse Act, 1774, 30–31
Madison, James, 11, 187–88, 194, 196, 201, 204, 211, 215
Malcom, John, 137
Martin, Joseph Plumb, 115, 119–21, 164, 165
Martin, Josiah, 107, 136
Mason, George, 61, 192–93
Massachusettensis, 86
Massachusetts, 5, 20, 31–33, 53–54, 55, 58–59, 60–61, 63–64, 65–67, 71–72, 78, 79–81, 82, 83, 85–86, 88, 92–93, 107–12, 115, 119, 125, 136–42, 143–44, 147–48, 149, 153–54, 155, 163–64, 170, 171–79, 183, 187, 198, 199–202, 203, 204, 225, 226, 237, 238, 239
Mather, Cotton, 5
Matthews, James Tilly, 25–27

Mauduit, Jasper, 53–54
Maynard, Malachi, 202–3
McHenry, James, 162–63
McKean, Thomas, 3, 4, 100–101, 121
medical metaphor. *See* disease metaphors
Monro, John, 7
Montaigne, Michel de, 19
Moody, James, 79, 94
Moravians, 95–97
Muhlenberg, Henry, 123
Murray, Judith Sargant, 221

Native Americans. *See* Indians
nature, state of, 18, 79, 144, 149, 163, 170, 221
Neilson, Archibald, 142
Neutrality Proclamation, 217–18
Newburgh Conspiracy, 166
New Hampshire, 82, 150, 177, 192, 193, 222, 236, 240
newspapers, 30, 66, 70, 176, 193, 196, 215
New York Restraining Act, 64

Observations on the Deranged Manifestations of the Mind, 8
Ockett, Molly, 5
Oliver, Andrew, 58, 59
Oliver, Peter, 31–32, 58, 62, 137
Osgood, Samuel, 163, 217
Otis, Jr., James, 24, 31–34, 59

Page, John, 204
Paine, Robert Treat, 67
Paine, Thomas, 121, 127, 150–52, 170, 183; anti-Quaker, 98–99
Paine, Timothy, 86
Palmer, Abigail, 124–25
pamphlets, 3, 23, 26, 29, 31, 40, 50, 51, 54, 56, 72, 78, 84, 99, 100, 148, 150, 151, 205–6, 215, 222, 237
Pargeter, William, 4
Paris Peace Treaty, 163, 183
Parsons, Samuel, 124

party rage, 186–89, 193, 239
Paxton Volunteers, 48–53
Penn, John, 48–49
Pennsylvania Hospital, 22, 25, 36–37, 236, 237
Pennsylvania Society for Promoting the Abolition of Slavery, 203–4
Phillips, Mary, 124–25
Pickering, John, 239–41
Pinel, Philippe, 21
Pitt, William, 55, 59–60, 113, 127–28
plunder, 95, 110, 121, 123–24
Porter, Roy, 23, 26
post traumatic stress syndrome (PTSD), 2
Preston, Thomas, 66–67
Price, Richard, 161–62
prisoners, political, 140–41
PTSD. *See* post traumatic stress syndrome

quacks, 5
Quakers, 7, 57, 97–101, 144; fighting, 97, 144

Ramsay, David, 170
rape, 96, 124–25, 127
Rawle, Anna, 101
reconciliation proposals, 125–27, 147
redemptioners, 36–37
Reed, Joseph, 114, 153
regulators, North Carolina, 67–70
Republican, party. *See* Democratic Republican Party/Democratic Republicans
Revere, Paul, 108–9
Richardson, Ebenezer, 66
Richardson, Experience Wight, 111–12
Rivington's New-York Gazetteer, 71, 83
Robinson, John, 32, 33
Rogers, Thomas, 98
Rosenberg, Charles, 6
Rothman, David, 21
Rowe, John, 67
Ruggles, Timothy, 85–86
Ruggles Covenant, 85–86

Rush, Benjamin, 5–6, 8, 22, 52, 162, 183–84, 204–6, 212

Sandy Creek Association, 68
Saxby, George, 56
schizophrenia, 25–26
Schuyler, Philip, 120–21
Scott, Joseph, 90
Seabury, Samuel, 78–79, 84
Sedgwick, Pamela, 200–202
Sedgwick, Theodore, 170, 173–74, 187, 199–202
Seidel, Nathaniel, 95–96
Seider, Christopher, 66
Sermon, Joseph, 98
Seven Years' War, 47, 96
Shays, Daniel, 171, 176, 177
Shays's Rebellion, 171–79, 184, 187, 191–92, 200
Short, William, 214–16
siege of Boston, 138–41
slavery, 9–10, 35–36, 69, 119, 149, 168–69, 175–76, 188, 196–97, 202–6; bar to insanity, 8, 35–36; metaphorical, 9, 17, 27, 30, 35, 52, 71, 98
slaves. *See* enslaved people
Smith, Jr., Isaac, 79–83
Smith, Samuel, 57, 58
Smith, William, 221
social contract/compact, 3, 19, 47, 85, 100, 141, 155, 178, 228, 230, 241
social memory, 19–20, 109, 125, 235
Sons of Liberty, 63, 64–65, 67
South Carolina, 36, 52, 56, 124, 126, 129, 167, 168, 170, 191, 194, 221, 222
Spank Town, Yearly Meeting at, 99
Sparhawk, John, 150
Sprague, Jenks S., 17
Spurzheim, Johann, 8, 20, 32, 236
Stamp Act, 52–61, 63, 192; Congress, 54; protest of, out of doors, 56–57, 68
standing armies, 64–67, 108, 138

St. Domingue, 205–6
Strachey, Henry, 114–18, 129
Strachey, Jane, 114, 117
straight jacket, 24, 34, 38, 39, 41, 51, 53, 54, 82, 91, 236, 238
Stretch, Peter, 79
Sugar Act, 31, 52, 91
Sullivan, John, 99, 128, 153–54
Sumner, Increase, 178

tar and feathers, 84, 87, 137
Tarleton, Banastre, 129
taxation, 34, 41, 69, 72, 89
Tea Act, 70–72, 94; resolutions, 70–71
Test Act, 97
Ticonderoga, 120, 143, 145, 146
Townshend Acts, 34, 61–62, 66
Trenchard, John, 18
Trumbull, Benjamin, 120
Tryon, William, 69, 124, 127
Twenty-Fifth Amendment, 240

unnatural, use of word, 85, 126, 149, 177

veterans, 162–67, 171
"A View in America," *122*

Walton, John, 188
Warren, Mercy Otis, 32, 33, 161–62, 184, 188–89, 190, 215, 228; *History of the Rise, Progress, and Termination of the American Revolution,* 70, 128, 130–31, 188
Washington, George, 5, 114–16, 120, 123, 129, 147, 164–66, 175, 185, 199, 211, 214, 217–18, 220, 221, 223–25, 227–29, 235
Watson, Elkanah, 184–85
Waxhaws, Battle of, 129–30
Webster, Noah, 174, 184, 220
Weedon, George, 120
Wells, Helena, 220
Wentworth, John, 150
Wesley, John, 6

western insurrection, 219–20
Wharton, Thomas, 101
Wheatley, Phillis, 161
whiskey, tax on, 219–20
whiskey rebellion. *See* western insurrection
White, Hugh, 66
Whiting, William, 171–74
Wilkes, John, 113
Wilkinson, Eliza, 124
Willard, Abijah, 86
Williams, Roger, 80
Willing, Thomas, 146
Wolcott, Jr., Oliver, 224, 226–27
Wolcott, Sr., Oliver, 211, 212, 226, 228–29
women, 22, 27–28, 39–40, 62–63, 92–93, 110, 124–25, 184–85, 191, 200–202, 220; female politicians, 185
Wooley, Thomas, 93
world turned upside down, 141, 175, 184
Wright, James, 88, 89–90
Wright, Matthew, 29

York Retreat, 7
Yorktown, Battle of, 130–31

Zoonomia, 2

About the Author

Dr. Sarah L. Swedberg is a professor of history at Colorado Mesa University where she has taught for 21 years. She is a regular writer for Nursing Clio, an open access, peer-reviewed, collaborative blog project focused on the history of gender and medicine. This is her first book.

www.ingramcontent.com/pod-product-compliance
Lightning Source LLC
Chambersburg PA
CBHW050900300426
44111CB00010B/1323